# THE
# LOSS
# OF
# SELF

# THE LOSS OF SELF

A Family Resource for the Care of
Alzheimer's Disease and Related Disorders

DONNA COHEN, PH.D.
CARL EISDORFER, PH.D., M.D.

W · W · NORTON & COMPANY · NEW YORK · LONDON

Published simultaneously in Canada by Penguin Books Canada Ltd, 2801 John Street, Markham, Ontario L3R 1B4
Printed in the United States of America.


The text of this book is composed in Avanta, with display type set in Weiss Series 1. Composition and manufacturing by The Haddon Craftsmen, Inc. Book design by Nancy Dale Muldoon.


First Edition


Library of Congress Cataloging-in-Publication Data

Cohen, Donna.
    The loss of self.

    Bibliography: p.
    Includes index.
    1. Alzheimer's disease. 2. Alzheimer's disease—
Patients—Home care. 3. Alzheimer's disease—Patients—
Family relationships. I. Eisdorfer, Carl. II. Title.
[DNLM: 1. Alzheimer's Disease—popular works. 2. Family
—popular works. 3. Self-Help Groups—popular works.
WM 220 C678L]
RC523.C65 1986     616.8'3     85–15515

ISBN 0-393-02263-3

W. W. Norton & Company, Inc., 500 Fifth Avenue, New York, N. Y. 10110

W. W. Norton & Company Ltd., 37 Great Russell Street, London WC1B 3NU

1 2 3 4 5 6 7 8 9 0

Throughout this book we tell the stories of patients and families who shared their pains and triumphs, their frustrations and hopes. In order to protect their privacy, we have changed their names and any identifying details. Dialogues, interviews, letters, and communications have also been altered to preserve anonymity.

---

To OUR FAMILIES

Who are infinitely precious to us.
They gave us the love and knowledge
To sustain a sense of self
And treat others as our own.

---

# CONTENTS

# PREFACE

ALZHEIMER'S disease, is now a familiar term. Over the past five years Alzheimer's disease has gone from being a little-known disorder to being a much publicized one. Although people may stumble over the name, most know what it means: a progressive brain disorder in which the victim experiences the slow deterioration of mind, sometimes lasting five, ten, fifteen, or more years. At this time there is no way to prevent the disease or reverse its course.

The aging of our society is perhaps the great bittersweet success of the century. That people are living longer is a tribute to science, medicine, better economic conditions, improved sanitation, and other public health measures. However, we face many challenges in dealing with some of the problems of an aging population. One of the most serious of these challenges is that of caring for the increasing numbers of middle-aged and older persons with Alzheimer's disease and related disorders. The brochure of the national Alzheimer's Disease and Related Disorders Association (ADRDA) refers to dementias as the silent epidemic of the twenty-first century.

Alzheimer's affects more than two million middle-aged and older

Americans, and the number is expected to more than triple in the next fifty years. Until recently, victims suffering from the disease and their families struggled alone, leading what one patient's husband called "lives of quiet desperation" trying to cope with the impact of the disease. Families had nowhere to go for help and little if any information to read. In one of the series of films we produced between 1975 and 1979, called *The Thirty-six Hour Day*, one daughter of an Alzheimer's victim declared emotionally, "Everywhere we went no one could tell us anything about it. Everything we learned about Alzheimer's disease we learned from living with it!"

Today, patients and their families have more help available to them. Research and clinical centers are developing throughout the country. Several books, pamphlets, and family handbooks on Alzheimer's are available, and features have appeared in newspapers, in magazines, and on television and radio. However, the care of Alzheimer's disease remains a challenge. Despite the increased publicity and public awareness and despite the growth of research activity, little progress has been made in changing the physical course of Alzheimer's disease or of the other progressive dementias. Nevertheless, we have found that a great deal can be done for the patient and family to maintain the quality of life at the highest possible level. Caring for the patient by working with the family, an approach which we adopted more than a decade ago, is the best strategy available. The latest evidence supports the idea that the patient's family, where available, is the key to truly helping the patient.

The powerful impact of the disease on the entire family was one of the most striking features we noticed in the early 1970s as we began our collaboration in studying the cause as well as the natural course of Alzheimer's disease. Our families showed us how to provide care for patients and helped us to help them in turn.

At the outset we were struck by the serious problem of the misdiagnosis of Alzheimer's disease. A surprising number of patients referred to us from across the United States had cognitive deficits which were the result of some reversible cause. Our studies and those of others have since shown that as many as one-third of the patients referred from the community for memory difficulties have a treatable and reversible basis for their problems. Depression, medications, and physical illness can mimic symptoms of apparent dementia. In those instances where we were able to reverse the dementia, the emotional response of the families was enormously gratifying.

At the University of Washington in Seattle we focused not only on issues of diagnosis but also on matters related to the management, treatment, and rehabilitation of individuals with dementia. Over and over again we had heard accounts from our families of diagnoses which were delivered in hospitals or clinic corridors or, worse yet, on the telephone with no time for any questions. Occasionally, the diagnosis came with the dire prognosis of a shortened life expectancy and the need for institutionalization in the immediate future. Often against the advice of physicians and with little help, families fought courageously to keep the patient at home. At that time many people in state and national governments were expressing concern that families were dumping patients into nursing homes. If anything, we saw the opposite. We began to wonder about how best to care for and help patients live their lives comfortably and meaningfully at home. And we asked ourselves how we could help families cope with the stress of living with the disease.

The country's first experimental treatment ward for Alzheimer's disease was established under a special program at the American Lake Veterans Administration Hospital and the University of Washington School of Medicine. Initially, all of the patients, who had to be veterans, were men, but subsequently a few women were also admitted. Psychologists, psychiatrists, nurses, and internists worked together as a team to maintain patients as free of medication as possible and to implement environmental and behavioral programs to raise the patients' level of functioning.

Once again we were impressed by the activities of the families. Most of our families had been caring for their "patient-relative" for years with little or no help from anyone; until this highly specialized unit became available, they had resisted any thought of institutionalization. Their chronicles of care reflected their long-term support of patients at home, and their energetic involvement sustained the patients on the ward and influenced the staff.

It touched us deeply that in the face of this tragic disease our families were doing things that defied the textbooks. Many had incorporated the patient into a full schedule of projects and activities, and some invented creative household regimes designed to support the individuals even as they become progressively impaired.

Our families persevered despite increasing isolation from other relatives and friends and little help from professionals in the community. We discovered, too, that although caring for a patient with dementia can be an exhausting and overwhelming experience, most of our family care givers did cope successfully most of the time, and for some it was an experience that led to enormous personal growth, during and following the ordeal.

Even before the experimental Alzheimer's ward was established, many families had begun to talk with each other in waiting areas while their relatives took part in a variety of research studies conducted by us and many of our colleagues. These studies involved sleep, electrical activity of the brain, changes in memory and mood, as well as the use of drugs to improve memory. These relationships and friendships among families deepened even after their participation in the research was completed. Over time a number of families, patients, and professionals began to meet and in 1976 founded the organization ASIST—Alzheimer Support Information and Service Team. The initial ASIST self-help group established additional chapters and rapidly expanded throughout much of the Northwest. Subsequently, ASIST became one of the seven founding chapters of the national ADRDA.

Our principal task was to help the family so that it could help the patient. We came to believe even more strongly that the family is paramount in the care of the Alzheimer's patient, even when the patient is institutionalized. We also came to feel that the principal role of professionals is to help the family maintain its own strength in the service of caring for the patient. Clearly, families make mistakes and need help in caring. Misinformation about the disease, the increasing isolation of the spouse or principal care giver, sexual difficulties, emerging legal and financial crises, the cumulative impact of emotional and physical fatigue on everyone, including children, the splintering of the family around issues like the need for institutional care, and the increasing ambivalence felt toward the patient—these were only a few of the issues we saw upsetting the family.

In order to help patients and families in the community, we organized the first outpatient geriatric family program in the country. It was established in the Department of Psychiatry and Behavioral Sciences at the University of Washington. The goal of the

Geriatric Family Service, as it was named, was to provide a comprehensive evaluation of the patient and to offer counseling, support, and advice to the families. The multidisciplinary staff initially included a psychiatrist, an internist, nurses, psychologists, social workers, and an architect. Soon afterward they were joined by a family-practice physician and a law clerk. The patient evaluation consisted of several visits, including one to the home, after which staff developed recommendations for patients and families. Among the treatment strategies implemented were appropriate use of medications, communication with the patients' physicians, use of community resources, physical changes in the home or in living arrangements, help in dealing with specific behavioral problems of patients, and family counseling.

In 1981 we moved to Montefiore Medical Center and the Albert Einstein College of Medicine in New York. Here we established the Dementia Family Health Care Program, focusing on the specialized evaluation and treatment of patients and families. The program's goals were to provide comprehensive assessment, treatment, and rehabilitation for patients and families. Although the program was based in a medical center, the treatment plan emphasized care in the home and in the community. The interdisciplinary geriatric team worked intensively with the patient and family members to develop and implement a comprehensive life care plan to maximize the health and the quality of life of the patient and family. The patient, the family, and the health professionals developed a treatment plan to carry out recommendations in many areas: physical health; emotional health; cognitive enhancement; patient rehabilitation; housing and the living situation; nutrition; legal and financial matters; transportation; household tasks and responsibilities; structured daily activities for the patient; family health and vulnerability to stress; marital issues, where relevant; family communication patterns; and organization of the family system around care of the patient.

We wrote *The Loss of Self* to help families and other care givers understand what their options are in caring for a patient. *The Loss of Self* reflects more than fifteen years of research and clinical experience; it was written to convey our approach to understanding and caring for the patient and family. The word "care" means many things, according to the dictionary—protect, provide for, watch over, love, like, cherish, treasure, and respect, to name only a few. In this context all who have a care-giving role with the Alzheimer's patient, whether at home or in a nursing home, face constant challenges to sustain both the patient and themselves.

This book offers practical information about how to recognize when memory problems are serious, how to get a comprehensive diagnosis, what to do after the diagnosis, where to go for help, how to work effectively with the patient, where to get financial and legal counseling, how to deal with sexual difficulties, how to care for your relative at home, when to institutionalize the patient, and how to find a good institution. There are many strategies to help patients and care givers adapt to and cope with the impact of the disease. *The Loss of Self* shares the personal thoughts and experiences of many of our patients and families, who showed us not only how to live with their burden but also how to prevail.

*The Loss of Self* also tries to help families organize themselves to provide new options like home care and to find other resources in the community. We provide information about the history and the financing of health care in this country, for it explains why services are not more available to support the family. The challenge to the family is to meet the many needs of the patient, to find resources in the community, and to be able to pay the cost of caring— emotionally and financially.

Caring and the value of human life are a part of our moral fabric. Given the increasing incidence of irreversible disease in our older population, already considered by many to be a drain on the productive capacity of the nation, the pressure to rethink our moral contract has attracted national attention. The challenge is to find effective and affordable ways to help the helpless and ease the burden on the caring family. It is to these families that we dedicate this work.

Ethical and moral issues cannot be ignored in caring for cognitively impaired and terminally ill patients. Our philosophy recognizes that caring is costly in time and to emotions and finances. It also generates a reward—one perhaps more implicit than explicit— but there is no personal human growth without stress and strain. Overwhelming stress can lead to collapse, but helpful interventions along with information and education can make the difference between becoming overwhelmed and dealing successfully with crises.

Working with our patients and families over the years has been a special privilege for us. Despite the pathos of a tragic illness, many of our patients and families have achieved enormous growth and developed a special intimacy we have been privileged to share. They have taught us to appreciate life and its inalienable dignity. They have touched our lives forever.

D.C. & C.E.

# THE
# LOSS
# OF
# SELF

# 1

# THE
# LOSS
# OF
# SELF

---

I am hungry for the life that is being taken away from me. I am a human being. I still exist. I have a family. I hunger for friendship, happiness, and the touch of a loved hand. What I ask for is that what is left of my life shall have some meaning. Give me something to die for! Help me to be strong and free until my self no longer exists.—J.T.

JAMES THOMAS, the man who wrote these lines in his diary, died at the age of seventy, having lived with Alzheimer's disease for more than eight years. Mr. Thomas began a daily journal shortly after he was diagnosed in an effort to come to terms with what he called "God's cruel joke." Many of the entries in the early phases of the dementia reveal courage, energy, and a sense of purpose as he, his wife, Jean, and his family struggled together to overcome his losses. Approximately a year after the diagnosis he wrote,

No theory of medicine can explain what is happening to me. Every few months I sense that another piece of me is missing. My life . . . my self . . . are falling apart. I can only think half thoughts now. Someday I may wake up and not think at all . . . not know who I am. Most people expect to die someday, but who ever expected to lose their self first.

James kept the journal daily with his wife's assistance. He named it "Song of Myself," after one of his favorite poems by Walt Whitman. James knew that everything would soon be lost from his memory. He wanted to record his granddaughter's childhood, his son's struggle to build a business, as well as the daily events that had meaning for Jean and him. As long as he could write or dictate to his wife, he felt a sense of worth. It also gave him great pleasure to read through the entries knowing that he could still hold on to some of his memories. Long after James could neither write nor talk, Jean would sit with her husband and write in his journal. Although he could no longer actively participate, the ritual remained part of their life until he died.

Alzheimer's disease is a cruel disorder. However, no matter how devastating it is, the essential humanity of the "person turned patient" remains. As the disease progresses, there is little or no hope of recovery of memory, but people do not consist of memory alone. People have feelings, imagination, desires, drives, will, and moral being. It is in these realms that there are ways to touch patients and let them touch us.* The millions of people who suffer from dementia, like James Thomas, have much to teach us about living and how to enjoy being alive even with a catastrophic illness.

In recent years the brain disorders of later life have become a personal tragedy in millions of lives throughout the world. Both the victim and the family suffer with the inexorable dissolution of self. Loss of sight, hearing, an arm, or a leg challenges a person to cope with significant change. However, the victim of Alzheimer's disease must eventually come to terms with a far more frightening prospect —the complete loss of self. And for the family, according to one daughter, "the death of the mind is the worst death imaginable." Family members share a life of emotional turmoil as they witness the disintegration of someone they love.

*See O. Sacks, p. 334.

However, a great deal can be done for patients and for their families to ease the burden of Alzheimer's disease and related disorders. Almost everyone who is willing can take an active role in treatment throughout the course of the illness. Resources and therapeutic strategies exist to meet many of the needs of the family and help it cope with the changes in its life. Without assistance the family's chronicle of care often carries it unnecessarily to the limits of physical and mental exhaustion.

After the diagnosis is made, an individual may live five, ten, or fifteen years or more. These are long human years. Therefore, it is important to set realistic goals, make plans together, find appropriate professional help, and prepare for the future and all the changes it will bring. If the patient and family are able to prepare themselves to deal with the future, there is time for them to live and love, despite the ravages of a progressive brain disease.

Jean Thomas describes a moving incident with her husband, James, and one of their grandchildren which occurred several months after James had been diagnosed as having Alzheimer's disease.

It was a Saturday morning, and I was working upstairs in my sewing room making a dress for Evelyn, the oldest grandchild, to wear in the school play. Evelyn sat in the yard rehearsing her lines as Juliet with James reading the part of Romeo. Even though James read slowly and had trouble pronouncing several words, he and Evelyn were very good together. I was proud of Ev for involving him. It was her idea for James to help her practice, and he enjoyed it thoroughly.

I remember calling down to Evelyn to take a break and try on the dress for me. While we were pinning the hem, there was a funny sound outside. I walked over to the window to be greeted by James climbing up a ladder. He placed his arms around me and spoke softly: "I wish I were the young Romeo, strong of body and mind, for I love you so." We both smiled, and then I began to cry, remembering that those were the exact words James spoke years ago on our first date when he climbed up a ladder to my window!

That night during dinner, James and I talked about what had happened that morning. It was a turning point in the way I thought about his diagnosis. Up until that time both of us had been upset and irritable. I was frightened and unable to talk with James. However, seeing him on the ladder and caught in the warmth of his embrace, I understood for the first time that my husband was still someone I could touch and love. And just as important, he could still love me even with the Alzheimer's. The disease would change him, but we still shared a life together and we had a future.

Throughout this book we tell the stories of many individuals with dementia and their families who have struggled with their fears, anxieties, and hopes. Many stories are heartbreaking, but many more are moving and profound testaments to the ability of people to transcend suffering and find meaning in their lives. Elizabeth Gold, the wife of an Alzheimer's patient, called the disease "life's last battleground." She went on to say,

I cannot believe that God let my husband survive Hitler to get this disease. He was the only one in his family not to be killed by Hitler's army. My Joe was a good man who lived for me, his children, and his congregation.

Now, even with the Alzheimer's disease, he still goes to worship each day. I do not know how many of the prayers he still understands, but of one thing I am sure. Joe finds inner peace and comfort there. One Saturday he came home and sat down with me for dinner. I prepared to say the blessing when he reached for my hand and kissed it: "My lips cannot say the words, but you know my spirit fights to speak. I must fight to worship in a silence that goes beyond words."

Our patients and families have taught us that there is life that transcends Alzheimer's disease and related disorders. It is important to see the individuals with dementia in the context of their family as well as in that of their personal needs and aspirations. Every patient has a history, complete with accomplishments and failures, relationships with other people, as well as dreams and ambitions for the future, however limited. Furthermore, patients and families need each other in very special ways, even in the later stages of dementia. Ironically, Alzheimer's disease forces people to deal with each other in a smaller time frame. The anticipated enjoyment and freedom of the later years are changed. However, our patients and families have taken the challenge valiantly, finding time to love and care for each other.

## The Myth of "Senility"

Alzheimer's disease and other forms of dementia afflict an estimated three to four million middle-aged and older persons in the United States alone and affect the lives of at least fifteen million family members. Perhaps 10 percent or more of the world's population over the age of sixty-five has Alzheimer's disease or a related form of dementia. However, Alzheimer's disease and similar disorders are not normal consequences of aging.

We all know of individuals in their ninth and even tenth decade of life who continue to be creative, productive, and in full command of their mental faculties. The list of older artists, writers, political figures, scientists, and other prominent persons is virtually endless. It is no longer rare to find college students in their sixties or individuals working productively at a job in their seventies. A historical search also reveals the contributions of older persons. Thomas Jefferson founded the University of Virginia at the age of sixty-five. Goethe finished *Faust* in his middle seventies. George Bernard Shaw began writing his first novel after the age of sixty. Verdi was nearly eighty when he composed *Falstaff*, one of his best operas.

As we improve our ability to deal with the diseases of later life, more and more individuals will be able to remain productive. One advantage of the growing number and proportion of older persons in our society is that all of us are getting firsthand experience with older persons who remain vital, effective, and involved with their world. Simply stated, people do not lose their minds as they age. When we see profound losses in older persons, these are in every sense the result of some identifiable problem or disease.

A large number of diseases cause memory loss in middle-aged and in older people. Among the very old, these conditions are seen so frequently that for many years they were confused with the aging process itself. The term "senile" was used to refer to older persons who were unable to function intelligently and care for themselves. If younger persons were affected with these conditions, they were identified as "prematurely senile" or "presenile."

The terms "senile" and "senility" are misleading. They have as much professional status as the word "crazy." Unfortunately, the idea that aging and "senility" go together has been a part of the mythology of our culture and literature for centuries. Shakespeare's "seven ages of man" relates the last part of life to "second childish-ness and mere oblivion, sans teeth, sans eyes, sans taste, sans every-thing." Toynbee in his book *Mankind and Mother Earth* proposes that mankind has a choice between death and senility. What sad nonsense! Advancing age is accompanied by a greater risk for disease and frailty, but aging itself is not a disease, and it does not cause dementia.

Unfortunately, the consequences of false beliefs about "senility" and its inevitability in later life have been tragic. Not only have these myths retarded our efforts to understand the causes of dementia; they have also influenced the way many professionals think about such patients and the quality of care and treatment individuals or families may receive. This leads often to the heartbreaking state-ment "Nothing can be done," which in some cases is accurate but in others is not.

Growing older does carry a risk that we may develop dementia. "Dementia" is defined in the dictionary as "a condition of being out of one's mind." It also is a medical term referring to decreased mental performance. Dementia is a "syndrome," not a disease. A syndrome refers to a group of symptoms, in this case the loss of many aspects of language, learning and memory, thinking and reasoning. A dementia syndrome may be temporary or permanent, but the symptoms occur as a result of a disease or an abnormal condition. The term "dementia" is valuable because it alerts us to look for the underlying cause of the mental disturbance, and it implies the exis-tence of medical and psychological procedures for the care of in-dividuals who exhibit such losses.

## Forms of Dementia

Since dementia is a group of symptoms, it should not be surprising that some of the conditions that lead to symptoms of cognitive impairment may be reversible. In such situations, if the patient is diagnosed and treated promptly, the dementia may clear without any long-term effects. Indeed, the conditions of as many as 25 to 30 percent of the individuals complaining of memory problems have a treatable cause.

A wide variety of conditions may cause dementia. They are thoroughly reviewed in the next chapter. Infections, diabetes, poor nutrition, heart disease, pulmonary diseases, depression, anxiety, and the use of alcohol and many types of drugs may cause transient periods of delirium as well as more-persistent confusion and memory problems. However, many other factors besides poor health have a significant impact on a person's behavior. Lack of motivation to perform, feelings of inadequacy about one's self worth and competence, financial insecurity, social isolation, recent losses like the death of a friend or family member, or any major life change can cause a reaction which may appear as a significant dementia. Although these issues are usually considered when younger patients are examined, they may unfortunately be ignored when an older person is the patient.

Not all of the disorders which lead to intellectual loss are reversible. These diseases include cerebrovascular diseases also known as multi-infarct dementia, Pick's disease, Huntington's chorea, Korsakoff's syndrome, Creutzfeldt-Jakob's disease, some forms of Parkinson's disease, and the most prevalent of all dementias, Alzheimer's disease. It is important to recognize that although these diseases may not be reversible as of this writing, there is nonetheless a great deal we can do for the patient and the family.

## Recognizing Dementia

The early diagnosis of dementia is crucial for two reasons. First, if there is a treatable disease or condition, the problem may be reversed, if detected soon enough. If too much time passes before diagnosis, that chance may be lost. Second, even if the dementia is nonreversible and due to Alzheimer's disease or a related disorder, early diagnosis leads to early intervention and treatment. When the diagnosis is made in the early stages of the disease, patients are in the best position to deal with the dementia's impact on their future. If an accurate diagnosis is delayed too long, the consequences may include emotional distress, family upheaval, and even physical harm to the patient or others.

However, an early diagnosis is often hard to make since it can be extremely difficult to decide when something is seriously wrong. A progressive dementia may go unrecognized for a very long time because the individuals may conceal it well or because they are protected by friends and family.

Men and women from all walks of life and all occupations have reported they knew something was wrong but found ways to cope for a while. They delegated more work to other people, talked less, wrote notes to themselves, or limited their activities to ones they could manage. A government official reported to us that he could not remember conversations or questions well enough to make decisions. He survived in his job for more than a year by insisting that all questions be submitted to him in writing, ostensibly to have a "paper trail," so that he could give a more studied answer. A senior pilot (not flying a U.S. commercial airliner) told us that for more than six months he had worried about his judgment while flying, although his copilots and engineers never suspected a problem. On days when he did not "feel like himself," he allowed the copilot to fly the plane. He felt confident about continuing to fly most of the time, but at the same time he experienced anxiety about getting lost in airports, driving home, or finding his hotel in another city. One night, after getting lost for ninety minutes while driving home, he finally decided to see a physician.

Often people who live and work with a dementia victim may consciously or unconsciously delay the recognition of a problem out of loyalty or denial. One president of a corporation functioned adequately for over a year with the help of his wife, secretary, chauffeur, and two assistants. It was only when he had a minor traffic accident one weekend that the disease became public. He forgot which direction to turn and stopped suddenly in the middle of an intersection only to be struck in the rear by another car. The police thought he was drunk or hurt because he seemed so confused and disoriented. A medical evaluation led to a more comprehensive set of examinations, and ultimately the diagnosis—Alzheimer's disease.

After the diagnosis it is always easy to look back and recognize that a serious problem was developing. Unfortunately, before the dementia is diagnosed, family members often feel something is wrong but cannot pinpoint the source of their discomfort. These feelings can become intense and often affect the family for a long time to come. It is not only a husband or a wife but children who feel and react to the strain. In the following interview Henry and Sandra Long describe the early frustration before they knew that Henry's dad had Alzheimer's disease, as well as their sadness that they cannot undo the past.

MR. L.:   We first noticed that Dad had a problem finding the correct words for a situation. He always had a tendency toward this, in my opinion, but it began to get worse.

It also became difficult to deal with him because he did not seem to listen. He would ask a question. We would respond to the question, and then he would ask it again a short time later. This was even apparent in telephone calls. It was so frustrating, and we would ask ourselves, "Why isn't he listening to us? Why is he doing this?" We didn't know what it was at that time.

MRS. L.:   We felt like he didn't care enough to listen. It was as if he really wasn't interested in me or in what I was doing. I realize now that was a faulty perception on my part. But that was the feeling then.

After we married, Henry and I moved away, and we had very little contact with his parents. However, we moved back five years ago, and it has been difficult to get close to Henry's dad.

DR.:   Even though you were never close to him, he had a powerful effect on you?

MRS. L.:   Yes, it has always bothered me, and now it's especially frustrating. I know why I was never able to get close to him. And now I never will. I can't go back and change anything, because he's not going to ever understand that.

DR.:   Mr. Long, how did you feel?

MR. L.:   Frustrated and irritated. Why wasn't the man listening to what we were saying? Why didn't he understand what we were saying? Was he too busy thinking about something else? Yes, I would get upset, and I would especially get angry because I didn't think he was listening to Sandra when I thought he should be. And I look back now and understand what's been happening. It's too bad. I wish I never got angry.

DR.:   You seem to be self-critical as you look back on it now?

MRS. L.:   Yes, a little bit. I lost my temper with my father when he had a problem that he couldn't do anything about. Now it's too late to say I'm sorry. He has deteriorated too much.

Husbands or wives often report communication problems or difficulties in the marriage at the beginning of the disease. Lois Neuman told us,

I thought my husband was having an affair. He seemed less interested in me for a while, but I thought it would pass. We had been married forty-five years, and you understand how people need space every once in a while.

But it didn't pass, and I began to get angry. We fought a great deal the year before the dementia was diagnosed. I didn't want to lose my husband to another woman. Now I have lost him to something much worse.

In the following interview, Greg and Tina Jenson describe some of the early marital discord before Greg was diagnosed with Alzheimer's disease three years prior to this interview.

MRS. J.: I think the first time it struck me that something was wrong was about five years ago. We began to bicker, and we couldn't understand each other. Our communication was breaking down. We even went to a psychiatrist. We had been married for over thirty years at the time, and our arguments were different from anything that had ever happened between us before. As I look back on it now, I understand, but at the time I was baffled. We thought it was because we had both retired the year before, and that we were both having difficulty adjusting to retirement. However, it wasn't that.

DR.: Greg, what are some of the difficulties that you experienced over the past few years?

MR. J.: We went through pretty much what Tina had told you . . . of not getting along after many good years. It just didn't seem right. We were getting on each other's nerves.

DR.: How did you feel you might be getting on your wife's nerves?

MR. J.: Oh, little things that previously wouldn't have bothered us.

DR.: Your wife had mentioned that you had both recently retired at the time the difficulty started.

MR. J.: Yes.

DR.: I also understand that you went to see a psychiatrist because you thought there might be some conflict in your relationship with each other?

MR. J.: Yes.

MRS. J.: And later we realized that the cause of our problem was Greg's memory losses. He would say, "Let's go with so and so to see such and such a place," and then forget what he had said. Then I would say, "You said we were going," and he would get angry. "You are putting words in my mouth. I never said that!" I couldn't understand what was happening. I didn't know anything about Alzheimer's disease, and I was completely baffled.

Another problem was the double bind. He would urge me to go ahead and do something and then say that he would worry about me if I did it. I was damned if I did and damned if I didn't.

DR.: As time went by, did you seek other help?

MRS. J.: No. We seemed to adjudicate this between ourselves. We were determined that we were going to get along well, and we did for a while. One of the ways in which we did this was to each seek separate interests. I took courses at the community college. Greg did work around the place. We left more spaces between ourselves.

Later we came up against other problems which eventually led to the diagnosis of Alzheimer's disease. We switched doctors. A new general practitioner examined us, one right after the other. I recall that Greg was seen first, and I went in second. The doctor said to me, "I'm amazed at your husband. He's younger than you, and yet he seems much older than you. He's aging very rapidly, and I must get to the cause of it." This was the first inkling I had that something was wrong. The doctor sent us to a neurologist and ordered an EEG.

DR.: And what were the results of the examination?

MRS. J.: The EEG showed diffuse dysfunction. I didn't get any written report, but the neurologist explained what was happening. I wanted to know the truth. He told me Greg probably had Alzheimer's disease.

It is not unusual for individuals to have difficulty communicating with each other. This is precisely what often makes the early recognition of dementia difficult. However, when these problems persist, losses in the ability to communicate with others weakens even the strongest relationships. When this disruption is also accompanied by personality changes, temper tantrums, irritability, and suspiciousness, the situation usually becomes toxic. Angry outbursts may be directed at almost anyone and for no apparent reason. This is particularly troublesome since most persons involved do not understand why the outbursts have occurred or why the patients are not able to control their emotions.

In the following interview, a physician talks with Jane Dombrowski and her three young daughters about the early changes in Mr. Dombrowski and how the disease affected them as a family. Mrs. Dombrowski was forty, and her three daughters from youngest to oldest include Suzie, aged seven, Jean, fourteen, and Margo, seventeen.

DR.:     Margo, when did you first begin to feel that something might be wrong with your dad?

MARGO:     It's really hard for me to say. I didn't live at home, and I didn't see him that often. I think one of the first times I noticed a problem was when I needed a ride to a job interview. It was far away, and my dad gave me a ride. We couldn't find the place, and he finally got so frustrated he said, "To hell with the job, to hell with the interview," and he took off. I don't think I've ever seen him madder. That was when I started noticing things were wrong.

DR.:     How would you describe him before he got sick?

MARGO:     Easygoing. He'd never get involved in arguments unless it got so bad he felt he had to stop it. He usually left the arguing to us.

DR.:     What happened after he got sick?

MARGO:     If he heard fighting, he would lose his temper and tell us to stop it.

DR.:     Did he ever start them?

MARGO:     With me, yes. I don't know about the other girls, but we got in some really terrible arguments. Once he got so mad we started hitting each other—which is something we had never done before. I had never hit my dad. I just got so mad at him because he started yelling at me and hitting me for no reason at all. I got fed up and hit him back.

What must it feel like to be stricken with Alzheimer's disease or any of the other progressive brain disorders? The "individuals turned patients" have much to tell us if we watch and listen. The chapters of this book should expand our vision of what both patients and their families can do to mitigate the effects of brain disorders. The tragedy of dementia challenges victims and family members to reaffirm their existence and redefine their lives.

The first challenge is to discern whether something is wrong and then to determine what is causing the symptoms. The next is to recognize not only that the future will be affected by what is wrong but also that early diagnosis can help in structuring a meaningful family life. The ensuing chapter will describe how one goes about obtaining the most accurate medical diagnosis, because the correct diagnosis is the beginning of the caring process.

# 2

# THE
# DIAGNOSIS
# OF
# DEMENTIA

---

IT is normal occasionally to forget names or facts at any age. "Where did I put my car keys?" "Where is the letter I left on the desk?" "I would have introduced you, but I couldn't remember her name." We have all had the experience of having a word at the tip of our tongue but being unable to get it out. Some of us have never been very good at remembering names, directions, or numbers, but we learn to live with the inconvenience, to rely on others, and often to joke about our lapses.

When do memory lapses signal dementia—the serious disturbance in mental ability indicating that we have passed the boundaries of normality and that the brain is not functioning adequately? In order to answer this question, it is helpful to know a few facts about memory and the other cognitive abilities which are necessary for us to function intelligently. The word "cognition" is derived from the Latin "cognoscere," which means "to know." When cognition is impaired to the point where individuals have difficulty knowing what, when, why, or how to do things in their life, an evaluation is necessary.

Memory is only one of many cognitive abilities controlled by the brain. The list of abilities is long and includes such skills as the recognition of words, objects, and people, thinking, speech and language, mathematical calculation, reasoning and judgment, attention, problem solving, and many others. Disturbances in any of these abilities make it more difficult for a person to remember and act intelligently. Furthermore, deficits in thinking, talking, remembering, or decision making are interrelated and affect each other.

In dementia, memory for recent life experiences may be impaired more than memories of the distant past. Learning new information may become a problem, while people, places, and events from the past are retained. As this happens, an individual in the early stages of dementia may begin to confuse the present and the past. If language disturbances are present, it may be difficult to express a thought, read a sentence, or understand what is said and answer a question. A change in our ability to concentrate and pay attention causes confusion, since we do not pick up important clues about what is going on around us. These clues are necessary to help us act appropriately in the environment. There are also many "higher order" mental abilities that refer to our ability to organize information, to think and reason, to solve problems, and to make choices between alternatives. These may also change as dementia begins to reveal itself.

Cognitive losses are the result of brain failure. The phrase "brain failure" can be used like that of "heart failure" or "kidney failure" to mean that a bodily organ is not able to do its job. This incapacity may have many causes—some of which are treatable and reversible, while others are not. Analogies are never ideal, but a comparison of brain failure to the breakdown of an automobile or any complex piece of machinery may be instructive. A car will not run well or will not run at all if the clutch is worn, the oil has leaked out, the fuel tank is empty, the carburetor is not adjusted properly, the electrical system is faulty, or any number of different parts fail.

The machinery of the human brain is exquisitely complex—certainly more complex than an automobile. When something is wrong, it affects not only mental powers but much of what the body does. The ability to walk, talk, eat, sleep, and make love may be disrupted by failure of the brain to function properly. The expression of emotions like anger, jealousy, happiness, and fear is often disturbed when a disease of the brain exists. Emotional control may be seriously affected, and strong feelings will be expressed for no apparent reasons, or the intensity may be totally out of proportion to the cause. Rage, anger, foul and abusive language, and even violent threats emerge where mild annoyance might once have been expressed. Emotions may shift quickly from one extreme to another for little apparent reason. Laughter or giggling will follow on the heels of crying or anger. Any or all of these may occur in association with a dementing illness.

Dementia evolves slowly but relentlessly. The changes may seem subtle until one day odd or atypical behaviors become distressing enough to upset or unsettle the family. An engineer or bookkeeper has serious trouble adding numbers at work. Grandmother asks to go out to lunch with Aunt Bessie, who has been dead for two years. A master's level bridge player loses his ability to play no-trump. Individuals forget how to organize and complete work assignments or household chores, and even such simple matters as shopping and dressing may be difficult.

Although the coordination individuals need in order to drive a car may not be affected in early stages, they may either forget where they are going or how to get somewhere, and as a result they may behave erratically behind the wheel. An excellent driver takes the wrong freeway exit five times before finding the way home. Sudden turns, driving in circles, traffic violations, and other problems related to the individual's confusion create dangerous situations and often lead to accidents.

The inability to adjust to new situations is a problem for many individuals, even early in the disease. Problems may become apparent on a vacation or immediately after a move into a different house or apartment. Travel may result in major family crises when the patient is unable to remember enough to orient himself or herself in a hotel or a new city. On a vacation in Hawaii a wife found her husband urinating in their hotel room closet. These startling and often heartbreaking examples are varied and numerous.

## How to Judge When Cognitive Losses Are Serious

In many cases the initial changes in mental ability are more subtle and difficult to pin down. How then do we know when forgetfulness or lapses in judgment become serious enough to require professional attention? The answer is that there is simply no clear line which marks the boundary between normal and abnormal mental ability. The border is a zone rather than a line, and careful assessment is necessary to decide whether a problem exists. We believe, however, that it is helpful to highlight several indications which should signal the individual and family that there may be reason for concern.

1. Changes in mental ability which are *unusual* for a particular individual are worthy of attention. Some people pride themselves on their memory for names, faces, abilities. When the loss of an ability occurs in an area of previous strength, as in the case of a bookkeeper who begins to make numerous mistakes in calculations or a mechanic who forgets the parts of an engine, it is, in our opinion, an important danger signal.

2. The mental changes *persist*. Although some days may be better than others, there is no improvement over weeks or months. It is human to have days when we feel sharp and on top of everything as well as others when we feel less alert. Occasionally our words slip out inappropriately or we mispronounce common phrases. When word-finding problems, unusual behaviors, memory lapses, or other language disturbances continue over time, your index of suspicion should rise.

3. The decline is *progressive*. There may be good and bad days, but things are clearly getting worse with the passage of time. The lapses appear to be getting more severe and to occur more often. It is the gradual nature of the changes which usually delays judgment about the seriousness of the problem, since day-to-day differences may seem subtle. Over time, however, the magnitude of the losses becomes evident.

4. The changes *disrupt* the routine of life. They affect job performance, marital communication, sexual relations, and family and social life—indeed almost all facets of existence.

5. The person shows unfamiliar or bizarre changes in *emotional* expression. Calm people may become irritable, excitable, edgy, and jumpy. Profanity erupts from someone who seldom used foul language in the past. Angry and aggressive outbursts or sadness and crying are observed in individuals who rarely express emotions in public. Emotional outbursts are a particularly suspicious

sign when they appear and fade rapidly for little or no obvious reason.

The presence of *any* of these signs is, we believe, important enough to be taken seriously, and it should lead one to seek qualified professional help.

## How Dementia Is Diagnosed

What types of tests and evaluations are done to reach a diagnosis of Alzheimer's disease or any of the related brain diseases? At this time there are no medical tests that can diagnose Alzheimer's disease with complete certainty during the life of the individual. Brain biopsies are occasionally done in Europe, but they are not performed in the United States solely to confirm a diagnosis of Alzheimer's disease. Such a biopsy may be done in the United States only when there is another medical indication, such as a brain tumor or abscess. Furthermore, the analysis of brain biopsy material does not always verify the diagnosis. The brain changes which characterize Alzheimer's disease do not occur uniformly throughout the brain. Thus, healthy specimens may be taken from the brain, and areas where neuronal destruction has occurred may be missed. A definite diagnosis of Alzheimer's disease can be established only after the patient has died and a careful postmortem study of the brain has been performed.

At the time of the diagnosis, a series of medical and psychiatric evaluations must be undertaken to determine what type of dementia is present, whether it is treatable and therefore reversible, whether it has a cause which is not reversible, and, if it does, what the most probable condition is. The conclusion we reach is known as a clinical diagnosis. On the basis of what is already known about others with the same or similar symptoms and of the clinical findings for the patient, we make predictions as to the reversibility of the disorder and the types of treatment needed. A great deal rests on the clinical diagnosis, which should be done as carefully as possible. About one-third of those individuals who are examined by a physician because of memory problems have an illness or problem which can usually be treated. If no reversible causes of dementia can be found (and these will be reviewed shortly), the diagnosing physicians must decide which one of the nonreversible dementias is present.

Differential diagnosis is the process of making a clinical diagnosis by deciding which of many possible causes is responsible for the patient's signs and symptoms. A number of laboratory tests may be performed to determine which causes may be eliminated or found to exist. Ideally, several clinicians should examine the individual. Currently, we arrive at the clinical diagnosis of Alzheimer's disease when we cannot find any other basis for an individual's symptoms. It is a diagnosis of exclusion; we go through the process of eliminating all other possible diagnoses.

The examinations and laboratory tests involved in making the diagnosis of Alzheimer's disease and related dementias are the following:

1. A complete *physical examination* should be carried out to identify all possible health problems, including that of poor nutrition. Many physical diseases may cause disorientation, difficulty with concentration, confusion, and the memory problems associated with dementia.
2. *Laboratory tests* are done routinely in conjunction with the physical examination. They provide additional information to help the physician assess the state of health or disease. Blood and urine samples are needed to analyze body chemistry, including the functioning of the glands. An electrocardiograph and X rays will also be taken as a general rule. If abnormalities are found in the routine tests, numerous special diagnostic tests may follow. If such special procedures are recommended by your physician, ask for a explanation of their value.
3. *Personal and family medical histories* are necessary for a good evaluation. The thorough physician will want to be familiar with the patient's previous illnesses, hospitalizations, and operations and will ask questions about a wide range of possible symptoms. The medical history of the family can provide extremely valuable information. Inquiries about previous work or even hobbies can help indicate whether an individual has been exposed to dangerous chemicals or toxins which may have caused brain damage. Information about exercise and eating habits, use of caffeine, and fluid intake is also important.
4. *An accurate history of recent medications and alcohol use* is

essential in order for the doctor to determine whether the individual is suffering from the effects of drug use or misuse. Often, older patients are taking many different drugs. Too much medication, the wrong combination of drugs, or the side effects of a drug can cause dementia. It is important for the patient and family members to inform the physician about all medications. This includes drugs purchased over the counter at a pharmacy or store as well as prescription drugs.

5. A *neurological examination* is important in the determination whether there is a specific disease in any part of the nervous system. The neurologist may repeat some questions about the medical history and even do a short physical examination again. A routine neurological examination will include tests of mental status and alertness. An examination to evaluate muscle strength, reflexes, and the ability to feel such different sensations as a pinprick, vibration, or heat or cold in different parts of the body will be conducted. The neurologist also gives special attention to a person's sense of smell, hearing, vision, and use of the muscles of the mouth and tongue. Language skills, posture, walking, and muscle coordination will likewise be examined.

The neurologist's tests are fairly simple, but if abnormalities are found, they can help locate the presence of lesions in specific areas of the nervous system. This information is extremely useful for the diagnosis of brain disorders other than Alzheimer's disease. With the exception of the appearance of cognitive impairment on the mental-status test, the neurological exam will usually be normal in the early stages of Alzheimer's disease. Abnormal reflexes appear as the dementia progresses, indicating an increasing degree of brain involvement.

6. A comprehensive *psychiatric examination* complements the neurological evaluation. The psychiatric interview is a carefully organized set of questions to determine not only whether the individual is suffering from a significant mental disorder but also what the nature of the disorder is. The answers are used to evaluate a wide range of thoughts and feelings as well as to weigh the effect of major life changes like the death of family and friends, financial problems, or family conflict.

A careful psychiatric interview with appropriate psychological testing can identify the type and severity of the mental disability as well as the presence of personality disorders, depressions, or other problems which may cause dementia or make it worse if the dementia is caused by other disorders.

7. *Psychological testing* is an important part of the diagnostic examination. A complete battery of psychological tests usually takes several hours. However, the information obtained will document the profile of intellectual strengths and losses. The results of testing also provide essential information for setting up a treatment plan.

8. *Special diagnostic laboratory evaluations* are used to reach an accurate clinical diagnosis. The electroencephalogram (EEG) is a record of the brain's electrical activity, which is picked up by wires pasted on the scalp, amplified, and recorded on a machine. The EEG can usually provide a good index of the general state of the brain's activity. Abnormal electrical activity may be seen on the EEG if there is a brain tumor or seizure activity or if a stroke has occurred. The EEG helps to determine whether other diseases of the brain are present, although it cannot specifically diagnose Alzheimer's disease. In Alzheimer's disease there may be evidence on the EEG for what doctors call "diffuse slowing." The recordings of the brain's electrical activity show the presence of lower frequencies and slow electrical waves.

Computerized tomography (CT) studies should be part of every dementia workup. The term "computerized axial tomography" (CAT) is also used. Thus, "CAT scans" and "CT scans" are equivalent terms. The CT is a special type of X-ray apparatus. It shoots a series of X rays through the brain, and a computer analyzes them to create an image of the inside structures of the brain.

CT scans are useful to identify abnormal structural changes and specific pathology like brain tumors or damage due to small strokes, which are known to cause dementia. When several CT scans are taken over time, brain changes may be seen which indicate Alzheimer's disease. If enough brain cells are lost, the amount of brain tissue shrinks and the size of the ventricles in the brain increases. The ventricles are spaces inside the brain which are filled with cerebrospinal fluid that bathes and supports the brain and spinal cord.

Enlarged ventricles and decreased brain size alone are not

diagnostic of Alzheimer's disease, since they also occur in the course of normal aging. However, when serial CT scans show progressively larger ventricles, when cognitive losses are worsening, and when all testable causes of dementia have been eliminated, Alzheimer's disease is probably the correct diagnosis.

9. *New technologies to image the brain* are on the horizon. Although they are not routinely used to diagnose dementias, they are being employed experimentally in the effort to learn more about what happens to the the brain in Alzheimer's disease. Perhaps someday we will be able to detect brain disorders much earlier.

Positron emission tomography (PET) is a new diagnostic research technology based on nuclear physics and computer science. It provides a picture of the brain somewhat analogous to that of the CT scan, but there is a major difference. The CT images are pictures of brain structure—size and shape. In contrast, the PET image reveals the metabolic activity of the brain. Specifically, it shows how the brain metabolizes or burns up its source of energy, a sugar called glucose. One way to conceptualize the image we get from PET scanning is to think about the pictures we get from infrared cameras. Supersensitive to heat rather than to light, they enable us to "see in the dark."

During a PET scan the individual lies on a padded table. His or her head is inserted into the doughnut-like hole of a large machine. Doctors then inject into the individual's arm radioactive glucose which makes its way into the brain. The most active parts of the brain consume greater amounts of glucose, and the concentration of isotopes is greatest in these areas. Inside the machine are many detectors which absorb the radiation and carry signals to a computer. The computer gathers messages from all of the detectors and creates an image of activity in the brain. Bright spots show exactly where the isotope has accumulated.

PET scanners are currently in an early phase of research and development. The experimental results to date reveal a significant reduction in sugar metabolism in different regions of the brain of the Alzheimer's patient. PET scanning may someday be a valued clinical diagnostic tool. At the moment it is an expensive experimental procedure. If PET research leads to diagnostic breakthroughs and if it becomes more available and affordable, it may in the long run revolutionize the diagnosis of Alzheimer's disease.

The NMR (nuclear magnetic resonance) machine, also known by the acronym MRI (magnetic resonance imaging), is one of the latest technological tools for obtaining a computerized image of soft tissue in the body. It provides a sharp and detailed picture of the tissues of the brain.

Again the patient lies on a padded table, which moves so that the body can be slid into a doughnut-shaped hole. The NMR or MRI contains a powerful magnet which changes the magnetic field of the body. The body is 97 percent water ($H_2O$), and the positively charged hydrogen in water reacts to the magnetic field. Computers are used as part of the NMR to create an image of the brain from the changes in magnetic field. Diseased areas of the brain will thus appear in sharp contrast to healthy tissue. If there is a lesion in a particular part of the brain, that area behaves differently in reaction to the powerful magnet of the NMR.

These newer imaging procedures are much safer and more revealing than the X-ray technology of only a few years ago. Since it was not possible to visualize the soft tissue of the body with the use of conventional X rays, we had to use such techniques as the injecting of dye into the blood stream to "see" the anatomy of the brain. Such procedures were not without risk and did not give us enough information in most instances. NMR (MRI) and PET scans are not invasive to the body and offer a great improvement in our diagnostic capacity.

During the series of careful examinations needed to obtain an accurate diagnosis of Alzheimer's disease or a related disorder, it is important to ask questions about any tests the doctor wants to conduct. The entire set of evaluations may cost $1,000 or more if done on an outpatient basis. Are all the tests necessary? The answer is usually yes. Up to 30 or 35 percent of all individuals who show symptoms of dementia have a condition which can be treated and is therefore potentially reversible. In many instances, prompt diagnosis and appropriate treatment will entirely reverse the dementia. Delay or failure to conduct a crucial test increases the chance that the patient may not fully recover from some reversible problem.

Helena Swanson argued with her children for six months before she and her husband, Oscar, visited a geriatric psychiatrist. She was embarrassed about his condition; furthermore, she did not see how a "shrink" could help. Oscar had already been diagnosed as having dementia for about eight months and had been growing increasingly despondent and withdrawn. After the examination, Oscar began a combined drug-psychotherapy program, and within six months not only had his depression cleared but his cognitive functioning improved dramatically as well. It soon became obvious that Oscar did not have Alzheimer's disease. His internist and neurologist had missed the depressive illness entirely. Obviously, not all visits to the psychiatrist yield dramatic results. However, depression is a frequent and unrecognized cause of memory problems.

Under the present regulations, not all diagnostic costs are reimbursed by Medicare. Perhaps 60 to 80 percent of the expenses will be reimbursed if the examination is done on an outpatient basis. Almost all costs are reimbursed if the patient is hospitalized for the diagnosis. In most cases, however, it is better to evaluate patients out of the hospital. For patients who are already mildly impaired, the hospital stay itself can be stressful, causing them to become more confused and disoriented. Hospitalization is usually necessary only if in addition to suffering the memory loss the individual is very frail and sick, or if the person is abusive and difficult to deal with at home.

## Reversible Causes of Dementia

Since the diagnosis is so important to the future life of the patient, great care must be exercised in an accurate initial evaluation. What are some of the common causes of dementia which may be treated if discovered?

### INFECTIONS

Infectious disorders are frequent causes of dementia. A major illness accompanied by a fever, regardless of the cause, may precipitate problems in memory and thinking in persons of any age. Infectious diseases change the body's metabolism, cause pain, and often affect the way an individual behaves. Older individuals with even modest infections may become confused and lethargic, eat sparingly, and find little pleasure in social activities. As a result of the withdrawal, they may ignore requests to do many things, refuse to answer questions, and generally communicate less effectively. This behavior gives the false appearance of progressive dementia when in reality the difficulties are a result of the infection.

## METABOLIC AND NUTRITIONAL DISORDERS

A number of physical disorders are the result of disturbances in the body's metabolism. Many of these diseases are capable of causing intellectual problems as well as physical symptoms. The cells and tissues of the body contain many substances, and innumerable chemical reactions must occur between them to sustain life. Metabolism refers to those chemical reactions by which the materials necessary for life are synthesized, utilized by the body, and broken down as waste products or for reuse. Many factors can disrupt metabolism— for example, the shortage of needed enzymes and minerals, dehydration, or poor diet. An individual with thyroid problems may feel run-down, have difficulty concentrating, and become forgetful. A disturbance in the body's electrolytes, such as sodium and potassium, may result from dehydration or too much fluid consumption, kidney problems, or the use of drugs like diuretics. Too much sodium or potassium, as well as too little, may cause a change in mental state.

Uncontrolled diabetes may also lead to behavioral disturbances and mimic dementia. Levels of glucose and insulin may fluctuate as a result of changes in diet, in exercise patterns, or in body weight. While this may seem obvious, subtle changes in exercise and nutrition occur in older people over time. Often neither the family doctor nor the individual will stop to consider the effect of these changes. For example, the diabetic patient who retires, travels, or changes lifestyle and physical activity will need to adjust his or her nutrition and insulin use.

Malnutrition will in time lead to significant metabolic changes which are often first observed as memory loss or other cognitive problems. It is important to find out what the older person is actually consuming rather than to accept what is reported. Vitamin deficiencies are common in older persons. It is estimated that at least 10 percent of all persons over the age of sixty-five are deficient in the following vitamins: thiamine, riboflavin, ascorbic acid (vitamin C), and vitamin A.

The diet of older persons may vary as a function of economic circumstances or social isolation, or because of problems with their teeth or mouth. Many older people have difficulty purchasing or preparing food because of poor access to transportation, limited mobility, or physical frailty. Eating is also a social activity. The same meals eaten night after night following the loss of a spouse or the death of close friends are lonely occasions. It is difficult and simply less enjoyable to prepare balanced meals for one person, and eating habits generally deteriorate. A significant change in eating habits is also an important sign of depression.

### CARDIOVASCULAR AND PULMONARY DISEASES

Diseases of the heart and lungs may also contribute to cognitive losses, depression, and other behavioral changes. The cardiovascular system acts as a "slave" to the other organs of the body. It not only delivers nutrients and other substances in the blood to all parts of the body but circulates blood cells and helps maintain a constant temperature in the body as well. A decrease in the working performance of the heart and blood vessels or impaired oxygen exchange in the lungs may affect the amount of oxygen and other nutrients that reach the brain.

Many vascular problems like high blood pressure, arrhythmias, severe heart disease, and arteriosclerosis in the blood vessels of the brain affect memory and learning. Although it is clear that not everyone with cardiovascular disease suffers from intellectual deficits, the potential vascular basis for a change in mental status deserves a careful evaluation. Some of these conditions can be treated successfully, thereby partially or completely reversing the cognitive changes.

### MEDICATIONS

Drug-related problems are probably the most common cause of cognitive impairment. If they are identified early and corrected, the disturbances can usually be corrected. What are some of the drugs that frequently have serious side effects? Diuretics used in the treatment of high blood pressure may cause an electrolyte imbalance and subsequent cognitive difficulties. Drugs like digitalis, hormone preparations like thyroid, and insulin are frequently taken over many, many years. Long-term use of certain medications can lead to problems in later life, since they have side effects which cause losses in cognitive abilities in some persons.

It is not unusual for older people to be taking more than one drug. Estimates are that persons over sixty-five living in the community are taking an average of five drugs each day and that those in nursing homes may take more than ten. Drug combinations can be dangerous because many drugs interact with each other, causing a wide range of physical problems as well as sedation, agitation, drowsiness, or memory loss.

The time invested to understand drug and alcohol use will pay off. What drugs is the individual taking? How old are they? Where did they come from—the doctor, the drugstore, the grocery store, or a neighbor? Are they being taken at the proper intervals? With or without food? Are they dangerous when used with alcohol? How many doctors does the patient have? Does each physician know what the other is doing or prescribing? Is the dosage too high or too low? Are the drugs really necessary?

As will be reviewed in Chapter 5, changes in the nervous system with advancing age affect drug action. Older persons are generally more sensitive to drugs. Smaller doses, perhaps from 20 to 50 percent of that for a young adult, are generally recommended. Large doses may actually cause a full-blown, dementia-like syndrome.

STRUCTURAL DAMAGE IN THE BRAIN

The brain is surrounded by several membranes and encased in the skull for protection. Although well-protected, it can be damaged by changes inside the skull as well as by external blows to the head, automobile accidents, falls, and other traumatic events. A thorough psychiatric and neurological examination, including a CT scan, should determine whether structural damage is causing the dementia observed in a patient.

Brain tumors and subdural hematomas are two common causes of structural damage. Brain tumors may not be detected for a long time, and the first sign of one in older persons—or in younger persons, for that matter—may be subtle cognitive losses and changes in emotions or behavior. A subdural hematoma is a blood clot underneath one of the membranes surrounding the brain, called the dura mater. The clot causes increasing pressure inside the bony structure of the head, and this affects the brain itself. Subdural hematomas can be caused by a blow to the head resulting from a fall or by anything else that ruptures blood vessels. A CT scan shows a subdural and should be done since patients may forget a fall and family members may not have observed it.

Normal-pressure hydrocephalus, also called NPH, is the name of an important structural disorder, which deserves special discussion. NPH is not a common problem. However, it has received a great deal of attention because it is sometimes reversible. There are two major forms of hydrocephalus—primary and secondary. In the condition called secondary hydrocephalus, the pressure of the cerebrospinal fluid within the ventricles of the brain is increased as a result of some problem inside the skull cavity, such as a brain hemorrhage (bleeding), head trauma, or meningitis (an infection). Cerebrospinal fluid is produced in the brain, and it circulates throughout the tissues of the brain and the spinal cord. A number of conditions, including head trauma, can block the natural flow of the cerebrospinal fluid and thereby increase the pressure. The pressure can sometimes be relieved by a procedure called shunting. This is a neurosurgical operation in which a tube is placed in the brain to allow the fluid to drain into other areas of the body, where it may be absorbed without harm.

Primary hydrocephalus is difficult to diagnose, and its cause is unknown. The use of the word "primary" before the name of any disease indicates that its cause is unknown. Primary hydrocephalus is also called normal-pressure hydrocephalus. The spinal fluid pressure appears normal, but the CT scan shows that the ventricles on both sides of the brain are very wide. Patients with primary hydrocephalus also usually show three very specific symptoms. First, they walk with difficulty, appearing to have forgotten how to do so and exerting great effort to move their arms, legs, and feet. Second, they are incontinent. Third, they give evidence of intellectual deterioration.

When a patient shows these three signs at the beginning of an illness—problems in walking, dementia, and rapid onset of incontinence—a careful neurological workup is necessary before a decision about a shunt is made. Neurosurgery to transfer cerebrospinal fluid from the brain area into a body cavity, such as the gut, has been reported to be effective in about 65 percent of patients with secondary hydrocephalus. Only 40 percent of patients with primary, normal-pressure hydrocephalus show some improvement. However, the mortality rate associated with this procedure has been reported to range between 6 and 10 percent. Furthermore, surgical complications and infections reportedly occur in more than 40 percent of the patients. In these instances, another operation must be done and a new shunt inserted.

The use of shunting as an "exploratory diagnostic procedure" in the case of the relatively unambiguous Alzheimer's patient is not justified. The neurosurgical procedure is not without substantial risk, and the patient becomes vulnerable to a variety of complications because of the operation itself. These, in turn, often make the patient's mental condition worse, and the emotional toll on the family may be profound. The risk-benefit ratio of the procedure should thus be considered very carefully.

Normal-pressure hydrocephalus is rare. With only about 5,000 cases a year in the United States, it is not a disease that will be seen very often. Although it is almost never seen in persons over sixty-five, it occurs in 5 to 6 percent of those under sixty-five suffering from dementia.

VISUAL AND HEARING LOSSES

Impaired sight and hearing have a significant impact on the ability of an individual to understand questions posed by an examiner. Older persons with sensory impairments, especially the very old and frail, may appear to be unable to answer questions. It is unfortunate that many people, including physicians, may underestimate the importance of sensory handicaps and assume the existence of a major memory problem. Hearing losses, which are often subtle and difficult to detect, significantly reduce a person's ability to communicate effectively.

DEPRESSION

It is well known that emotional disorders may impair thinking. Often it is a diagnostic challenge for the physician to determine whether a severely depressed or anxious person has an irreversible brain disease or a severe but reversible emotional condition. Many depressed individuals are apathetic and often do not respond to what goes on around them. Others appear very restless and agitated. In most cases memory is affected, and most activities of daily living are performed with greater difficulty. The longer these conditions persist, the harder they are to treat.

Depression is not the same as sadness. Depressed persons are indeed sad, but their problem goes far beyond the sadness all of us experience in our lifetime. Clinical depression affects thinking, memory, sleep, and appetite and interferes with daily life. The term "depression" can be confusing, because it is used to describe many different, albeit similar, conditions. The word can refer to a normal mood in the lives of healthy people. This mood is characterized by feelings of sadness, usually over a loss or in response to some memory. The clinical term "reactive depression" is used to describe a sudden shift in mood which is moderately incapacitating and lasts for a few weeks as a result of some crisis, usually a severe loss. The death of a close relative or friend, the loss of a job, the occurrence of physical disorder, or any of a wide range of life changes can trigger a reactive depression. This is a normal response to such changes.

The word "depression" also applies to a major class of psychiatric disorders characterized mainly by sadness but also by many other symptoms. In some individuals with clinical depression, sadness is not even reported; the patient may just feel "empty." Appetite usually changes, resulting in a significant weight loss or weight gain. Sleep is disrupted; affected persons may wake up early in the morning and sleep fewer hours, or, alternatively, they may lie in bed and sleep too much. Loss of interest in pleasurable activities is another characteristic of clinical depression. Irritability and restlessness or the opposite—decreased energy and fatigue—may be present. In addition, physical problems like pain, personal expressions of worthlessness or guilt, difficulty in thinking, a sense of hopelessness, helplessness, and worthlessness, and thoughts of death or of suicide are also frequently associated with clinical depression.

Depression is not always "obvious" to the observer. Among the aged it is perhaps the most unrecognized and underdiagnosed psychiatric disturbance. Older persons often complain about physical problems but say little about their feelings. Thus, when no medical reason can be found for a complaint and the person is not a hypochondriac, the possibility of depression should at least be considered. Physical diseases, personal losses, and the use of alcohol or a number of drugs can produce some depressive symptoms, making the diagnosis difficult even for the doctor.

## ISOLATION AND SENSORY DEPRIVATION

Social isolation and sensory deprivation are also major causes of dementia-like behavior. Being with other people—talking, shopping, working, and otherwise interacting socially with them—creates a sense of well-being and fulfillment. A deprivation of human touch, activity, and excitement is experienced by many older persons who live alone or are homebound or institutionalized. The lack of meaningful human interactions and warmth has a potent effect. The human spirit withers. The mind may become dull or forgetful or confused.

This effect should not be surprising. Little has been written about the impact of the loneliness of old age, when family, friends, and companions are absent or the intimate circle is constricted. There are, however, situations to which all of us may relate. A long bout of illness which confines us to bed for days or perhaps weeks keeps us from our routine and severs most relationships with the outside world. When we recover and resume daily life, our body and mind may feel sluggish, awkward, and clumsy. Interactions with other people may seem strange and disconnected. Thoughts and words do not come easily. However, these experiences are transient; as we feel better and get back into the swing of things, our behavior becomes normal again.

Life apart from other people may create a major problem after enough time has passed. Just as a mirror shows us how we look, other people reflect whether our behavior is appropriate, acceptable, and desirable. Without rewarding relationships, our behavioral field is restricted and our behavior changes. The initial withdrawal may be subtle, but eventually it leads to confused and disoriented behavior. An extensive body of literature on sensory deprivation documents what isolation can do to human thought and behavior.

## Diagnosis Takes Time

As should be apparent, a good diagnostic evaluation for intellectual deterioration takes time. Indeed, several months may pass, and doctors may repeat a number of tests before they are in a position to confirm a diagnosis. The symptoms may be baffling. If medical disorders, drugs, or depression are suspected as the probable cause of the dementia, it will require some time to observe whether deficits improve with treatment. It is also possible that patients with Alzheimer's disease have coexisting reversible physical disorders which make the dementia much worse and prompt a trip to the doctor in the first place. In such instances a partial reversal of dementia may occur as the secondary cause is eliminated.

Even though an individual and a family may be concerned enough to request professional help, the results of the examinations may be inconclusive. The mental-status testing may show only the mildest of deficits. Repeated examinations several months in the future may be necessary before it can be ascertained whether the deficits are becoming worse. Remember, Alzheimer's disease is characterized by gradual, progressive, and hidden changes. A diagnosis of Alzheimer's disease should be rendered with the greatest of care. If the physician tells you and your family that he or she is unsure, wants you to return in the future, and assures you he or she will be available if something happens before the next appointment, you are probably in good hands. A premature and incorrect diagnosis can have unfortunate and often irreversible psychological effects.

## Nonreversible Causes of Dementia

When reversible causes of dementia have been ruled out, the differential diagnosis between Alzheimer's disease, cerebrovascular diseases, and other brain diseases with dementia may be easy or quite difficult. Although Alzheimer's disease is the most common irreversible dementia, cerebrovascular dementias rank as the second-most common. Cerebrovascular diseases, those conditions which result from problems involving the circulation of blood to the brain, are discussed in some detail in Chapter 12.

Small strokes may occur in as many as 15 to 20 percent of all those persons with nonreversible dementias, and it is these strokes, and the resulting reduction in the flow of blood to parts of the brain, which lead to loss of memory. Since this condition involves many small strokes, it is called multi-infarct dementia. "Infarct" is the technical term for an area of cell death resulting from the blockage of circulation.

Although individuals with multi-infarct dementia may seem very much like Alzheimer's patients to the family, there are subtle but important differences (see Chapter 12). Furthermore, since multi-infarct patients have circulatory problems rather than an unknown disease of the nervous system itself, there exist medical approaches which may help—at least to slow the progress of the condition (see Chapter 12).

## How to Find a Good Doctor

Obtaining a careful diagnosis may not be easy in many places. However, throughout the country more physicians are becoming informed about these diseases, and in many major medical centers and hospitals health professionals have developed special programs for the dementias. The appendixes to this volume identify organizations and services throughout the United States which can help identify local clinical resources. For families fortunate enough to live near one of these sites, knowledgeable and caring professionals are usually available. The problem is what to do when these resources are not available.

There are several approaches to the search for caring medical professionals. Ask doctors and nurses in your community whom they would consult if someone in their family had a similar problem. Perhaps the best way to find professional help is through other families who have a relative with Alzheimer's disease. (See Appendix 1 for a list of local groups in the United States.) These organizations are extremely valuable for many reasons. Their members may have information about good doctors and health resources as well as community services and agencies. Referral lists available from local medical societies or hospitals are often outdated and may or may not be useful. A telephone call to the physician will confirm whether he or she is interested and cares about older patients.

## The Qualities of a Good Doctor

How do you identify competent, knowledgeable, and compassionate physicians? Ask them questions, listen to their answers, and trust your own judgment. You might ask them such questions as "What causes memory loss in older people?" "What do you think causes Alzheimer's disease?" "What research is being done?" or "What can be done to treat the disease?" The answers to these questions, the willingness of the doctor to spend the time to talk about these problems, the content of the answers, as well as the tone of voice reflect a great deal about the person. If the doctor seems uninterested or distant, or if you feel uncomfortable, you should find someone else. The objective is to find a doctor who is technically up-to-date and also cares about the suffering of the patient and the family.

Your internist or family-practice doctor will refer you to specialists in psychiatry and neurology. Find out whether the "specialist" is "board eligible" or "board certified." "Board eligible" means that the doctor has completed specialty training beyond medical school in an approved residency program. "Board certified" means the doctor has also passed a national examination and has been certified in that specialty. These examinations are not mandatory and are not required for physicians to obtain a license to practice. Although passing the specialty-board examination is not always the sign of better physicians, it does mean that they have at least had the minimum required training and experience in the specific area of medicine in which they "have their boards." You should try to make certain that the specialist you choose is at least "board eligible."

It is important that you feel comfortable with your doctors and sense that they know the patient, the disease, the family, and what is available in the community. You will soon discover whether they are willing and able to provide you with the care and support you need. Let your informed feelings help guide you.

## Do Victims Recognize They Need Help?

Long before professional help is sought and a diagnosis established, individuals with cognitive problems and their families usually recognize that something is seriously wrong. Often, however, patients, as well as relatives and doctors, falsely attribute these changes to the normal aging process, to problems at work, to stress, or to other life problems. The results of one study suggest that family members are more accurate than patients in identifying a problem and that affected individuals are more likely to underestimate or deny their problems.

Unfortunately, many individuals are so reluctant to recognize they have a problem that to even suggest that something is wrong may provoke indignation and angry denial. Ann Sylvester and her husband had spent summers at their cabin on the lake over the past ten years. This summer Arthur had noticed that Ann seemed more irritable and less interested in entertaining their friends. This withdrawal from social activities was disconcerting to Art because over the years they had both become very attached to the area and especially to their friends. Ann and Arthur had developed special friendships with four other couples, having become virtually inseparable.

When Ann first seemed detached and bored, everyone was supportive. Ann was a talented artist; Art and the others had grown accustomed to her periodic mood swings. However, this summer there was a raw edge to her personality. She argued over the simplest things—the amount of salt to put in the soup, the number of coals for the barbecue, the hour they had to leave in order to arrive at a concert on time, the type of mayonnaise to buy. Indeed, Ann would become deeply insulted and pout if Art bought a different brand of mayonnaise. Ann not only argued with her friends over trivial matters but even began to turn down opportunities to do things together.

Their friends shared their concerns with Arthur and each other. They had even begun to evolve a plan for confronting Ann with their belief that something was wrong and to ask her to see a doctor. However, it was Ann's sister Maria who finally questioned Ann about her behavior one evening as they sat together by the fire. Ann's response was as swift as a bolt of lightning. She asked Maria to mind her own business and even suggested that Maria could leave that weekend if she did not like her company.

More than two months passed before Ann saw a doctor. She fought with everyone and denied that anything was wrong. Finally, Maria called an old family friend who also was an internist and begged him to help get Ann in for an evaluation. Ann found many excuses and broke several appointments. The family decided to meet together for a Saturday evening meal and "gang up" on Ann. Arthur, their three children and their families, and Maria and her husband spent over four hours trying to persuade Ann to get a checkup. It was a stormy evening, but everyone was unrelenting. They gave Ann the room to be angry, continually reiterated how much they loved her, and insisted that there was no way they would let her go on like this. Everyone, including the grandchildren, emphasized how important she was to all of them.

The comments of her six-year-old granddaughter, Mary Jane, brought the arguments to an end. Ann reached over to hug Mary Jane who ran to her mother and began to cry. "I'm afraid. Nana scares me sometimes." Ann finally gave in to her family's pleas to see a doctor.

Clearly, the individual's inability to recognize that a serious problem exists delays the diagnosis of the problem. Furthermore, in such instances, the family members may fight so hard to get the individual to see a doctor that they are unable to see when their relative becomes more accepting of help. As a result, families may continue to argue with their relative and escalate conflict rather than work with him or her more cooperatively and supportively.

Family members usually make the initial appointment for the diagnostic evaluation. Several factors appear to deter the "patient" from contracting the doctor personally even when the individual is aware that something is wrong. However, in many situations one or more family members work together to pressure a loved one to see a doctor; then, once the individual has agreed, they set up the appointment without letting the patient take any initiative. Some family members become so overprotective that they not only arrange all the appointments but also talk with the doctors on their own and effectively exclude the patient from active participation in the entire diagnostic process. It is important to give patients opportunities to participate as much as possible. Let them help set up appointments and talk with the doctors on their own if they wish.

The exclusion of the patient is sometimes reinforced by professionals who seem unaware of the insight the patient has into his or her own condition and who are more comfortable talking directly to family members. In meetings with professionals it is important to include the patient as well as available family members and to involve him or her in understanding the diagnostic process as early as possible.

### Preparing to Hear the Diagnosis

Once the examination begins, ask the doctor to explain the steps in the diagnostic process as well as the signs or results that are being looked for. If your doctor does not do this, press for the information, but recognize of course that it may not be useful to demand the results of each individual test until the entire evaluation is over. Many individuals displaying symptoms of dementia can be puzzling diagnostic problems, and careful health professionals may need time to think and discuss their findings with knowledgeable colleagues.

There is something very specific you and your family can do during this period. Bring the family members together and develop your own plan of action for the day you meet with the health professionals to hear their conclusions. Ask your doctor to give you an approximate date when the tests might be concluded, and tell him or her what the family is doing. Decide who wants to be present. Does the identified patient want to meet alone with the doctor first, before the spouse or other family members join the conference? As the agreed-upon date for the conference draws near, remind each other, especially the patient, several times. This tactic is a way of allowing the patient who wants little or no information to say so. This is extremely important when the patient lives alone and other family members are trying to help. Although most people want to hear the diagnosis, this is not always true. Well-meaning relatives should not impose their views on the patient.

When Marlene Van Dyk was told that she probably had Alzheimer's disease, she was alone with her doctors, at her request. Even though her husband and daughters had accompanied her to the various appointments and had met the doctors, Marlene had been adamant about meeting with them first: "I knew something was terribly wrong. I wanted to hear the verdict without my family present. Yes, I even knew it was Alzheimer's before they told me. I was afraid when they said the words I would cry, and I needed to cry before I could face my family."

Not all people want to be alone when they hear the diagnosis. Craig McCarthy sat around a conference table with his wife and children when the doctors summarized the results of his examinations: "When I heard 'Alzheimer's disease,' the words struck me like a thunderclap. My heart began to ache, my knees trembled, and my body was numb. I felt like a gurgling whirlpool was sucking me down. I remember looking around the room—at my family and the doctors. I needed them all to get my bearings again. Without them I would drown."

Receiving bad news is never easy. If you are fortunate, your doctor will spend the time you need, answer your questions, and listen carefully to what you say. The next chapter discusses common reactions to the diagnosis as well as what you can do to help the patient and yourself after the diagnosis has been made.

# 3

# REACTIONS
# TO
# THE
# DIAGNOSIS

A sense of utter helplessness swept over me when the doctor said that I probably had Alzheimer's disease. The very words "Alzheimer's disease" sounded harsh and unreal. I wanted to believe that he was talking about someone else—not me.

I remember asking a few questions. Was he sure? Could it be something else? What could he do for me? I remember how he leaned forward and stayed close to me when he answered, but I don't remember what he said. I did not want to listen.

I wanted to talk; but I didn't want anyone to know how scared I was. I had always imagined myself to be a strong person who could face anything. But now I was afraid of a disease I did not understand. How was I going to live the rest of my life and take care of my family? All I could see was darkness.

WHEN given the opportunity, many individuals will discuss their thoughts and feelings after receiving the bad news—shock, anger, disbelief, fear, despair. Jan Prescott, whose words open this chapter, was aware of word-finding difficulties several years before she finally submitted herself to a full battery of medical tests:

My memory lapses were humiliating. I couldn't depend upon myself anymore. Mysteriously I was changing. I knew about this Alzheimer's disease, how it destroys intelligent behavior in bits and pieces, but I was afraid to think that it was happening to me. When the doctor began to talk to me in the office, I began to get very nervous. I wanted to run away. It may sound absurd, but I thought if I didn't hear the words then I couldn't have the disease.

How do you tell someone he or she has Alzheimer's disease or a related disorder? There are no right ways, but there are some wrong ways. Too often doctors deliver the diagnosis quickly and then offer a brief statement that little or nothing can be done. They tend to speak to the family members and leave to them the job of informing the patient. Frequently, all those involved—professionals and family members—are uncomfortable and do not know how to talk or listen to the person who had been diagnosed. Listening carefully and actively to the "person turned patient" provides important clues about what the patient is prepared to hear.

In most instances once the individual and the family receive the diagnosis, all go home and are left alone to live with the news. One woman told us,

We lived in an atmosphere of silence. The doctor said that Jim had Alzheimer's disease. We didn't know whether to be thankful that the disease had a name or to be afraid. Jim would not talk about it. Sometimes at night, he would sit at the desk with his head in his hands, staring at a book. One evening I found him downstairs by the furnace, with a can of peas in his hand. He was crying, but turned quickly away when I entered. I pretended not to notice. He walked past me and pressed the can into my hand. "Choose a wine for dinner. I don't know whether to have red or white." And then I realized he had forgotten where the wine cellar was located. He had gone to the pantry instead.

The tragedy of the situation is repeated over and over. Individuals do not in fact have to suffer alone, but they often need help in voicing their emotions and coming to terms with them. By providing opportunities for dementia victims to talk and then listening supportively, one can aid the evolution of initial grief and despair into acceptance. However, talking and listening are not always easy, because much of what patients say is painful for the listener. Jim Evans spoke the following words several months after the wine cellar episode:

Alzheimer's disease is worse than death. It leaves bone and flesh intact while it erases judgment and memory. I could live with death. Death is a part of the cycle of life. It's like spring, the end of winter. But this disease —it's unnatural. It's the end of hope.

However, Jim and his wife, Dee, conquered his initial hopelessness and desperation. Dee learned to listen to Jim supportively when he felt sad, but then she always found ways to say how much they could still do together which brought them both pleasure.

After the diagnosis several important questions arise: When should individuals be informed about the full impact of the disease? Should patients see and associate with others suffering from more-advanced phases of the disease? It is, of course, not possible to answer such questions categorically. As this chapter shows repeatedly, each family and patient deals with these issues on an individual basis. The rule of thumb is to *hear* what the patient wishes to learn, and then to make responses tempered by the patient's reactions and perhaps by what you are able to endure.

If we pay close attention, patients will usually tell us how much they want to know. One patient, a retired longshoreman, listened carefully to an explanation that he probably had Alzheimer's disease. His gaze shifted to the window for a brief moment; then he looked back at his wife, the rest of his family, and the doctor and surprised them with his response: " 'More light.' These are the words Goethe said when he was dying. I want to know more. I need to prepare my family."

Although it may be emotionally difficult for you, it is valuable to share information with the patient as he or she is ready to receive it. Do not withhold information when asked a direct question. Listen very carefully and gauge your response according to the question. Sometimes you may not have to say very much at all. You may only need to show that you are ready to talk, and the patient will say a great deal. Confronting the disease gently and slowly is often the beginning of a successful treatment program which involves patients in discussions about their future. Alzheimer's victims have the right to determine how they will live their remaining years while they still have cognitive capacity in the early stages. Realistic discussions about the nature of their illness are the basis for plans for the future, before they become incapacitated.

One of the most difficult challenges after the diagnosis is to deal with patients who seem upset and agitated but are unable to express personal feelings. Patients are quite often afraid of upsetting other members of the family and wish to protect them. Some individuals, generally men, may never have spoken much about their feelings. The thought of becoming a burden on their wife or children may be too difficult for them to bear, and raising feelings about their dementia is contrary to a lifelong pattern. Here the family must show its strength and gently create openings over time which may allow for the expression of unpleasant feelings. If this does not work, counseling by a minister, physician, or other professional may be the best approach.

Discussions are also likely to occur in the context of the legal and financial planning which should be done soon after the diagnosis. A lawyer or accountant may be instrumental in helping the patient begin to address the problem of planning for the future. Although the role of these professionals is not to focus on feelings, legal and financial issues often evoke emotions. The simple act of developing a legacy for members of the family may begin with financial and material matters, but it often evolves into the more significant emotional legacy which patients may need to express.

Marie Edwards told her lawyer that the disease had forced her to find a new meaning in life. Marie had been a successful business-woman preoccupied with money, achievement, and constant activity. In order to face her dementia, she constructed a philosophy that measured her life in terms of values rather than time and money. She decided to concern herself with what gave her life meaning rather than with the number of years she had left. Her children were important to her, and she decided to visit them more often. She spoke with them about her desire to leave something for them to remember her by. One day she announced that she wanted to arrange the many hundreds of family photos into albums. With the help of her children, over a two-year period, she reviewed fifty years of photographs and seemed to become more contented emotionally. Mrs. Edwards felt that she had finished an important task with and for her family before the progressive dementia left her in oblivion.

## Understanding the Patient's View

The period following the diagnosis is the time when patients must deal with their feelings and begin to incorporate the disease into their lives. George Christos describes it to his doctor in the following dialogue:

DR.:     How did you feel when you were told that you had Alzheimer's?
MR. C.:  I was angry. I was confused. I was fighting against the diagnosis. I felt like it shouldn't happen to me.
DR.:     Are you still fighting?
MR. C.:  Yes, I'm still fighting, but not against the diagnosis. I am resigned to it. Now I am fighting to live each day. I'm fighting to live as it comes. I am fighting against my fears. Every morning when I wake up, I have to ask myself who I am. I am afraid of the day when I will not know who I am. But until that day the world will know that George Christos is alive!

Some patients do not seem to understand the diagnosis, whereas others admit to being at a loss as to how to deal with it. Many say that they feel as if they have been given a death sentence. Death and loss are frequent themes, which surface early in discussions with certain patients and families. Often the issue of death begins as a reaction to the diagnosis. The labels "Alzheimer's disease" or even "dementia" convey the idea of profound loss as well as that of an incurable and life-shortening disease.

Such concerns reach deeply into an individual's emotions at a time when abilities are still largely intact, and many patients are capable not only of understanding what is at stake but also of feeling and reacting to their frustrations. The victim of the disease is in the position of having to catch up psychologically with the consequences

of the disease and what it means for his or her future life. In reaction
to the diagnosis, one patient told us, "Death wasn't knocking on my
door. Death kicked the door in to show his face."

Early in the disease many patients are desperate to talk about what
it means for their future and for their family. They will often confide
in a compassionate friend or health professional. They have questions to be answered and need patient support to overcome their
anger, fears, and anxiety. Cognitive losses as well as speech and
language problems often make this difficult for everyone. One patient spoke hesitantly about how difficult it was for her children and
husband to talk with her. She knew how much love filled her family,
but she lamented their fear of her disease and the breakdown in
communication between them. One day, her eyes filled with tears,
she quoted these lines from the poet Theodore Roethke: "Like the
half-dead, I hug my last secrets. . . . I fall, more and more into my
own silence. In the cold air, the spirit hardens."

Reactions of professionals and family members to the patient are
important. The task is to be honest with the patients and inform
them as much as possible about the nature of their disease, the
prognosis, and the willingness of clinicians and family to help. Care
givers should work carefully with the patients, giving them information as they are ready to accept it. This is made difficult by the
patients' deficits and emotional response as well as by the care givers'
own emotions. It also requires time and repetition. In the end, this
sharing may foster the acceptance that allows patients to live with
themselves.

In the following dialogue, Albert Johns, aged sixty-two, describes
what he remembers feeling both at the time he was diagnosed and
at the time of the interview:

DR.:     When you were told that you had Alzheimer's disease, could you
        talk about the diagnosis easily with your wife?

MR. J.:   No. I had trouble. It's an inevitable sort of thing, so you have to
        accept it. That's all. I didn't want to accept the truth then. Now
        I hope for the best and help other people who are going through
        the same thing—give them a little hand up.

DR.:     Does that make you feel better?

MR. J.:   Sure it does. You bet.

DR.:     Do you think you and Dorothy have become closer?

MR. J.: Since working together on this? I think we have.

DR.: Do you ever feel very angry and frustrated?

MR. J.: Well, I suppose we all go through this. It's a continuing thing, but let's put it this way: I think I'm coping with it better now than I was a year ago.

DR.: What makes you say that? Why do you think you're coping better?

MR. J.: Well, maybe it's because I have more time to think about it and I realize what I'm doing wrong, where I'm making my mistakes. I won't say that I'm curing them, but I like to think that I'm on the right track.

DR.: Do you think very much about the future and what might happen as time goes by?

MR. J.: Yes.

DR: Do you worry about the future?

MR. J.: Yes, but I am resigned. I know more about what's going to happen to me now than I did a year or two ago. A year or two ago I was shaken up quite a bit more. Now I can accept the situation. I might also say I am curious. I'm interested in what's on next.

DR.: What do you think is next?

MR. J.: Wish I had a clue.

Patients have a great deal to teach us about living with the anguish of what one man called "a living death." Jerome Lambert and his wife, Irene, invited us to their home to talk with them approximately two months after Mr. Lambert had received a diagnosis of Alzheimer's disease. Mr. Lambert had some difficulty finding the right words, but he spoke slowly and effectively for several hours. He even gave us a small notebook to read. Together with his wife he had written a daily diary describing the changes in their lives as a result of his illness.

Mrs. Lambert cried several times and spoke of the anger she felt that her husband should be suffering such a cruel and senseless disease. He put his arm around her whenever she cried and once said to us, "My brain is an attic, a place full of junk, but my shoulder is strong." Throughout the afternoon Mr. Lambert was enthusiastic about continuing to live. He was committed to telling his family what he wanted to do before he was incapacitated by the dementia.

Perhaps the most important concern of many patients is the need to participate as actively as possible for as long as possible. They want to have the information to make decisions relating to what is happening to them. Often patients voice this concern because they feel excluded from the families' decision making too soon. They want to be involved in plans dealing with their future and the changes in their lives. A frequently expressed desire of many, though not all, patients is that heroic measures not be used when they are in the terminal phases of the illness. Firmly expressed, too, is the desire to avoid a nursing home, a wish that often comes back to haunt family members if institutionalization becomes necessary. Finally, most patients tell us that if indeed there is no cure, they want the primary goal of living to be "comfort" for themselves and for their family.

Many Alzheimer's patients share their fear and sadness that as the dementia progresses their confused mental state will deprive them of the ability to relate to their family and themselves with dignity and self-respect. Although answers do not flow easily when these conversations occur, the act of letting the persons express themselves is itself valuable. One way to respond may be to acknowledge that you understand their wishes and will help them with whatever happens in the future. It is important for family members to try to accept the reality of the future if the patient is to be able to do so. The emphasis should center on the present and what can be done to maximize comfort, pleasure, and meaningful activities. The focus should be on the patients' strengths. Challenge them to discuss with you how to use the time most valuably.

The courage of our patients and families is remarkable. Arthur Roberts, a successful writer, told us that he, his wife, and his family were living a life of "tranquil heroism." Mr. Roberts knew there was no cure and that the disease would slowly leave him unable to function as a husband, father, writer, and man. But he was determined to fight to live. He regarded his wife as a heroine who had the courage to accept his limitations and continue to love him as a man who still gave her life a special quality. Mr. Roberts needed to feel that his wife, children, and friends would let him remain part of their lives. Although he was afraid of the future, he was helped by sharing that fear with them. For him it was the only way he could live, and die.

One man, a physician, told us that he wanted to develop "the courage to make a series of silent retreats." He spoke of his need to gain power over his disease and to die a little each day without losing the desire to live. Other persons speak little about death. Some have quite forcefully told us that they simply do not wish to think about it. One man, a clergyman, shared his reflections with us several months following the diagnosis. He quoted freely from the Scriptures in early discussions, but as the disease progressed over several years, he remembered less and less. However, he retained one important passage which he always quoted when asked how he was doing: "I am content. For all creatures, death has been prepared from the beginning."

Sometimes individuals are reluctant or afraid to talk openly because they are embarrassed, ashamed, or frightened. In other cases, the individual will open up and overwhelm the receptive listener. The content is often surprising and unpredictable. Victims of the disease are middle-aged or older adults who have had a rich life filled with events and people behind them. In order to plan for the future, one must carefully explore the patient's attachments to family, friends, places and life activities. Although the losses in Alzheimer's disease and the related disorders are unique, there is a parallel for the patient and family in the reaction to terminal illness, such as late-stage cancer. In fact, there is a valuable literature which may be useful in learning how to deal with Alzheimer's patients (see references).

With improved medical care, patients are living longer. It is almost impossible to gauge the life expectancy of individual patients at this time. Some professionals may not be well informed, but rather than confess their ignorance they may give patients and families incorrect information. Alex Georgio vividly recalled what he was told at the time of his wife's diagnosis: "She'll be in an institution within six months and dead in eighteen months." He repeated this often during the years following the event, and both he and his wife took particular pride in proving these words of doom wrong. He often emphasized that planning for his wife's demise as predicted by their neurologist was inappropriate. For years both he and his wife remained convinced that physicians knew little about the disease or its management: "What we learned about Alzheimer's we found out for ourselves."

## Dealing with the Patient's Denial

What do you do when the patient flees from information? What tactics do you adopt when a close family member refuses to acknowledge what is occurring? The answers are complicated, and we can offer only guidelines. Most people need time to adjust to severe stress, and some simply require more time than others. Dealing with the formidable diagnosis and prognosis of irreversible dementia brings up profound feelings. Some individuals may never be able to face the reality of their disease. And in these instances, family members may have to develop a lifestyle which supports the patient as well as his or her denial.

The family can take some very specific steps. First, family members should sit down and put their heads together to formulate a plan. If health professionals are available, they may be able to provide some valuable insights and assistance. If this form of help is not available, bring in a clergyman, a trusted friend, or an outsider who may help you see the world a little more objectively.

Jesse Barker received a diagnosis of Alzheimer's disease at the age of forty-six. His wife and children described him as a gentle, quiet man. He had not only worked hard to provide for his own family but also supported his brother's wife and two small children. His younger brother, Bill, had been killed in a hunting accident.

Mr. Barker refused to admit that he had Alzheimer's disease. He would sit through family meetings and listen attentively to others, but he would say very little. His sister described him as silently amused by the way everyone behaved. Jesse had always been a tolerant man, and nothing seemed to upset him. No one could remember him crying, even when his brother was killed. And whenever the family would reminisce about Bill, Jesse would seem not to listen. After Bill's death he took a second job and never complained about the long hours, even to his wife. But Mrs. Barker wrote us several times about the family's frustration with Jesse's denial of his condition.

Dear Doctor,

Jesse goes about his days, business as usual. He quit one of his jobs last week. He just came home Friday and told me he would not drive a cab anymore. He said there were too many taxis for a town this size and business was slow for him. He had better things to do. There would be less money for a while, but he would find something else.

I called my daughter. I did not want him to take another job, and I also did not want him to continue in the second job. I am afraid he will be fired someday soon. He can still do his job as a salesman, at least with his old customers. But the new ones are a problem. We had dinner with his boss last week. Gerry told me that Jesse forgets appointments occasionally, and it had started to happen more frequently. Some of the customers have even started to complain. Although Jesse has been sick for almost a year now, we never told his boss or his friends at work. We wanted Jesse to be able to continue working as long as he could.

Doctor, I think the time has come for him to stop working altogether. I do not want him to be embarrassed by a pink slip. On the other hand, I am ashamed to tell his boss he has Alzheimer's disease. Each night I help him with the receipts because he cannot itemize the daily sales and deliveries. However, I cannot go out in the car with him. Someday he may forget to file an order for a big customer or he may have an accident. He hides it well, but I don't know how long he can go on like this. And I'm at the end of my rope.

Can you help us find a way out? When the kids and I talk to Jesse he listens but ignores us at the same time. He makes me so angry.

Several meetings were held with the members of the family to convince them they had done everything they could. Mr. Barker's denial of his symptoms was consistent with his personality style. From all we could tell this was the only way he could deal with the illness, just as it had been his only way of dealing with his brother's death.

The employment issue was settled when Jesse was fired. However, Mrs. Barker, with the encouragement of her family, explained the situation to her husband's boss. The head of the company allowed Mr. Barker to retire with disability compensation.

With time Mrs. Barker, the children, and the rest of the family became more comfortable with Jesse and his dementia. To fight him was ineffective and senseless. Jesse continued to live at home for five years before being institutionalized. The following excerpt is from a letter Mrs. Barker wrote after her husband died.

Dear Doctor,

I still think about Jesse every day. I did everything I could to care for him. He was my life, and now that he is gone I feel lost. Jesse was such a fighter. The entire time he was sick he stayed active. I always got the strangest feeling that he was determined to make it through every day, even towards the end. He never accepted the fact that he was sick, and he was determined to live. In his mind nothing has changed. In his own world he seemed so happy, so content, even though he appeared so confused to us.

I remember one time when he seemed to know what was going on. Last Christmas I visited him at the nursing home. In fact, it was Christmas Eve. We sat together in the day room for over an hour opening up his gifts. As the children and I prepared to leave, Jesse touched my check and he began to cry. He spoke slowly, "I guess I will never have a Christmas at home again."

Everyone was surprised. And everyone cried . . . me, the kids, and even the nurses. The children had to drag me out of the nursing home, and they brought me to their home for two weeks. I still think about that incident every day.

Jesse has been dead almost ten months now. We had so many wonderful years together. I am happy that he seemed not to know what was happening most of the time. I like to think that he died happy. Doctor, he lost his self with that disease, and I pray that he did not know what was happening.

How do you know when it is better to support rather than continue to confront the patient's denial? How do you deal with a patient with a strong denial system? The preceding example illustrates how important it is to analyze and understand the patient's reactions to severe stress in the past. If the patient's personality style has been to respond to stress and crises by avoidance and denial, it may be appropriate to quietly support the individual's denial and strengthen it.

There are strategies for working around the denial in certain crucial situations. Psychologically trained professionals may be successful in conjunction with appropriate attorneys to help families deal with specific problems involving financial assets and other legal issues.

Eleanor Samuels turned to a psychiatrist and a lawyer to help her resolve an upsetting problem with her husband, who had recently been diagnosed as having Alzheimer's disease. Ronald Samuels had just been hospitalized because of internal bleeding. Mrs. Samuels was distressed by her husband's condition and by their financial straits. Mr. Samuels had a small business firm with several partners, and his wife thought the contract specified that all assets went to the firm when any of the partners died. Mr. Samuels completely denied that he had Alzheimer's disease and thus insisted that there was no need to deal with the matter. His wife was concerned about her ability to protect their assets.

The following conversation illustrates how the doctor was able to talk with Mr. Samuels and successfully work with him.

MR. S.: It is very nice of you to visit me, but I am doing quite well, thank you. I didn't ask to see a psychiatrist. Why are you here?

DR.: Your internist, Dr. Hanks, asked me to see you. He is a little worried about you and thought that I might help.

MR. S.: What do you mean? I am in perfect health except for this bleeding in my stomach. When they find out what's wrong, I will be out of here and back to work.

DR.: Mr. Samuels, I know you think everything is fine. However, both Dr. Hanks and I are worried about you. You have Alzheimer's disease. And there are several things we can do to help you.

MR. S.: Doctor, I do not have this Alzheimer's disease. My wife believes anything a doctor tells her. My memory is fine. I forget a few things now and then, but everyone does when they get older. It is nothing to get excited about. Everyone is making far too much fuss about this. Please leave me alone.

DR.: Mr. Samuels, I will leave you alone in a little while. May I ask you a few questions before I go? It would be very helpful to me.

MR. S.: Sure, go ahead.

DR.: How long have you and your wife, Nancy, been married?

MR. S.: She's my second wife. I think it has been twenty-six years now.

DR.: How would you describe your marriage to her?

MR. S.: (Silence) She is a wonderful woman. There is nothing I wouldn't do for her. Nancy is part of me, and I could not live without her devotion.

DR.: Has Nancy spoken to you about what the two of you should do to fight this Alzheimer's disease?

MR. S.: Doctor, nothing is wrong with me. Nancy wants me to talk with my partners. She says I have no life insurance and that I may lose my assets to the firm. I have plenty of money, and I intend to live a long and happy life with her. I will take good care of her. She deserves everything I can give her.

DR.: Ron, please I must interrupt you. May I call you Ron and talk to you man to man?

MR. S.: Yes, you may call me Ron. What do you want?

DR.:     If you love your wife as much as I suspect you do, why not talk to a lawyer with her. It will make her feel better and put her mind at rest.

A series of meetings took place between Mr. and Mrs. Samuels, the attorney, and the psychiatrist. Mr. Samuels never acknowledged that he had Alzheimer's disease. However, since he had such a strong relationship with his wife, this love became the key with which to open discussions about the business. In this instance, there was no need to confront him with the reality that he had Alzheimer's disease.

We have a great deal to learn about denial and how it helps or interferes with dementia victims' ability to cope with their illness. For some patients denial may be an adaptive reaction to the need to survive; others are capable of mastering their painful emotions and of overcoming denial in dealing with their disease. However, the work must begin in the early phases of the illness, and the objective must be to do whatever brings the patient the greatest comfort, peace, and functional effectiveness.

Honest discussions after the diagnosis do not mean that the patient will not later deny the truth. Ivan Hackett asked his doctors endless questions about Alzheimer's disease during the diagnostic conference. The next day he told his wife that he didn't know what was wrong with him. The next week in the doctor's office he did not want to ask questions, and he told everyone that he was in good health. A week later he informed his doctor that even though he did not like it, he was going to die from this Alzheimer's disease. Ivan vacillated this way for several months. His family and doctors supported him by listening to him when he wanted to talk. Eventually, Ivan accepted the diagnosis.

## Family Denial: A Common Reaction

In view of the many strange and disturbing incidents families experience before the diagnosis is finally made, it is startling to learn that the most common immediate response to the diagnosis itself is denial. Reactions vary, but expressions of surprise are typical. "No, it cannot be! It can't be happening to me, my husband, my mother." The same questions are put to the doctor, particularly when younger patients are involved. "Are you positive? Are you sure there's no mistake?" "Are you sure there's nothing we can do? Is there someone else who could help us?" These are all frequent queries—and for some families the doctor's answers are not satisfactory.

The denial can extend to some, if not all, people involved with the patient—spouse, children, in-laws, brothers, and sisters. Feuds may even develop if the reactions of different family members cannot be reconciled. Or the denial of family members, often living far away, will reinforce the reactions of the spouse or primary care giver, sometimes resulting in a search for a better diagnosis.

John Harriman first had difficulties at work. Although John could still sell a million dollars' worth of insurance a year, he could not fill out the forms correctly, if he remembered to do them at all. His wife, Bertha, would patiently organize the papers and calculate the premiums. His bridge game deteriorated to the point where he could not compete and members of the bridge club politely refused to be his partner. The final blow came when he received a new watch for his birthday. The wristwatch, a gift from his family, had small diamonds at four positions but no numbers. He could not tell the time. Finally, he and the family recognized that something was seriously wrong and that it could not be ignored any longer.

Almost on the heels of Mr. Harriman's evaluation, the situation seemed to deteriorate rapidly. His wife, a strong and articulate person, began to take over. She arranged for a second diagnostic examination, then a third, a fourth, and even a fifth. By this time she was well known in the medical community, and everyone concurred about the nature of the problem and the completeness of the evaluation. Her relatives and friends urged her to put him in a good nursing home. He would receive expert care, and she could have a life of her own again.

Mrs. Harriman shrugged off all advice concerning the diagnosis and about the need for institutional placement. She took her husband everywhere, involving him in many activities. Mr. Harriman's brother, however, insisted from 2,000 miles away that something more could be done. Out-of-town trips to more doctors and clinics were arranged. Finally, they found a physician who felt that a neurosurgical shunt should be tried as "a last resort."

John was operated on, placed on high doses of sedative medication, and then sent back home for care. This was more than seven years after the initial diagnosis. His condition had become aggravated by the postoperative complications of the neurosurgery. He was hospitalized and clearly could no longer be managed at home. Even then Mrs. Harriman fought bitterly against his placement in an institution. She brought him home from the hospital, but three weeks later consented to let her doctor put him in a nursing home. At home he had struck her many times and yelled obscenities. It was only when he stabbed at her with a kitchen knife while she was preparing dinner that she let him go into a nursing home.

John Harriman's experience illustrates both the positive and the negative aspects of denial. The family's early refusal to follow medical opinions favoring institutionalization doubtless was appropriate for them. Keeping John a vital part of the family, challenging him to the extent possible, and relating to him in as normal a way as possible was helpful not only to Mr. Harriman but also to his wife and children, all of whom remained close.

On the negative side were the emotional crises during the multiple diagnoses, the costs involved, the family feuding, and the anger at physicians, hospitals, and clinics for failing to deliver a more optimistic diagnosis. This in turn led to needless surgery and its complications, forcing the use of medication to control postsurgical agitation, and finally to an increasing complexity of care which required that he be hospitalized and then institutionalized. Furthermore, the reactions of geographically distant relatives strengthened Mrs. Harriman's denial system. Her brother-in-law's insistence that something had been overlooked and that she seek further help from real specialists forced the diagnostic issue to be reopened. It was almost to prove a point to relatives not involved in his daily care that Mrs. Harriman sought additional evaluations which eventually led to the neurosurgery. Dealing with the denial in the very beginning would have saved a lot of grief and resources and possibly would have improved the quality of life for the patient and the family. Sadly, the situation of John Harriman, his wife, children, and relatives is not rare.

The best way to begin to deal with your reactions to the diagnosis and to plan for the future is to understand exactly what examinations the doctors have conducted and to ask for a complete explanation of the results. If possible, the patient should participate in meetings with the doctors. The patient should not be excluded or made to feel that information is being discussed behind his or her back. Family members may also feel the need to have personal time with the doctor to ask for special help. If this is the case, let the patient know why you want to speak to the doctors privately. Explain briefly that you are worried about yourself. The patient may not understand your needs, but at least this gives him or her the courtesy of a brief simple explanation. Then too, the patient *may* understand.

Often the patient and family become engaged in a "silent battle" of which they are unaware. It is a battle over the control of information. Talking about Alzheimer's disease and what it does to the individual is painful. Everyone, patient and family, is uneasy, and whatever is said is usually done in a way that consciously and unconsciously restricts discussion about the future.

This is an emotionally loaded process. Difficulty in dealing with mental deterioration and death is a basic cause of communication problems with the patient. The attempt to control what is discussed undermines family members' efforts to communicate with each other. This is also an area where professionals are not always immune to blame. Too often they control the way information is exchanged about the disease because of either their own feelings or their fear of upsetting the patient and family. Their discomfort tends to become a barrier to a caring and effective relationship with the family. If you cannot talk openly with your doctor or if you feel that he or she cannot speak easily with you, perhaps you should find another to help you.

When something is unpleasant, people unconsciously respond by denying what is painful to them. The process of denial keeps information about Alzheimer's disease a "secret." More often than not the patient and the family are trying to keep the "secret" from each other, in the hope they can spare each other the pain. Sadly, many families are out of sync, working against each other rather than with each other.

In an effort to protect one another, family members sometimes consciously try to withhold information from the patient, or they communicate in a way that says very little. It is easy to spend time with a person during the day or night with little or no interaction —watching television, reading, writing, shopping, or listening to music. Nor is it unusual for family members physically to isolate themselves from the patient. People can control time by frequent business trips, shopping, meetings away from home—anything that precludes being with the patient.

Carroll Houck was unable to face his wife's illness, but he still managed to provide her with a high level of care. Kathleen Houck had begun to deteriorate in her late fifties. She was a beautiful, engaging woman who prior to the onset of Alzheimer's disease had enjoyed a successful business career. After its diagnosis Carroll began to live what his oldest daughter Karen called an "imitation of life." He could not face Kathleen's illness and spent long hours at the office, including business dinners each night of the week. Since it was well within his financial means, Carroll hired a suitable and attractive companion to live with Kathleen in their summer home. Since Kathleen loved to jog, swim, play tennis, work out in the gym, and lie in the sun, this life would be perfect for her. He would visit at least once a month. The other family members would visit less frequently but whenever they could.

The family carried out these plans, and Mrs. Houck was happy to live in the villa. What Carroll and his family did not anticipate was her insistence on speaking with each member of the family on the telephone several times daily. Her questions were always the same. When would they come to visit? This was a query she repeated with the regularity of a broken record. It was as if she had no recollection that she had ever asked the question. The usual family response was to answer her question the first time it was put and to tell her they would see her next month. On subsequent questioning, they would simply ignore the query and tell her about whatever was going on at the moment, assure her of their love, and end the conversation . . . until the next phone call. Within a few months each of the family members had installed an answering machine.

On the surface it appeared that the family was in control of the situation, that Kathleen was secure and happy, and that the family members were organized and healthy. On one level, the family and the so-called patient were doing extremely well. The players, all family members, were engaged in their own lives. They spoke with one another and seemed to have a plan in which everyone was assuming a certain amount of responsibility.

Although the surface was calm, the deeper life of the family was in turmoil. The family members eventually sought professional assistance, and during severals sessions they began to discuss the critical problem which they had been successful in ignoring. They could not accept the fact that Mrs. Houck had Alzheimer's disease. They wanted her to be comfortable. They wanted her to be happy and busy. Most important, they wanted her to be away from them, so that they did not have to see her and face the reality of her condition. Was the family doing the right thing? There is no right or wrong answer to this question.

Denial helps people deal with various aspects of their life in the face of potentially overwhelming emotions. There is, however, a paradox. The process of denial which helps people deal with emotionally charged information by limiting the amount they handle may also blind them to information and feelings which can help. If you can recognize what is happening to you, the patient, and other relatives and if, even more important, you get help early, you will be in a better position to deal with your feelings as the disease progresses.

## Genetic Vulnerability: Who's at Risk?

One of the most common reactions to the diagnosis of dementia is the fear on the part of other family members that they or perhaps their children are at risk. Some adult children even express concerns about having children of their own. It is important to emphasize that most dementias are not genetic. However, in some families several closely related individuals have been affected (see Chapter 12), and the fear of inheriting the disease is a legitimate source of concern. At the moment there are no diagnostic tests to identify who is at risk. In instances of multiple family members with dementia, it is helpful to make an appointment with a knowledgeable professional who specializes in genetic counseling.

Usually, a geneticist will be able to give no more than the probability of the risk for the family in general. What tends to emerge as impressive in these cases is the courage of the family. Although it is usual for family members to express anxiety, it is also common for many to live with a sense of humor and perspective.

Richard Todd, a forty-two-year-old accountant, had a father as well as three uncles with Alzheimer's disease. All four had developed serious symptoms between the ages of sixty and sixty-five. Richard and his two brothers and two sisters lived close together and had shared the responsibility of caring for their father.

None of them seemed especially afraid of developing Alzheimer's even though their risk appeared to be reasonably high. Interviewed one evening on a local news channel, Richard described the burden of the family caring for relatives as part of a fund-raising campaign. After the broadcast, people in the studio stood around asking questions for several hours. Several individuals were in tears. Finally, someone asked Richard whether he worried about the prospect of getting Alzheimer's disease and whether he noticed any similarities between himself and his father and uncles. Richard appeared very serious as he answered, "Yes, I think my father, my uncles, and I are alike in one very important way. We are all oversexed!" The television crew began to laugh with him as Richard broke through their somber mood. Although Alzheimer's disease was possible, he could not afford to waste precious and happy years waiting for something that might or might not happen.

## Guidelines for Developing Coping Strategies

What happens during the time immediately following the diagnosis affects the way patient and family deal with the disease and each other for years to come. Open, honest, and careful communication can minimize the difficulties ahead. A number of general guidelines may help the family deal with the situation right after the diagnosis.

1. *Go back to your doctor or see another professional who is knowledgeable about dementias.* The meeting in which you learn about the diagnosis may be so emotional that much important information may be poorly heard, understood, or missing. A return visit is very valuable to the family. It should focus on informing you what you can do. Find out whatever you can about the disease and ask for help to understand what the disease means. Inquire about the location of Alzheimer's support groups in your area. If the doctor who makes the diagnosis is not the one to help you and the rest of the family understand the future, ask the doctor to recommend a knowledgeable professional with whom you are comfortable. Often a psychiatrist, psychologist, or

social worker may be the person in the community most experienced with the disease and best informed about the resources
available in your community which can be of help.

2. *Ask, "What does the diagnosis mean to the patient (my husband,
   wife, father)?"* Hearing the diagnosis and understanding and
   accepting it are two different situations. It may be emotionally
   difficult to think clearly for a while. The diagnosis affects the
   entire family and everyone who cares about the relative or patient. One of the most important jobs facing everyone is to come
   to grips with what Alzheimer's disease really means in emotional
   terms for the patient and the family.

   Patients have the right to learn all the information they are
   prepared to handle. Ask for help if you need it to educate your
   relative about the nature of the diagnosis. Remember, it is usually
   easier for people to express anger than sadness—and anger once
   expressed is often misdirected. Like buckshot, it covers too much
   area and is very hard to control. Do not be hurt or frightened by
   the early outbursts of anger even if directed at you or someone
   else blameless. Understand the cause of the patient's anger. It is
   important to allow people to blow off steam and then to deal with
   them rationally and constructively rather than to become guilty
   or to return the anger.

3. *Ask yourself, "What does the diagnosis mean to me?"* It is important to try to separate our own feelings about the diagnosis from
   what you think your husband, wife, or relative may feel. This may
   sound simple, but is usually extremely difficult. The bad news
   requires that all family member look inside themselves. Just as the
   patient has strong reactions, so will those close to the patient.

4. *Do not say anything to the patient that is not true.* Although many
   patients will have difficulty accepting the diagnosis, methods can
   usually be found to educate them as they are ready. However, do
   not mislead them. Do not tell them that it is simply their age or
   that they have nothing to worry about. Trust is essential in the
   management of the disease; once broken, it is hard to restore.

5. *Talk with the patient but do not argue with denial.* Since it is
   characteristic for patients to deny the situation, do not argue or
   confront them too aggressively regardless of how illogical their
   denial appears. Patients will "hear" the message when and if they
   are ready to deal with it. The denial is serving a short-term

purpose by giving them more time to deal with the problem psychologically. It may be sufficient for a while just to inform them that Alzheimer's disease is the diagnosis and that things won't get much better.

6. *Do not lose hope.* Alzheimer's disease and related disorders do not cripple the individual overnight. Work with health professionals to understand your relative's strengths, needs, and desires. After the diagnosis there is often a great deal of time to fulfill a number of personal and family goals. Living one day at a time has become an important strategy for many families to cope with the disease successfully. Sharing becomes the key to dealing with the future. A sense of humor and perspective also helps.

7. *Help yourself.* Recognize your own needs, fears, or anxiety and seek help. Living with a relative with the disease is a personally demanding burden. Finding a friend, clergyman, or professional to help you deal with your own feelings and reactions is a major step to helping your relative. Making a life for yourself in the midst of the tragic situation can also be crucial. Time out of the house—visits to friends, a movie, a restaurant, or a class—to take a break from the ceaseless problems at home not only are good for your physical and mental health but are even essential if you are to continue to provide care for your relative. Remember that if you break down, the patient suffers.

Putting life in order after a diagnosis is difficult. It is a time for everyone to come to grips with what one woman described as the "permanent uncertainty" of the diagnosis. Many changes and crises lie ahead. There will be days of fear, anxiety, and worry, and there will be times of tenderness, intimacy, and even humor. The next chapter offers some specific strategies for coping with the challenges of Alzheimer's disease.

# 4

# SETTING GOALS AFTER THE DIAGNOSIS

---

I am starting to lose control of myself. I feel robbed. I wish there were some way I could be repaired. Some of this brain must be good—or is it all rotting away? Must I disappear into oblivion? How much time will I have?

Last night my granddaughter Nydia sat on my lap watching television with me. My son walked into the room and reminded her that it was time for bed. Nydia began to cry and buried herself in the chair close to me.

Dear God, I can't get her words out of my mind. "Please don't take me away. I want to stay with Grandpa. You said that someday he will get so sick that he will not be able to take care of himself. You said that you don't know what to do. I know! I am going to stay and take care of him."

My son sat down next to me and began to cry. I cried too. We all held each other for a long time. I wish I could spare them my pain.

—J.T.

WE have offered some general suggestions about how to begin to deal effectively with the many psychological reactions of living with dementia, but understanding and doing are very different. Perhaps one of the most difficult challenges for everyone is to live daily with the suffering and work to overcome it. James Thomas's diary entry not only exposes his inner turmoil but also gives us a sense of his personal courage. Nydia's behavior moved everyone and impelled the family to talk to a doctor about concrete strategies for dealing with the impact of dementia.

There are no drugs or life-saving machines for Alzheimer's disease or other progressive dementias. However, there are many ways of maximizing health and comfort and of helping the patient adjust psychologically to the dementia. Alzheimer's disease challenges the patient and family to continually find new ways to cope with the patient's progressive disabilities and incapacitations.

The challenge is to struggle to continue to care about living. It is important to determine the preferences of the patient so that you can help your relative live as independently and comfortably as possible. As the disease progresses, consultations with professionals, exchanges of information about the patient's progress, regular check-ups, and frequent discussions about family difficulties will help families and patients exert control over their lives.

## Dimensions of Caring: Setting Emotional Distance

Care giving is not easy. The challenge of caring is to be close to the patient and distant at the same time. You have to regard your relative as a loved one who is suffering and as a patient with a disease over which neither of you has any control.

Developing at least a modest amount of emotional distance is helpful. It allows you to keep yourself psychologically more in control so that you can make decisions about the patient and about your personal and family life. If you are unable to separate yourself from your feelings about the tragedy of the situation, you will easily become overwhelmed with anger and with a sense of hopelessness or helplessness. As you learn to compartmentalize your feelings, you will be able to care for your relative more effectively and also protect yourself from total exhaustion.

Walter Eliot retired from his managerial job at the age of sixty-two. He looked forward to a life of travel and the "golden years" he had struggled to achieve. Within a year, though, he noticed his wife behaving very strangely. Evelyn would wear coats and sweaters inside out and forget to put on earrings, belts, or stockings; once she dressed casually for a black-tie affair and refused to change into an evening dress. On several occasions she served Walter sandwiches and beer for breakfast and fed the cat rice or cereal instead of Friskies. Within eighteen months he was stunned by the diagnosis of Alzheimer's disease and the neurologist's comment "Sorry there's nothing we can do—she'll have to go to a nursing home."

Walter decided that this would not be. He tried to get help from an unresponsive community and was determined not to burden his children. Evelyn deteriorated quickly, and a succession of housekeepers were hired and fired. Evelyn did not sleep well at night, and Walter was up at all hours trying to keep control of the situation. Growing more and more upset, he began drinking heavily—a problem he had dealt with decades before—and became an alcoholic, as he himself admitted. Only then did his children move in and force Walter to get help.

As he began to cope with his drinking problem, the overwhelming feelings about his life and Evelyn's condition emerged. Walter needed to find a way to care for Evelyn and also to have time for a life of his own. It took many months to control his drinking, and only when he became an active leader in a local Alzheimer's support group did he begin to deal more effectively with the situation at home. The support group had recommended a day-care center where Evelyn could spend five days a week, giving Walter the opportunity to be on his own. For Walter it was important in developing his emotional separation to keep Evelyn at home and also invest his energy in the local support group. Obviously, this is not everyone's solution.

Nancy Avery's friends made her "get out of the house." She did not want to join a support group or talk with anyone about the problems at home. She went to museums, where she could spend a few hours several days a week and focus on something else. For her it was "the pause that refreshed." Since she and her husband had always enjoyed collecting fine things, it gave her a feeling of "wholeness" in an otherwise difficult life of selfless and devoted care. Nancy felt guilty when she was away from her husband, but she achieved the recognition that the physical and emotional separation of a few hours each week improved her ability to care for him when they were together.

The enormous commitment which is involved in caring for individuals with progressive dementia requires that you develop a special relationship with the patient. You must understand and deal with his or her needs as well as yours in a way that does not emotionally, physically, and financially bankrupt you and the rest of the family. The process of evolving a special helping relationship has a technical name—approximation. Approximation is the process of forging a flexible or changeable relationship in which the care giver must continually make decisions balancing the patient's needs with his or her own. There are numerous daily opportunities to make decisions—whether or not to be physically present, to do certain things, to react, to talk, to inquire, to inform, or to express feelings. The pattern of decisions and actions creates the unique relationship in the home and sets the tone for future decisions.

Clearly, approximation is not easy to achieve or to maintain. Regardless of the personality, professional training, or background of the care giver, it is hard to be close to the patient for long periods without feeling uncomfortable. Learning how to distance yourself—not to avoid the patient or be insensitive, but to separate yourself on the basis of your knowledge of the patient's needs and your own —is helpful.

How do you learn the skills required for controlled distancing, which usually come with the professional training of clinicians? Here are seven guidelines we can offer.

## 1. Find competent and compassionate mental health professionals.

Sometimes there is no substitute for individuals with special knowledge and skills to help you and your family share the burden of caring and keep from becoming overwhelmed. The feelings engendered by caring for the Alzheimer's patient become awesome (see Chapter 8). Like the patient, the care giver may also feel abandoned and lonely and experience a profound loss of control. These feelings may occur early on, or they may not surface for a while. Finding appropriate assistance after the diagnosis may prevent future problems.

"Compassionate" derives from the Latin word meaning "to suffer with," and there is a healing power in having someone to suffer with you. Having trained care givers available will help you care for the patient and yourself by understanding the intensity of your emotions and their potential for disrupting or enhancing care. In years of training, mental health professionals have learned how to develop therapeutic relationships with patients, family members, and other care givers.

Asking for assistance is often difficult; moreover, many individuals are afraid of psychiatric help. The fear of the stigma of having mental illness prevents them from contacting precisely those professionals who are skilled in dealing with the difficult problems the patient and family encounter.

Unfortunately, many family members have serious misconceptions about the value of psychiatrists and mental health professionals. The couch and "talking therapies" are not the only tools of the psychiatrist. Psychiatrists are physicians with specialized training who are perhaps the best qualified to deal with human behavior and the many changes which affect the patient and the family living with Alzheimer's disease. They are also experienced in caring for people over long periods of time.

It is important to be forthright and ask the professionals you contact whether they can help you. Ask them to tell you about their interests, training, and experience with dementia. Their initial response will let you know immediately whether they will be helpful to you.

## 2. Find a confidant.

Mental health professionals are not always available. Friends or confidants are probably among the best aids to help you measure off the distance between you and your relative. Friendships are stabilizing forces. Sharing feelings and experiences with someone you trust may simply make you feel better. Talking about your frustrations often helps you see the world a little more objectively. A trusted friend may also be a helpful critic who is able to compliment your stamina and courage and simultaneously urge you to be a little selfish and think of your own needs some of the time.

This seemingly simple advice may be difficult to follow. Many people are afraid to let their friends know that a husband, wife, or family member has dementia. Some families have the financial resources to isolate the patient comfortably on an estate or in a luxury environment, hiding him or her away from the rest of the world. Although these arrangements may be done with the best of intentions, the isolation may in the end only create more problems.

Arnold Sands was stricken with Alzheimer's disease in his early fifties, ending a brilliant artistic career. His wife, Julia, and the children were devoted to him and financially able to construct a physical and social environment to simulate the activity of his previous existence. A chauffeur drove him to his studio. Young artists were employed to carry out the technical work associated with the production of his sculpture. Everything that money could buy was done to re-create his art world. Openings were even staged to show off new pieces at a local gallery.

As Mr. Sands grew more impaired, he became unable to participate in any part of the artistic process. However, he was happy to watch the activity around him and continued to spend many hours each day in his studio. Julia Sands found it emotionally impossible to be with her husband as he deteriorated. Although she cared deeply for Arnold and took great pride in what the family did to keep him happy and comfortable, Julia had set up an emotional barricade between herself and Arnold after the diagnosis. She instructed her sons and daughters not to tell anyone what was wrong, and she withdrew from all of her friends, making excuses that the business was consuming her time and energy.

The entire family was concerned about her inability to accept the diagnosis and "go public" by letting her friends know about the Alzheimer's disease. Gradually, Mrs. Sands became more irritable, drank heavily, and withdrew from many of her responsibilities in the family real estate business. Her children were able to take over at work, but they worried about her alcohol abuse. One evening Julia had a car accident while driving under the influence, injuring herself and a pedestrian. When she recovered, the family insisted she see a psychiatrist.

After several months of therapy Mrs. Sands was able to deal honestly with the situation. Her fears of rejection were unrealistic, and her friends and family surrounded her with support that continued until her husband's death.

*3. Hold regular family meetings to discuss how your relative is functioning and try to anticipate future changes.*

As long as the patient lives, the family will be caught emotionally between two different and changing worlds. One consists of memories of a time when the patient was an active, productive, and responsible member of the family or marriage partner. The second is the world of the present, in which the patient is changing and has diminished capacity to do many things. Families can help themselves by meeting to discuss the future needs and rights of various family members. Caring for someone with dementia changes the time family members have for other personal and social responsibilities. Meetings are the forum for relatives to begin negotiating their needs with one another and the patient.

Children should not be excluded from family discussions, but some may not wish to participate. The best way to proceed is to ask them and then accept their wishes. When they are included, they often show remarkable insights. Marion Talbot had been diagnosed with dementia for more than three years. Her husband and children were devoted to her, and together they did everything possible to keep Marion active and happy. Even Tim, her five-year-old grandson, showed a special involvement with his grandmother, visiting three or four days a week. On weekends, when Tim often spent the night, Marion would read him bedtime stories. As Marion's word-finding difficulties increased, Tim's father tried to prepare him for the changes in his grandmother, by explaining that grandma could not read his books anymore, because she had a disease which affected her ability to read and talk. Tim replied, "That's all right, you or Grandpa can join us. She can still hold me in her lap while you read the story to both of us! I like being with her."

Family cooperation in problem-solving activities around patient issues is not always easy. The larger the number of family members involved with the patient, the greater the room for family disagreements and arguments. These conflicts are not abnormal; indeed, they are necessary as different members voice divergent opinions and observations. The crucial variable is the family's ability finally to agree on solutions which represent the best interests of the patient and the family. By resolving problems together, families can achieve a sense of control over the situation. There is no way to control the dementia per se, but it is possible to achieve an internal sense of limited mastery which emerges from knowing that you have done everything in your power to deal with an impossible situation.

## 4. Try to sustain or develop a sense of humor.

Humor is a healthy way to handle problems, and there are those who believe that it is better than any medication or elixir. Many daily circumstances and conversations elicit smiles and laughter. The ability to laugh at yourself and the world around you is therapeutic.

Larry Weiss had been diagnosed with Alzheimer's disease for about one year. He lived at home with his wife, Barbara. Both enjoyed living in their cottage on the lake. Larry could fish, work around the boat shed, and visit with friends at the marina. In the evenings when they did not entertain or visit friends, they would sit and read or watch television.

Each morning on rising, they would take a walk together around the lake. In the evenings when the weather was good, Larry would take Barbara out in the flatboat and row until he tired. Their time together had become even more precious since the doctor had told them that Larry probably had Alzheimer's disease. They were fearful of the uncertainty of the future, but they were both determined to enjoy their lives together as long as possible.

One evening in the fall Larry and Barbara were getting dressed to go out on the lake. When Barbara entered the boat shed, she saw Larry standing with his hunter's vest on upside down and the life vest backward. He was struggling to put on a rain slicker, which would not fit over the life preserver. She burst out laughing, and within minutes both of them were laughing uncontrollably in each other's arms. Later, in the boat, Larry asked her what had been so funny. He had been unaware of what he was doing, and as Barbara described his actions, he became troubled. This was the part of the disease that scared him—that he could not do something as simple as dress himself.

Barbara admitted that she, too, was frightened but said that they could fight this disease together. For the moment and for the foreseeable future, they could still enjoy each other and find happiness and laughter.

Later, as they walked along the sandy beach near the dock, they watched a small puppy pull a large log along the beach. Larry walked over to the dog, dropped down on his hands and knees, eye to eye with the animal, and began to push the log with his head. Barbara froze in horror as she watched her husband. Within a few minutes Larry stood up and smiled broadly. She relaxed as she heard him say, "You're right, Barbara, it's good to play and be alive!"

*5. When you talk with your relative, it is sometimes more important to listen and observe than to speak.*

Part of the process of emotional distancing is to learn how to act like a paraprofessional. Since patients often have great difficulty with language or in remembering what happens around them, the understanding of their needs and wants often requires you to become an "active listener." Observe and listen carefully. Sometimes it is helpful not to talk at all, but give the patient time to speak what is on his or her mind.

Even the most devoted families may lose their ability to understand the patient and need help to rebalance their perspective of the patient's capabilities. Doris Watson had been caring for her husband, Alex, for more than ten years. Despite the dementia, she had kept him physically active. They walked six miles together each morning before breakfast. They played tennis and golf four or five times a week. They also went cycling and swimming every day at the health club. As Alex's dementia worsened, he could utter only a few words and required assistance with bathing and dressing. Doris began to leave him at home and did more activities on her own. Alex became less active, gained weight, and began sleeping longer in the morning.

Their friends continued to visit them at home, and several invited Alex to play tennis or golf. Doris discouraged their invitations, saying that Alex could no longer play well. However, Alex could still hit the ball and seemed thoroughly to enjoy the exercise. Doris refused to watch Alex play, insisting that her friends would grow tired of playing with him. They in turn were gently insistent that he was still a good partner. In the beginning Doris was insulted that her friends would challenge her ability to understand her husband. However, with time they were able to convince her that although Alex had changed they still enjoyed his company, and he theirs. Alex lost his excess weight, slept less, and regained his zest for living. Doris was grateful to her friends for helping her see Alex for the man he still was and for what he still had to give others.

## 6. *Honesty is the only basis for a relationship with your relative.*

Being honest is the first rule for treating a relative as a human being and a patient. Family members who learn to share the emotional burden of Alzheimer's disease with the patient can decrease the stresses and strains of daily life. Sharing the burden means working together and honestly accepting what the future brings, taking it one day at time. Unfortunately, it is common for many family members to withhold the diagnosis or information from the patient, often for many years, or to refrain from answering a question many individuals ask—"Will I get worse?"

Being dishonest or avoiding answers creates psychological tension. Most, if not all, patients sense the discomfort or dishonesty on a nonverbal level. Some may respond by social withdrawal or retreating emotionally under the false assumption that this will make the family more comfortable. The patient's fears and anxieties then go unresolved and result in frustration, rage, and even violent acting out by the patient as well as the family.

Some patients place care givers in a difficult position when they insist that no one outside the family be told about the dementia. This often forces the husband or wife into a stressful double existence—a social world where problems are denied and a personal and family world where problems are real. However, in both worlds tension increases because there is no basis for honest transactions in the family.

When the patient and family visit friends, shop, attend social events, or eat out, the family may be overprotective and make excuses for the patient rather than be honest with friends. However, as the dementia progresses, families may withdraw from social and leisure activities and become openly angry with the patient in public.

John Santini took his wife, Sonya, out to dinner four or five times a week because she enjoyed what had been a lifelong social pattern for them. Sonya had been diagnosed as having Alzheimer's disease but still enjoyed an active social life with her husband. And for many years after the diagnosis she had been a companion at business dinners. However, Mr. Santini was ashamed to tell anyone about the Alzheimer's disease. On those occasions when she had problems, he dismissed it with the excuse that she had had too much to drink.

As the disease progressed, John was becoming increasingly uncomfortable with his wife at business functions because of the way she dressed and acted. Sonya had begun to talk more at dinner and to giggle inappropriately, and sometimes she played with her food. One evening John exploded at his wife and stormed out of the restaurant when she insisted on pouring everyone's wine back into the bottle.

The Santinis' son, Frank, was successful in getting his father and mother to see someone. Frank was distressed that most of his father's friends thought his mother was an alcoholic. After several months the members of the Santini family were able to successfully confront the Alzheimer's disease and also to do shuttle diplomacy with their friends and dispel the image of alcoholism.

*7. Just as parents provide consistency, love, security, and a sense of order for children, so do family members provide a stable emotional environment for the patient.*

Hundreds of books have been written about infant and child development and caring for children. Until recently, little published information was available about aging and caring for older adults with health problems such as dementia. Many families are traveling in uncharted regions, trying to do the best they can, often walking a narrow trail between knowing and not knowing what to do. Sometimes they stumble onto answers by trial and error; sometimes knowledgeable experts or other families provide useful advice.

Patients with dementia often fear being isolated, rejected, and abandoned. This fear may be present even in the early phases of dementia and in the strongest of family relationships. Consequently, when care givers have difficulty with their own emotional reactions and become so overwhelmed that they withdraw or avoid interactions with the patient, they cause reactions in the patient.

Jim Ricci and his wife, Gina, had been married for over forty years and raised ten children, all of whom were grown and married. After Jim was diagnosed as having Alzheimer's disease, Gina insisted that she was able to assume the additional responsibilities of the family business she and Jim had run together as partners. The children tried to persuade their parents to interview candidates to help them manage affairs, but neither would hear of it.

During the first year following the diagnosis, Gina and Jim quarreled more. Mario, the oldest son, and Anne Marie, the oldest daughter, who lived closest to their parents, had stopped by the store frequently throughout the years, and both became concerned about the increasing tension between their parents.

Mario and Anne agreed that the first tactic was to talk with their parents separately—Mario to their mother and Anne to their father. Afterward they would compare notes and plan accordingly. It was immediately obvious that Gina was frustrated and confused by her husband's behavior. She wanted to ask him to do things at the store, such as stock the shelves and inventory the items, and although Jim would agree to her request, he would then do something else. It was not his making mistakes in occasional confused periods that upset her; it was what she described as his deliberately doing something else to make her angry.

Jim was slow to confide in his daughter, and it was not until both Mario and Anne cornered him at the store alone that the story began to emerge. Jim was deeply concerned about his memory losses and afraid that Gina would want to sell the store if she knew how much his difficulties troubled him. Jim was reluctant to do many tasks around the store because he was afraid of making errors, when in fact he was quite capable. The many lapses were sporadic, and Gina was so sensitive to these periods that she would simply take over. Jim was embarrassed and ashamed that his wife would have to see him helpless and incompetent. He also secretly feared that she might begin to reject him.

Jim admitted that it was perhaps foolish for him to imagine that Gina would suddenly stop loving him after so many years. But he was beginning to dislike himself, and if he felt this way, she certainly could as well. Because he was so uncomfortable, Jim, rather than talk to her, simply walked away from many tasks. This triggered arguments which were becoming more frequent. Jim admitted to being ashamed, and since he was angry at the whole situation, he exploded at Gina. He felt trapped.

Mario and Anne invited their parents to dinner and afterward spoke of what they had seen happening to their parents and expressed their desire to help. Both Gina and Jim were relieved by their children's intervention, although they admitted embarrassment that their own children could discern what they could not.

Gina and Jim continued to work in the store for several years. Jim became more comfortable asking for help, and they both agreed to hire someone to manage the store as well as a few salesmen, so that they could get away and travel as long as Jim was only mildly affected.

Alzheimer's disease can threaten even loving family ties that have existed for many years. Patients may consciously or unconsciously test the strength of their family bonds, somewhat in the way adolescents test parents. This analogy with children is used not to infantilize the patient but to emphasize the strong reactions and needs of individuals after the diagnosis. Some may repeatedly express a wish to die or a desire to kill themselves, a tactic reminiscent of many teenagers. Other patients may become angry and irritable and argue over trivial issues to get attention. If a relative is behaving in unusual ways, it may be difficult to determine whether there is a psychological explanation for the behavior or whether it is a result of the dementia. Discussing a relative's behaviors with a professional may be helpful in seeking to understand disturbing threats and behaviors. A verbalized desire to die is deeply disturbing to the care giver. However, it may be a way for the patient to get a loved one to say that he or she is needed and wanted.

As the dementia progresses, many of the cognitive losses and behavioral changes cause extreme embarrassment for the patient. Even patients with advanced dementia may be angry and ashamed. This anger may be expressed in strange ways because of the dementia and thus be misdirected at the care giver.

It is hard to be supportive of someone who is difficult to live with. Sometimes the task may seem impossible. Remember, the patients are adults who experience shame and hurt when they cannot finish a sentence, complete routine tasks, or do things which once came easily. Whereas babies must feel great relief when they wet their diaper, adults who have an accident and need help can only be deeply ashamed. Dealing with the humanity of shame and anger is one of the toughest challenges for families.

Although strong infant-parent bonds develop with the feeding, dressing, changing, holding, and playing as the child grows, different feelings and obligations may arise out of the daily activities of helping an impaired adult. The bond may be slowly broken by the demands of caring. Or a new intimacy may be achieved as the patient and care givers adapt to different roles, which may be demanding but also fulfilling. The setting of goals is an important step to maximize your well-being and that of your relative.

## Setting Goals

The patient with Alzheimer's disease has many needs—physical, emotional, and social. The belief that patients cannot participate in their care and are untreatable often leads to an exclusive reliance on drugs and a failure to use other techniques which can be effective.

So where do you begin? Perhaps the first step is to define a clear set of plans. The process of establishing goals is helpful because it enables you to think of your relative both as a patient with specific disabilities and needs and as an individual who can make certain contributions to the family.

### Goal 1: Evaluate the Patient's Ability to Work as Well as Your Own.

In the beginning the "patient" can manage alone or with minimal help around the house or even at work. When Alzheimer's disease strikes a middle-aged or older adult who is still employed, the individual is usually not able to continue on the job. Indeed, the cognitive losses which ultimately bring about the diagnostic evaluation have usually disrupted the individual's ability to perform effectively, despite ingenious attempts to compensate for and hide these losses. Although the patient may be able to continue part-time work, this often requires an extremely supportive network of friends. Some individuals have worked as salesmen in a store or as volunteers in a hospital, social agency, or library, and some have even continued to tutor children in music and other school subjects.

The patient's continued ability to work needs to be carefully evaluated in terms of safety and competence. What is the nature of the individual's work history, accomplishments, and motivations to continue any type of work? What resources or opportunities are available for the creation of a viable structured work situation for the patient? How acceptable are any arrangements with current or prospective employers?

In many instances it is imperative to discourage the individual from working, whereas in others there may be merit in supporting continued employment. In many jobs impaired individuals cannot perform the work safely or the level of impairment is so high that adequate performance is not possible. However, in some situations individuals can go to their place of work and feel that they have a place, when in reality they can no longer work. Many businesses, schools, law firms, and even factories have supported the presence of an impaired partner or former employee.

Patients and families may find it very difficult to deal with the dilemmas of retirement from work. Virginia Rich and her husband, Dale, both aged fifty-five, lived together in a small town. Dale had recently been diagnosed as having Alzheimer's disease, after the completion of the full series of diagnostic evaluations in another state. He and his wife deliberately flew out of town to hide the situation from their friends and from Dale's employer. Mr. Rich was determined to continue to work as long as he was able to drive safely and handle his accounts. Virginia helped her husband with the paperwork in the evenings, but she was concerned about his ability to continue to drive safely as the dementia progressed. Fortunately, Dale was senior enough that he did not have to take on any new accounts, and at least for a while he was able to handle all of his old clients successfully.

Dale and Virginia decided that they would take each day as it came. Dale agreed to see a psychologist and have his ability to drive evaluated by a series of tests. As long as he passed these examinations, he would continue to drive. And as long as he felt comfortable talking with his old clients and with Virginia's help on the books, he could keep going.

Although Dale continued to work for more than a year after the diagnosis, Virginia began to feel more and more frustrated. She worried about the future and became increasingly distressed, because she felt isolated, having no one with whom to share her concerns. She could not speak with her friends or even join the local Alzheimer's self-help group, because Dale's diagnosis was a secret.

How could they balance Dale's need to continue working and to feel worthwhile with Virginia's need to support her husband and also be supported in her care-giving role? Two years after the diagnosis Dale finally retired voluntarily. He had to do so, because his speech and memory problems had worsened, and it was dangerous for him to drive. When he failed his last driving test with the psychologist, Virginia and Irene urged him to retire. They wanted him alive, and the risk of a car accident was too great.

A number of other serious work dilemmas may emerge. A husband or wife may continue to work until the needs of the patient force him or her to stop. If the care giver is fortunate enough to be financially capable of paying for home help, he or she may continue to work. However, even in these situations the emotional toll affects the productivity and efficiency of the healthy spouse in the work role.

Children involved in the care of their parents or relatives may lose time from work and feel torn between loyalty to their parents and the need to support themselves and their family. The oldest daughter or daughter-in-law seems to inherit or assume the role of primary care giver when a parent is affected. The combined pressures of parent caring, family, and job can be intense.

Jean and Armand Ansel had been struggling to build their own lives and to care for their parents over the past nine years. Armand's eighty-five-year-old mother had a history of strokes over the years, and Jean's seventy-year-old father had Alzheimer's disease. They had placed Armand's mother, a widow of fifteen years, in a nursing home six months earlier because she could no longer live at home. The cost of a twenty-four-hour home attendant had depleted their resources, and another stroke had further debilitated her. Jean's father, Pierre, continued to live alone in his cooperative apartment several miles away from his children. Since he was one of the few men in the apartment complex where he had lived as a widower for more than ten years, several lady friends and a few men formed a tight group of friends who helped him get along each day.

However, as Pierre's condition began to deteriorate, Jean and Armand found themselves making daily visits in the evening to check on Pierre. Furthermore, without Armand's knowledge Jean began to visit Pierre's apartment over the lunch hour and also called him several times daily. Jean's distress began to interfere with her performance at work.

Jean was an administrative assistant to the president of a large corporation. She was brilliant in her job and was able to keep up with her work and with Pierre—at least for a while. After several months Jean's boss invited her to lunch to find out why she had begun to have so much trouble on the job. Jean had made significant errors in his calendar and in travel arrangements. Business files were incomplete for administrative meetings, and she was neglecting several important projects. Jean's boss suggested she take several weeks off to deal with her family problem and find another living situation for her father-in-law.

To avoid problems at the office or job, it is often helpful to sit down with your boss or supervisor, apprise him or her of the situation, and, if necessary, ask for some time off to get family affairs organized. Time invested in planning after the diagnosis will pay off later. The amount of time off from work is necessarily limited, and you will have to juggle work deadlines with the immediacy of family demands.

## Goal 2: Choose the Primary Care Giver.

Although this may sound strange, it is important to decide who the primary care giver or givers will be. Even in situations in which the patient has a living husband or wife at home, the spouse's physical and mental health may limit his or her capacity to be responsible for the patient on a daily basis. Family discussions should focus on this topic. The primary care giver lives with demanding daily responsibilities, and even a healthy, dedicated spouse will need help. It is not unusual for small groups of people in the family to function as primary care givers, such as a daughter, son-in-law, or several children. Primary care givers may also change with time. In some families in which the patient is alone, children and other relatives may decide to rotate caring responsibilities in order to give each person time off on a regular basis.

## Goal 3: Assess Whether Disturbed Family Relationships May Disrupt the Routine.

A number of family problems may surface if the Alzheimer's patient has had a strained, disturbed, or severed relationship with a spouse, son, daughter, brother, sister, or any other significant relative or friend. Conflicts, arguments, and disagreements occur in every relationship. However, marital problems, separation, and divorce, intense sibling rivalry, angry relationships between parents and children, or any combination of emotionally discordant relationships among family members can stand in the way of helping the patient.

Caring for an Alzheimer's patient can be complicated by any number of disruptive situations. When a husband or wife separates or divorces a patient, conflict with children and other family members may result. Children and spouses from previous marriages of the patient may be excluded from contact with the patient by the present family. An estranged adult child of the patient may refuse to visit the patient and cause additional emotional distress for the entire family. A trained professional or clergyman is a valuable source of help for the entire family in dealing with these situations.

## Goal 4: Establish a Structured Daily Routine.

The development of a structured daily routine is perhaps one of the most important tasks to be accomplished. Since dementia gradually impairs the patients' ability to plan activities and do things for themselves and others, an organized schedule keeps them active and involved to the limits of their abilities. Furthermore, a structured routine helps maintain the patients' abilities and develops a sense of security and accomplishment.

Setting up a routine requires an accurate analysis of the patients' capabilities as well as of the family's resources. Unfortunately, many families and their physicians encourage a premature dependency and reinforce a helplessness which often leads to the "one-person nursing home." It is natural to worry about relatives' safety and their reliability in carrying out various tasks. The mistake is to allow these feelings to interfere unnecessarily with individuals' freedom to function and express themselves. These are tough decisions. The patient has the right to continue to live as independently as possible. Likewise, the patient is only one member of a family system in which other individuals also have legitimate rights and needs.

Negotiations regarding the patient's limitations arouse feelings of discomfort in care givers and feelings of anger and sadness in the patient. The patient has losses which require alterations in lifestyle. Just as an individual with a broken neck or back is restricted in many activities, the individual with dementia must deal with the reality of undeniable limitations. Facing these life changes is painful, but one can deal with these feelings by implementing a plan of action and by living one day at a time.

Since the patient will change over time, the daily routine will inevitably need to be altered. If changes are anticipated in advance and alternative solutions prepared, the patient and family members will feel more in control of changes as they occur.

A psychological evaluation by a professional will determine the patient's strengths and weaknesses, assets and liabilities. This information is the basis on which to recommend life and work roles for the patient. Although memory and attention losses often make the successful completion of such household tasks as cooking, cleaning, and shopping impossible, individuals may nonetheless be able to perform some portion of these tasks. An impaired adult may be incapable of doing the weekly shopping but may derive enormous satisfaction from running a simple errand, such as buying a loaf of bread or a quart of milk. Cognitive testing highlights the skills an individual retains during the progression of the illness. It also gives the family or care givers a realistic baseline for what to expect from the patient, whether at home or in the institutional environment.

Remember that dementia is often a slowly progressing disease. In most cases not only are the losses gradual, but a number of intellectual skills are preserved for years. Individuals are not immediately and totally incapacitated. Furthermore, many everyday activities require little in the way of higher-order reasoning and thinking. Some of the most important and rewarding experiences in our lives are the special times we share with those we love by simply being together.

Amy and Archie Thompson had lived together for more than thirty-five years. At the age of sixty Archie began to complain of memory problems. He also had trouble finding words and finishing his sentences. This went on for six years before he and the entire family decided that a complete speech and hearing evaluation was in order.

The results documented what Archie and his family already knew. Now there was a technical report that described his language disturbance as an aphasia. Archie's internist, who gave him a clean bill of physical health, insisted on a neurological examination. The neurologist informed them that Archie probably had Alzheimer's disease. The entire family was deeply concerned, except for Archie.

In a subsequent family meeting Archie tried to tell everyone that he was coming to grips with the dementia. Yes, the day he heard the diagnosis he felt numb. However, as he walked to the car after leaving the neurologist's office, a trivial event occurred which had a special personal significance. A bright red leaf fell in his hand. Its simple beauty was overwhelming. Archie stumbled over his words as he tried to tell his family how he identified with that leaf. He and the leaf were both old. It was autumn and the leaf had aged, turned color, and was dying in resplendent color. He, too, was growing older, and now he had a disease that would someday affect him greatly. But for now he simply felt rich and proud to be surrounded by his family. "If only I could turn a bright color and you could look at me and say, 'How beautiful!' "

Archie was able to live with his speech problems. There was much he could still do. He and Amy lived in a small country town. He enjoyed working in the yard and also derived special pleasure doing carpentry in the basement workroom. His great love, however, was his personal computer, and he would spend hours in the den. Although Archie had difficulty with some of the computer programs, he still enjoyed many of the computer games, especially the airplane cockpit simulations. He had been a pilot in World War II and the Korean War, and his hours at the computer brought back memories of times past.

## Goal 5: Establish and Maintain a Program of Physical Exercise for the Patient.

Physical activity is important. A simple daily program including walks, jogging, gardening, exercise regimens, or even dancing can maintain the patient's physical condition and contribute to a restful night's sleep. Exercise may reduce the need for sedative medication and will also help the patient maintain a healthy appetite. Sports like golf, tennis, and swimming can be especially therapeutic for individuals who enjoyed such physical activities before the onset of the illness.

Some patients and families have arranged the entire day's schedule around exercise. Although Karen Hart, aged fifty-eight, had been diagnosed six years earlier, she and her husband, Calvin, continued to play golf and tennis together daily throughout the year. What changed after the diagnosis was the amount of time devoted to physical activity. Each morning they did thirty minutes of calisthenics before breakfast, and after eating they jogged and walked two miles around the neighborhood. This was followed by a tennis game or golf. In the afternoon they went to the health club to work out on the equipment and swim. This was also an opportunity for Calvin to leave his wife for a few hours and have some time alone. He had met with the health spa staff after the diagnosis and informed them of his wife's problem. From the beginning everyone was supportive, and indeed amazed at her physical endurance and stamina.

Not everyone can afford a health spa or tennis club, but there are many other ways to get exercise—watching exercise shows on television, gardening, riding a stationary bicycle, and taking long walks. Even when the patient has had dementia for years and is severely impaired, physical exercise and walking should be programmed several times a day, ideally after each meal. This is not only conducive to good physical health but also gives the individual a sense of personal achievement. As cognitive powers diminish, many patients report taking great pride in physical accomplishments. Feeling good about yourself is a cognitive act.

## Goal 6: Monitor the Patient's General Health.

Keeping physically healthy is an important aspect of care. Patients who are as comfortable as possible will be much more able to function at their best. Since many patients cannot explain aches and pains and other physical problems, the care giver must be attentive to the their physical well-being.

Francis Coco had been hospitalized for over a year. None of the local nursing homes would admit him, because he screamed much of the day and was a difficult patient to manage. Mr. Coco had a multi-infarct dementia but had originally been admitted to the hospital a year earlier when he fell and broke his hip. Multiple medical complications had developed in the intervening months.

It was in the tenth month when Mr. Coco became a "screamer," raving whenever someone entered his room. In the course of each day, the screaming decreased in the afternoons and evening as he became hoarse. The yelling was especially intense when his wife, Kathy, visited. The only way to quiet Francis was to give him his Bible or prayer book. However, there were days when this did not console him either.

Mrs. Coco insisted that something was wrong with her husband, but everyone—the doctors, nurses, and social workers—insisted that his screaming was part of the disease and that they hoped to get him into a good nursing home. Finally, Mrs. Coco was successful in locating a geriatric specialist for a consultation.

On the day of the visit, Mr. Coco had just finished lunch before the doctor entered the room with his wife. The doctor sat down and introduced himself, whereupon Mr. Coco began to scream, showering the doctor with food and saliva. Mr. Coco continued to yell, but the doctor said nothing and wiped the food from his face. After a few minutes the screaming stopped, and Mr. Coco only stared hard at the doctor. The doctor began his examination with Mr. Coco's quiet consent. It was not until he moved Francis's leg that Francis screamed in pain. A review of the chart revealed that Francis had a history of phlebitis, and further tests revealed that it was clearly a current problem. Psychological studies also revealed that Mr. Coco was capable of reading and writing and that he retained skills which nobody had imagined because of his difficult behavior.

Mr. Coco's phlebitis was successfully controlled, and the staff members were able to maintain some limited conversation with him. The screaming stopped, and for the first time Mr. Coco seemed happy. However, placement in a nursing home was still necessary because of the heavy nursing care he required. Within a short time an appropriate institution was found, and Mr. Coco lived out the next two years comfortably.

Patients with Alzheimer's disease become more susceptible to infections and other illnesses because of a weakened immune system. Regular checkups with the family doctor will avert many types of health hazards. The patient's health program should also include good hygiene, a suitable exercise program, dental care, and a balanced diet. A carefully managed health program may avoid an unnecessary drop in functioning as a result of problems with vision, diet, or teeth or of any other problems otherwise unrecognized.

In the early stages of Alzheimer's disease, patients do not appear to be physically less healthy than the rest of the older population.

In its later stages, though, especially when patients are long-term residents in nursing homes, multiple physical illnesses incapacitate them and often severely limit their activities. However, certain exercises can be done in bed or a wheelchair to maintain body tone and circulation. Several books on special exercises are included in the reference list.

When the patient does become ill, he or she should be treated with at least as much care as other members of the family. Care givers should never feel shy about using the medical profession when needed. It is important to remember that a commonplace illness can be more dangerous for persons with dementia than for a healthy person.

## Goal 6: Monitor the Patient's Vision and Hearing.

Sight and hearing should be tested at least once a year. As the dementia progresses, it will become more and more difficult for an ophthalmologist and audiologist to evaluate vision and hearing because of poor cognition and unreliable responses. Patients are not always capable of answering the questions posed by the examiner: for example, "Is this sound higher or lower than the last sound? Can you hear this sound?" or "Which letters are clearer—the letters on the right, or the letters on the left?" Alert the doctor to the problem. Ask him or her to make the procedure and the questions as simple as possible. Inquire about the availability of special tests designed for young children. Consult with specialists in your area who work with autistic children or developmentally disabled children, since special procedures developed to test sensory acuity in learning-disabled children may be modified for the adult with dementia.

## Goal 7: Monitor the Patient's Emotional Health.

Many people lead relatively functional lives for years after the diagnosis. They find their own ways of coping with the dementia and with the major changes that occur in their personal and family lives. Others, however, develop emotional disorders. Depression and anxiety, which lower the individual's ability to think clearly, are the most common ones and are usually treatable. Successful treatment of emotional problems does not correct the intellectual losses caused by

Alzheimer's disease, but it often helps the person function at the highest possible level.

Rebecca Hunt became extremely agitated when she was unable to dress herself or when she forgot her thoughts in the middle of a sentence. Her husband and children tried hard to help and comfort her, but Rebecca usually burst into tears and ran from the room. "I just seem to go to pieces. . . . I feel so awful," she said in a family interview. "Sometimes I feel good, and then, when it gets to be too much, I go all to pieces, and I want to die."

Mrs. Hunt was successfully treated by her physician for her anxiety. In addition, she and her family identified a number of tasks which were not too difficult for her to perform. As time went by, Mrs. Hunt became more comfortable asking for help. She and her husband even rehearsed together what they would do if she forgot her thoughts when they were out in public. This anticipatory coping gave them both a sense that they were at least prepared to deal with the future.

When symptoms of anxiety and depression occur, they should be treated as soon as possible. They may include loss of appetite, irritability or apathy, hyperactivity or a marked slowing in behavior, changes in sleep pattern, and often a noticeable drop in cognitive status (see the sections on depression in Chapters 2 and 5). If you think your relative might be suffering from serious depression or anxiety, seek help from a psychiatric clinic, community mental health center, or mental health practitioner. If there are no professionals knowledgeable about geriatrics in your community, contact a self-help group near you or the national ADRDA office for information (Appendix 1).

## Goal 9: Make Living Areas More Accessible in Your Home.

The home environment may have to be rearranged, or in some cases even remodeled, to make the living space more usable by the patient. Many activities—dressing, eating, bathing, resting, doing housework, or playing—can be hampered without these alterations. Changing the environment also allows the patient to exert more direct control over his or her world and be as independent as possible. Take time to examine the physical environment of your home, room by room. If available, an architect or home designer may be useful (although perhaps costly) to help you identify ways to make the physical environment more accessible. Chapter 7 provides some guidelines for evaluating ways to change your home to make it barrier-free and more comfortable and safe for the patient.

The following case illustrates the dramatic impact of certain simple environmental changes even in later stages of dementia. Harold Jacobs had been diagnosed as having Alzheimer's nine years earlier and lived with his wife, Angela, in a small house along a ship canal. Angela left him at home while she went to work each day, and neighbors would check on Harold during lunch and in the late afternoon. He enjoyed sitting in the backyard watching the boats or gardening.

They had managed well together until he began to deteriorate more in the ninth year. Angela came home one day to find some neighborhood children in front of their house making fun of her husband, who was shrieking at them and striking the fence with a small garden tool. She chased them away angrily. Angela was deeply shaken to see her husband act like a wild man. She was afraid to unlock the gate.

A neighbor and close friend heard the disturbance, and brought Angela to her home, where together they watched Harold from the window. After he calmed down, they went outside. Harold waved to them and seemed not to remember anything that happened. He lay down to sleep for several hours while Angela talked with her neighbor.

It was time to get help. Angela did not want to place Harold in a nursing home, but there seemed to be no choice. She had to continue working to pay the bills. The neighbors were willing to watch over Harold, but his violent behavior was frightening. Angela was also scared, angry, and embarrassed. She was troubled by the change in Harold's behavior. Angela did not understand his rage until her neighbors told her about some experiences their children had had while checking on Mr. Jacobs. Three teenagers had taken turns looking in on him over the years. Recently, on several occasions they found Mr. Jacobs clinging to the front gate, shaking it violently. They were afraid to enter the yard because he acted so crazy. The day Angela discovered them, several strange teenagers had begun to tease Mr. Jacobs.

A plan emerged one weekend when several neighbors were visiting. Harold's closest friend and neighbor, George, noticed that over the last few months he had become more restless. Harold paced around the yard and appeared lost and scared. George suggested that he would build a porch on the back of their house and enclose it with glass. The sunporch would give Harold a comfortable place to sit and watch the boats, and perhaps he would feel more secure in a more structured environment.

The solution worked. For the next year Mr. Jacobs seemed happy to sit on the porch, which gave him a magnificent view of the water. Mrs. Jacobs was able to continue working with the close support of her neighbors and friends. A year later Harold died peacefully in his sleep at home.

## Goal 10: Examine Your Financial Situation and Get Help to Plan for the Future.

Financial planning is often the last issue with which family members want to be bothered after the diagnosis. The newly diagnosed Alzheimer's victim will usually still be competent to handle money matters and may remain so for some time. In these cases family members may feel uncomfortable talking about money matters. However, as difficult as this may be, financial concerns should be taken up as soon as possible, while the patient is still capable of participating in the decision making. If financial planning is delayed, the family could find itself in economic trouble when it is too late to do anything.

Since caring for the patient usually becomes more of a burden than care givers can handle alone, home attendants or a nursing home usually become necessary at some stage. Both home care and nursing-home care are expensive and inevitably drain the family's resources. Chapter 13 includes a discussion of what Medicare and Medicaid will and will not cover; it also reviews the usefulness of Medigap insurance and other health insurance alterations. With early financial planning, the family may be able to arrange its finances so that it can feel confident of paying for a relative's care and having a more secure future (Appendix 4).

Because the legal and financial problems are complex, families should get legal advice to make the best decisions for their particular situation. Patients also have a right to make decisions about their assets, and this can be done only while they have the capacity to sign legally binding documents. Planning ahead and taking action before the dementia incapacitates the patient and before crises occur will prevent unnecessary emotional distress, protect assets, and avert needless legal proceedings.

There is some basic information you can gather even when it may be difficult to talk about money matters. At the very minimum you should know these things:

1. where the patient keeps his or her will, bankbooks, insurance policies, stock certificates and bonds, and other important papers
2. Social Security and Medicare numbers
3. name, address, and phone numbers of his or her lawyer, insurance agent, and accountant
4. names and addresses of banks, numbers of checking and savings accounts, and location of safe-deposit box
5. names of life, health, and other insurance companies as well as numbers of the policies
6. with whom he or she has a pension plan, IRA, Keogh, or other retirement plans

You may be able to work out an arrangement whereby you help the patient organize his or her financial matters and pay bills. Consider the following:

1. Arrange to have access to the safe-deposit box so that you can get important papers in the event your relative is hospitalized.
2. Consider a joint bank account so that you can get cash for the patient's emerging needs.
3. Arrange to pay insurance premiums so that policies will not lapse, and make sure you know what terms are in effect when the patient dies.
4. Find out when bills are due—rent, mortgage, utilities, charge accounts—and offer to sit down once a month to help write out the checks.
5. Make sure Social Security checks, interest checks, and other sources of income are deposited in the patient's account. The easiest way to ensure that Social Security checks are not lost is

to have the patient sign Form SF-1199, authorizing the Social Security Administration to send the check directly to the bank.

It is frightening when you first realize that your relative is making financial errors—losing or not depositing checks, writing large checks that bounce, forgetting to pay bills. It can also be upsetting to try and work with your relative to handle financial matters as he or she becomes more impaired. However, it is vital to monitor the income and outflow of money and to manage assets to protect the patient and yourself.

How do you judge when it is time to intervene with your relative? This is a difficult philosophical and legal issue, as well as a personal one. However, it is better to discuss this question in the family, including the patient when possible, rather than to let the courts decide it after the patient has significantly deteriorated. At some point your relative may become unwilling and unable to manage money or to do what is necessary to protect assets. The result may be harm to your relative or to others or lack of proper maintenance of his or her life. Remember, help in these instances provides crucial protection.

There are several ways of dealing with financial problems. Each involves giving to someone else a degree of control over the patient's assets. This may be a member of the family, a close friend, or an institution. The crucial variable is that this be someone who is trusted. Furthermore, expert advice is necessary because the alternatives available vary from state to state. Appendix 4 describes some of the alternatives available in different parts of the country. Regardless of which option you choose to pursue, it is important that you recognize the need for examining the choices open to you.

## Goal 11: In Addition to Publications on Alzheimer's Disease and Related Disorders, Read Other Literature.

Edith Shelley, who at the age of seventy-five had been diagnosed for sixteen months, spoke about the impact of reading Eudora Welty's "A Worn Path" and One Writer's Beginnings. "A Worn Path," the story of a grandmother's love in spite of poverty and frailty, helped Mrs. Shelley talk to her grandchildren about her fears of rejection.

However, the book *One Writer's Beginnings* troubled her because it evoked sad longing for the life that was being taken away from her. But after laboring to read the book several times, Mrs. Shelley spoke insistently about an important message for Alzheimer's patients in Welty's work:

The book has helped me to review my own childhood, my relationship with my parents and to think about those moments in life that are precious to me. It also allowed me to gently face my eventual loss of memory and still dare to live. My memory is the treasure most dearly regarded by me. Eudora Welty helped me put my losses in perspective: "Memory is a living thing, and it too is in transit. But during its movement, all that is remembered joins and lives—the old and the young, the past and the present, the living and the dead." As you know, I am a woman who, like Ms. Welty, came of a sheltered life. "A sheltered life can be a daring life as well. For all serious daring starts from within."

Several books, monographs, and articles have been written about dementia and its impact on the patient, the family, and society. The references at the end of this book offer a selected reading list. In early phases of dementia the patient may want to read what has been published. When small print, poor vision, or limited reading skills make this difficult, read to the patient or summarize some of the material for him or her.

Although handbooks on Alzheimer's disease contain information about practical problems and solutions, it is important to read other material—adventures and mysteries, romance, science fiction, short stories, commentary, drama, and poetry. Literature provides a resource for reflecting on the personal challenge of growing older and living with Alzheimer's disease. Reading is also an escape, a hobby, and a source of great pleasure to many. It may remain an important part of the patient's life. For those with visual problems, there are talking books, and many books are available on cassettes or records.

Alzheimer's disease changes everything in the patients' life, forcing them and their family to live what one patient called a "speeded-up version of life." Max DuBois responded to the diagnosis of dementia by making a list of everything he wanted to accomplish before the dementia made these goals impossible. Mr. DuBois wanted to live the good times left to him by keeping busy and conducting his affairs as usual: "I do not want to live an imitation of life just because I have this disease. There are books to be read, plays and movies to be seen, and time to be spent with my wife, children, and grandchildren. I also want to go to London one more time . . . to say good-bye."

Mr. DuBois traveled to London with his wife, Jean, and on his return began to collect every book he could about the city—travel guides, photography books, even novels about London. His library expenditures became part of the family's weekly budget, and even when Max could no longer read his books, he seemed to enjoy collecting them. Jean reported that in later stages of the illness, when he became agitated, she would sit with him in the library and read excerpts from a "London book." This calmed him, and often he fell asleep next to her. Mrs. DuBois seemed to derive great comfort from feeling that Max had lovely dreams about the city, where they had first met and married.

Many books are not only entertaining and inspiring but also tools for understanding and coping with the future (See "bibliotherapy" in the reference list). Patients and families who have seemed to adapt best are those who anticipated many of their future problems and conceived alternative solutions. Many also attributed their successful coping style to the growth and self-awareness that came from reading. Books helped them focus on the challenge of finding joy and pleasure and meaning in their daily lives. Reading became an outlet for private emotions and fantasies, a way to reassess their own nurturing needs.

The choice of reading material depends on many factors—health, educational interests and preferences, as well as special needs for tapes and recorders. A number of resources are available in many community libraries, community centers, and hospitals, and senior citizen organizations may offer special guided-reading programs. Many hospitals and long-term-care institutions have programs in "bibliotherapy" for patients who are hospitalized or institutionalized. Bibliotherapy is the use of selected reading materials and specific techniques to help individuals deal with personal problems. Here a trained librarian, teacher, or counselor evaluates the individuals' literary needs and involves them in private or group reading sessions. Even illiterate patients can be brought into group reading sessions.

Bibliotherapy proved to be a valuable addition to family-therapy sessions with the relatives of Harry James, an Alzheimer's patient who had been institutionalized for six years with dementia. Harry and several members of his family were Holocaust survivors. Everyone in the family had strong feelings of isolation and great difficulty in accepting Harry's extended deterioration. The institution's librarian suggested that Harry's grandson Hy read *Mr. Sammler's Planet*, by Saul Bellow. The novel shows how Mr. Sammler, a seventy-two-year-old Holocaust survivor, successfully adapts to the alien environment of Manhattan in the 1960s. After Hy read the book, he suggested that the entire family do so, and that became the focus of discussions about Harry and their own feelings of disassociation. Even though Harry himself was bedridden with advanced dementia and unable to participate in family sessions, the members of his family found that their reactions to the Bellow novel allowed them to sort through their feelings as individuals and as a family and to deal emotionally with Harry's psychological death and the pending physical death.

## Goal 12: Locate a Family Support Group in Your Area.

Alzheimer's family-support groups exist all over the country. Most of them are chapters of the National Alzheimer's Disease and Related Disorders Association (ADRDA). Information about the national organization and local chapters can be found in Appendix 1. The ADRDA can put you in touch with a local group or even help you organize one with others near you.

The experience of participating in or organizing a family support group is a valuable one. Groups provide the opportunity for families to discover others with common problems. Members provide essential support and help each other cope with the many changes in their personal and family life. The following excerpt from a letter describes one wife's experience with a group of care givers:

I am thankful for the family group. When I first joined I felt hope for the first time. It may sound strange, but seeing others with the same problem gave me hope for the future. Their strength gave me the confidence to face my own problems. I knew that I was no longer alone.

Some people were worse off than I was. I realized that I could reach out and help them—and I felt better. It was as if I could make part of me whole again by helping others.

With time I came to appreciate the group more and more. I was able to talk freely. I did not have to hold anything inside. They understood my anger and my sadness. I could cry and not feel ashamed. And whenever I felt down I could call someone.

The group has given Jim and me a sense of being connected again. I used to feel alone and abandoned—like a sailor who had fallen overboard during the night.

Groups are a safe place to talk. Family members can express many complicated feelings and not be afraid that others will misunderstand or think unkindly of them. For example, it is common to feel anger toward the patient or even wish that he or she were dead. This is the kind of feeling that may be shared with a clinician, who will try to support the care giver by saying that such feelings are normal. Hearing this same message firsthand from others in similar situations is even more powerful. Learning that such feelings have been experienced by others whom you respect as good and caring people, like yourself, has a remarkable effect.

Groups help families retain a sense of hope for the future. "Hope" may sound like a strange word in this setting, but it often emerges from a sense that others are in this with you and are prepared to be of help.

Groups provide practical information about Alzheimer's disease and related disorders. Most groups establish good relationships with local health professionals who offer lectures and seminars about the latest clinical research in the field. Larger groups publish newsletters with updated information about current issues on the national and local scene as well as about clinical progress.

In support group meetings family members are encouraged to ask questions freely. Factual information can remove misconceptions about dementia and often relieves anxiety. Relatives who have lived with an impaired family member can teach each other many things by drawing on their own experiences—for example, what personality and mental changes may occur, how to evaluate the needs of the patient and the rest of the family, how to minimize or alter distressing behavior, how to adjust expectations, and how to maximize the quality of life for the patient and each other. There is the added value of knowing that the family will hear about scientific advances as soon as they are made.

Groups also develop a sense of cohesiveness and social belonging. Cohesiveness refers to feelings of belonging that are so important to our mental health. Group membership often decreases the social isolation experienced by dementia patients and their families. Many families are surprised and pleased to find that their group becomes an extended family.

Groups allow family members to help society as well as themselves. The support of research into the causes, prevention, and cure of the disease becomes a significant goal for many families. There is also much value in acting together to deal with problems of government health policy, long-term care, and reimbursement and organization of services (see Chapter 13). These are important issues for the relief of those suffering with dementia. Through group efforts individuals may derive a genuine sense of accomplishment that we are moving a step closer to controlling or eradicating dementia, and thus benefiting future generations as well as our own.

## Goal 13: Identify Resources in the Community.

A number of programs and services available in many communities are focused on the aged and may be useful to families caring for relatives with dementia. An important organization is the Area Agency on Aging (consult the white pages of your telephone directory). If it is not located in your immediate community, you can find out where it is in your region. Refer to Appendix 3 for the addresses of your State Agency on Aging.

The Agency on Aging should help you identify several programs and areas of assistance:

- your eligibility for income maintenance programs
- health and mental health services
- transportation services
- legal assistance
- nutrition programs
- employment and volunteer programs
- multipurpose service centers
- housing

- adult day-care programs
- in-home services
- long-term-care institutions

Sometimes resources are difficult to find, especially when you do not live in a large city or if your relative lives far away from you. Chapter 6 includes a detailed discussion of various programs and various ways to go about finding them.

## Goal 14: Become an Advocate for Reforming Policy on Alzheimer's Disease.

Learn what is happening at the national, state, and local levels. Get the names and addresses of your U.S. senators and congressman, and your state assemblyman, as well as of appropriate state, county, and city officials, including your governor and mayor. The current chairmen of the House Select Committee on Aging and the Senate Committee on Aging are listed in Appendix 2.

Write and tell them about the needs of patients with dementia and their families. Educate them about your needs and problems and seek their help. Inquire about the existence of any pending bills to support research, about tax exemptions for families caring for a relative at home, and about community-based home care and day-care programs. Work with ADRDA, which has an active public-advocacy program.

## Goal 15: "Go with the Flow."

Obviously, the way patients and families cope with the impact of dementia is influenced by many factors—the course of the dementia and the severity of the losses, the availability of family members and friends, the technical competence of professionals, the family's life-style and philosophy of life. One daughter of a patient, Iona Fleming, admitted that her job became easier and the household calmer when she was able to adopt a strategy "to go with the flow." It took time to accept the complexity of dealing with her father's needs and safety as well as those of her family and herself. Although there were times when she imposed certain limits, such as not allowing her father to drive the family car, do the weekly shopping, or baby-sit with the children alone, she found ways to involve him, respecting his need to contribute something to daily family life. There were days her father could barely cope with the world around him and required constant help. There were others when it was hard to believe anything was wrong. Mrs. Fleming said she had to get over asking herself why and to live day by day with the changes.

## The Future: Living and Caring

Living with Alzheimer's disease or related dementias is a herculean task for everyone—patients, family members, and other care givers. However, the odyssey of care can be made less stressful if one identifies goals and implements plans. There are no specific rules for providing the best care as the disease progresses, but families can do a great deal to break through what one patient's wife called a "cycle of despair." Norma Hull told us, "For months after George was diagnosed, I felt beaten. I wanted to retreat from everybody and everything. However, one day I watched George in the garage carefully organizing his tools, and the truth became clear to me. With some help I could do a lot for us. We had each other, our home, and our future."

# 5

# DRUGS: HELPFUL AND HARMFUL

---

*The Search for a Cure*

AT this time there are no known drugs which can stop or reverse the destruction of the brain and the intellectual losses which occur in Alzheimer's disease. For several years, intensive research effort has focused on the study of drugs which might increase the amount of the neurotransmitter acetylcholine, which is deficient in the Alzheimer's brain (see Chapter 12). Replacement of that substance should theoretically help the patient. However, acetylcholine does not get into the brain when taken directly. It can be introduced only through substances like lecithin and choline. These substances, when taken orally, are broken down in the body to form acetylcholine, which is then able to enter the brain. Unfortunately, at least to date, lecithin and choline compounds have not been beneficial in patient care.

Clinical trials attempting to measure whether replacement of acetylcholine could improve memory in Alzheimer's patients originally created a great deal of excitement among scientists, clinicians, and families. The hope was to repeat the success achieved with drug replacement therapy in the treatment of parkinsonism, another brain disease whose primary causes are also still unknown today. Patients with Parkinson's disease have uncontrolled tremors, body stiffness, problems in walking, changes in facial expression, and a number of other neurological problems. No cure is known, but drugs have provided a modest degree of relief for some patients with the disease. In parkinsonism the neurotransmitter dopamine is diminished in specific areas of the brain. Dopamine given directly also cannot enter the brain, but the compound L-dopa (levodihydroxyphenylalanine) taken by mouth eventually does reach the brain. There it set offs a chemical reaction increasing the production of the needed dopamine. L-dopa has been used successfully to manage the tremors and rigidity of Parkinson's disease in about 75 percent of the patients treated and has thus changed their lives dramatically. However, the other disabling symptoms, which may also include dementia, are not relieved, and the course of the disease is basically unchanged.

No drug has yet been discovered which directly controls or reverses any of the symptoms of Alzheimer's disease. Although a number of drugs influencing acetylcholine and other neurotransmitters in the brain are still under active investigation, as yet there have been no major breakthroughs in the direct treatment of the cognitive deficits of Alzheimer's disease. However, researchers are accelerating their quest for new compounds which may someday prove to be effective medications.

## Psychological Needs of the Patient and Family

When someone you care for has Alzheimer's disease or a related disorder, it is almost impossible to accept the idea that there is no cure. We live in an era when medical miracles are reported in the newspapers every day, including the transplantation of vital parts of the body, new cures for other diseases, and important scientific discoveries about the body or the world we live in. Each story evokes the painful reaction "What is being done for us?"

Because Alzheimer's disease affects so many persons and has received so much national media attention, any new lead, no matter how unsupported, is widely publicized, giving grounds for optimism to families and clinicians alike. So far, the result has been that misleading information in the newspapers is later explained in the scientific literature with a full and accurate story. Meanwhile, the family rides an emotional roller coaster from excitement and hope to despair. This only aggravates the problems of caring for the patient.

Individuals living with incurable illnesses face a difficult psychological problem—how to live with optimism and hope when a cure seems unlikely in the near future. The reality is painful, and although progress is being made in understanding diseases like dementia and cancer, useful knowledge develops slowly. Rational thinking is often distorted when someone has a devastating, incurable illness. It is natural for patients and families to hope for a miracle, and for some the pressure to search for one is intense. Families desperate for a cure are easy prey for individuals, whether truly believing or self-serving, who promote new but unproven treatments. The vulnerability of Alzheimer's families to quacks and charlatans is extraordinarily high. The family may go on a frantic search for a miracle, often losing emotionally as well as financially in the process of running down yet another blind alley. As truly difficult as it may be to accept, we should at this time stress again that there are no medications or other approaches which will stop or reverse the brain changes which result from Alzheimer's disease or related dementias.

However, medical treatments can be helpful in dealing with many aspects of Alzheimer's disease, and these interventions can make the burden of caring a little easier for the family. Close contact with an informed and caring physician who takes a real interest in the patient and family is essential to everyone's physical and mental health. Doctors with good clinical judgment appreciate three elements: the patient, the disease, and the illness. Families should feel that the doctor understands the lifestyle, personal goals, and special needs of everyone—the patient as well as individual family members. Doctors obviously need to be knowledgeable about the disease and to be aware of the latest scientific developments. Finally, physicians must recognize that the illness, which refers to the way the disease affects the patient, may not be the same in any two individuals with an identical diagnosis. It is particularly important in Alzheimer's disease, about which we still know so little, to recognize how the illness will vary from one patient to another.

Although medications cannot cure Alzheimer's disease and related disorders, certain drugs are safe and effective in the treatment of specific disorders and conditions, such as depression and anxiety, to which patients are vulnerable. When used in conjunction with psychological therapies, drugs may be useful to help manage a range of behavioral problems which often make the patient difficult to care for—agitation, hostility, overt suspiciousness and paranoia, and sleeplessness. Drugs used to treat behavior are called psychotropic medications. Like all medications, these drugs can be harmful as well as helpful. If not used properly, they can make patients more confused and more agitated, lead to loss of sleep, and even cause physical harm.

This chapter is intended to help families develop a general understanding about how drugs work, what their side effects are, and how they may interact with other medications. It describes how drugs are absorbed and broken down in the body and the ways they act differently in older persons. It discusses the major classes of psychotropic drugs and indicates their use, appropriate dosages, and side effects. However, this chapter is intended as a general reference, not as the final word about the efficacy or dosage of a specific drug. Pharmacology is a complex specialty in science and medicine, and there is no substitute for a knowledgeable physician.

## How Drugs Affect the Older Patient

Since most patients with dementia are over the age of sixty, it is useful to review how changes in older persons affect the way drugs act in the body. Whether they are taken by mouth (orally) or by injection into a muscle (IM) or vein (IV), medications usually spread throughout the entire body. Therefore, although a drug is most often intended for a specific purpose in a particular region of the body, it may also affect parts of the individual unrelated to the disease and have a number of side effects.

Psychotropic drugs, for instance, affect behavior or mood because they work primarily by influencing the brain. However, they may also influence the heart, blood pressure, the liver, the stomach and intestines, and muscles. Indeed, the range of possible side effects of many drugs is extraordinary. Fortunately, as a result of the careful procedures used in developing new drugs established by the FDA

(Federal Drug Administration), side effects do not occur very often, or, if they do, they are usually not serious enough to cause the patient major discomfort. However, in some instances drugs may lead to problems worse than those being treated in the first place. For those unlucky patients and families, there is little comfort in statistics showing how rarely the side effect is reported.

Many changes in the aging body affect drug action. With advancing age, after the mid-forties in men and after menopause in women, there is a change in the body's structure. People have more fat and less protein, and this increase in fatty tissue influences the way the body handles some medications. Most psychotropic drugs are attracted to the fatty tissues of the body. They are lipophilic, that is, attracted to lipids—the technical term for fat. This attraction means that the medication is absorbed into body fat, leaving less to circulate to the brain or other target intended to be reached with the drug. The storage of drugs in fatty tissues also means that it may take our body longer to eliminate drugs from our system after we stop taking them.

The bodies of older people, especially of those with medical illnesses, are less efficient than others in metabolizing drugs. Most medications are broken down by the body into less active or inactive compounds. This is usually done by enzymes produced in the liver. After this process occurs, drug by-products or the parent drug itself passes from the body through the kidneys, the gastrointestinal system, or through the lungs. Dementia patients with diseases involving the liver, kidney, or lungs will have trouble deactivating or eliminating drugs from the body. In such cases, very low dosages must be used to prevent undesirable side effects. However, these low doses may in turn have a less intensive effect.

The sensitivity of various parts of the body to a given drug also varies with age. The older brain, and especially the Alzheimer's brain, appears to be more sensitive to medication. As a consequence, relatively low doses of a drug can have powerful effects not only in the brain but also in the rest of the body.

All of these changes clearly make management of medications complicated, but a working partnership of the patient, family, other care givers, and physician can go a long way toward resolution of the complexity.

## Guidelines for Care Givers

Drugs must be used appropriately in order to have the desired effect. They should be taken at the times listed on the label of the bottle. However, the high cost of drugs may lead to an attempt to be thrifty by cutting down on medications. Or in the hustle and bustle of the daily routine, drugs may be forgotten. Furthermore, when individuals take several different medications at various times of the day or night, it is common for them to forget a pill or to take one at the wrong time. Special pill boxes can be purchased at the pharmacy which allow you to store pills by the day and the time. Remember, a change in the prescribed use of a drug without the doctor's knowledge may create a serious set of problems.

One drug sold over the counter is worth particular attention—alcohol. Alcohol has significant effects, including the way it changes the body's ability to handle other drugs. The use of beer, wine, and whiskeys should be carefully regulated and discussed openly with the doctor. In almost no instance can Alzheimer's patients handle large amounts of alcohol without complications. Small amounts of alcohol, a beer, cocktail, or glass of wine at lunch or dinner, may be quite enjoyable and even desirable if there are no medical contraindications.

When alcohol use has been a regular part of the patient's social activity, social drinking is often pleasurable, but sensible judgment is important. For some households it is better to restrict the amount of beer, wine, or liquor kept in the home or perhaps to eliminate it altogether. Sometimes patients will drink themselves into a stupor, not because they are alcoholic but because they forget how much they have consumed.

Frequently, several different drugs are used by the same patient, and this can become a serious problem because drugs affect each other. Family members should question their family physician about the possible interactions different drugs have with one another. Drugs prescribed by different physicians, the use of old drugs which are not discarded, drugs "borrowed" from other people, or mixtures of drugs, alcohol, and over-the-counter preparations used together are all responsible for these "drug-drug interactions."

The manner in which drugs are taken can also be important.

Injections are generally the fastest way of getting drugs to act in the body, but this is not always true. Most medications are taken orally. The absorption of drugs from the stomach and the rest of the gastrointestinal system may be affected by the contents of the stomach—such as the presence of food recently eaten (especially fatty food)—the availability of certain enzymes or lack of them in the digestive system, the size of the meal, or the person's emotional state. Inadequate fluid intake, the use of laxatives, and irregular eating habits also have an impact on how drugs are absorbed from the stomach and intestines.

The giving of drugs can be a problem. Some patients will spit out pills and capsules or simply not swallow them. Others may resist going to the doctor if a shot is involved. If this is a problem, check with the doctor prescribing the medication. Is it available in liquid form? Can the number of times per day be minimized? Can the number of pills or capsules be reduced? Can the patient tolerate a drug-free day (or weekend)? If you show an interest, the physician will be far more likely to work with you on creating an optimal program. Physicians are usually happy to accommodate if it means the medications are more likely to be used correctly.

The following checklist may be helpful:

1. Keep a written list of the names of *all* drugs the patient is using.
2. Make a daily chart of times for which drugs are prescribed. Check off drugs as given.
3. Check with the doctor to determine whether a specific drug should be taken before or after meals.
4. Make sure *every* doctor prescribing drugs knows *all* of the drugs being taken.
5. Keep a record of any drugs that have caused a problem in the past. Be prepared to report this to doctors, nurses, hospitals, and other medical professionals.
6. If the patient is taken off of a drug, throw out the pills, capsules, or liquid remaining in the medicine cabinet. The temptation to use them again may be too hard to resist.
7. If you feel that the drug is too expensive, tell your doctor. If you cannot afford the cost of medication, there may be ways of reducing the expense. Physicians can often save you money if

they prescribe alternative forms of the same medication. In some states this is automatic, while in others you may need to discuss this with your physician or a pharmacist. Be honest with your doctor. No competent physician will be offended if you explain your problem. If your doctor is irritated by such a discussion, you may wish to consider changing doctors.

8. Remember that many of the drugs sold without a prescription can affect the patient. Among the most dangerous of these over-the-counter drugs are alcohol and sedatives (sleeping pills). It is generally a good idea not to use over-the-counter drugs without letting the doctor know or getting his or her advice. These drugs often alter the action of prescription drugs. This even applies to aspirin or similar drugs.

## Deciding to Use Psychotropic Drugs

The loss of brain cells and the other bodily changes that occur with dementia have a significant impact on the way drugs work. As a result, not all patients respond as expected to drugs. For example, some drugs which usually reduce agitation may have the opposite effect and cause patients to become even more agitated. The decision to use drugs with a patient requires careful consideration. Psychotropic medications are usually effective and helpful when used properly, but they should be considered only after several other steps have been taken.

First, it is worth remembering that individuals with dementia often have medical problems, and these conditions may themselves cause confusion, agitation, or other behavioral problems. Second, changes in the patient's physical or emotional environment often cause distress, making patients upset and agitated. Therefore, it is important to evaluate the patients' medical status as well as environmental conditions and changes in their personal life before simply assuming that the dementia is worsening. A careful evaluation should be done before the initiation of drug treatment. In addition, psychological interventions should be considered before medications are used, or they should be used along with a medication program.

The term "psychotropic" is applied specifically to those drugs primarily designed to influence the brain, emotions, and behavior. It is a mistake to think of psychotropic drugs only as tranquilizers. There are several major classes of psychotropics, each of which has a specific purpose. We have organized them into five groups. These include antipsychotic, antidepressant, antianxiety, sedative-hypnotic, and cognitive-acting medications. The remainder of this chapter reviews some basic information about each of the major psychotropic drug classes. Our objective is to help family members judge when drugs may be used appropriately and effectively to help the patient function at the highest level possible.

The information in this chapter is intended to help you understand the different types of drugs and ask questions of your doctors. It *cannot* be a substitute for the care of a trained physician, nor should it be seen as the final word about the safety of the drugs mentioned.

## Antipsychotic Medications

Antipsychotic medications are used for the treatment of disturbing behaviors like severe agitation, irrational violence, and bizarre thoughts, including hallucination and paranoid states. At times these drugs may also be used for other conditions, among them restlessness and irritability. In small doses they may be used quite effectively to eliminate the confusion which is noticed in some patients in the early evening. This is frequently called the "sundown syndrome." Thus, sometimes the agitation, irritability, and hostility frequently seen in dementia may be controlled by medication if treated by a knowledgeable and careful physician. On the other hand, regular exercise and meaningful activity are also extremely effective in the managing of restlessness and irritability. Drugs are a poor substitute for regular physical activity.

Table 1 lists some of the most commonly used antipsychotic drugs and their usual adult doses. Older persons, and especially those with dementia, usually require much lower doses. Antipsychotic medications affect the activity of several neurotransmitters in the brain— dopamine, norepinephrine, and serotonin. There are five major chemical classifications of antipsychotic drugs: (1) phenothiazines, such as Thorazine, Prolixin, Stelazine, and Mellaril; (2) butyrophe-

Table 1. COMMON EFFECTIVE ANTIPSYCHOTIC MEDICATIONS

| Generic Name | Brand Name | Usual Adult Daily Dosage* |
|---|---|---|
| Chlorpromazine | Thorazine | 30–1000 mg |
| Fluphenazine hydrochloride | Prolixin | 0.5–10 mg |
| Haloperidol | Haldol | 0.5–2 mg 2 to 3 times a day |
| Molindone hydrochloride | Moban | 50–75 mg a day increase to 100 mg in 3 to 4 days<br>maintenance dose—as low as 5–15 mg 3 to 4 times a day to 225 mg a day |
| Mesoridazine | Serentil | 30–400 mg |
| Thioridazine hydrochloride | Mellaril | 50–100 mg at first, then 50–800 mg per day |
| Thiothixene | Navane | 2 mg 3 times per day |
| Trifluoperazine | Stelazine | 2–4 mg |

*Older patients with dementia usually require less.

nones, such as Haldol; (3) thioxanthenes, such as Navane; (4) molin-dones, such as Moban; and (5) dibenzoxazepines, such as Loxitane. All of these drugs are powerful and, consequently, may also have powerful side effects.

It is important to keep in mind that antipsychotic drugs will not improve or reverse memory loss or other intellectual problems which characterize Alzheimer's disease or multi-infarct dementia. Although these medications often help with the management of problem behaviors associated with dementia, they are not always successful in treating them. One reason for this is the difficulty in regulating the dosage in older persons with dementia. Adjusting the amount of medication may be a delicate matter, requiring patience from everyone—patient, family, and doctor.

DOSAGE

Once a drug is selected, it is important that your doctor use the lowest effective dose. The usual procedure is to start low, to look for side effects, gradually increase the dose to an effective level, and then adjust the daily amount slightly until the best apparent level is reached. When individuals do not show the expected response to a drug, doctors often wish to test the level of the drug in the blood. There are laboratory techniques to determine whether individuals have a "therapeutic dose" of a certain drug in their body. Finally, after an antipsychotic drug has been used for a while, ask your physician whether it is advisable to stop the use of the drug for a short period—over weekends, for example—to determine whether it is necessary to continue treatment.

In general, the antipsychotic medications all seem to be equally effective. However, they do differ in their potency and the specific side effects they produce. Some antipsychotic drugs have a greater sedative effect than others. Mellaril and Thorazine are examples of drugs that the physician could use to treat sleep disturbances in certain agitated patients with dementia. However, because sedation causes clouded consciousness, the more sedating antipsychotic drugs may also cause slightly more daytime confusion and disorientation in the patient. Thus, observing and understanding the patient and knowledge about drug action are essential to help the patient and minimize the number of medications.

SIDE EFFECTS

Side effects to drugs are by no means universal, but they are not rare. When one administers antipsychotic medications, it is as important to watch for the appearance of side effects as it is to monitor the beneficial effect on the behavioral problem. When side effects are harmful or make the patient extremely uncomfortable, the drug should be withdrawn.

Among the most common side effects are sleepiness, dry mouth, constipation, blurred vision, and bladder problems. Patients taking antipsychotic medications may also have problems like stiffness of the joints and occasional drooling. In extreme cases, regular use of antipsychotic drugs will produce parkinsonian symptoms. When such problems occur, as they may in 20 to 30 percent of patients, the use of another class of medications (antiparkinsonian drugs) may reverse these symptoms. However, this causes the patient to use two drugs in combination and therefore increases the possibility of other side effects.

Different side effects may occur with antipsychotic medications. These include the lowering of the blood pressure and a sensation of being dizzy or light-headed, particularly when the patient moves from a seated or lying-down position to standing upright. This condition is known as postural hypotension, that is, a drop in blood pressure as a result of sudden changes in posture.

In some patients a surprising effect may occur with antipsychotic medications. A patient who is agitated and given antipsychotic medication may become more agitated. If this happens, the dosage should be decreased or the use of the drug should be stopped altogether. Agitation may be caused by many factors. Patients should be carefully examined to determine whether they are in pain or uncomfortable as a result of medical conditions. Supportive psychotherapy may also be effective. Even when patients are severely impaired, simply sitting and talking with them (even if the conversation is nonsensical) may calm the agitation.

There is one last side effect which deserves careful attention—a condition called tardive dyskinesia. This is a disorder associated with the long-term use of antipsychotic drugs. As many as 15 percent of individuals who have been treated with large doses of antipsychotic medication over several years develop uncontrolled and exaggerated movements of the mouth, tongue, and jaw area. At the moment the best approach is to recognize these signs early and stop using the drugs. Regular examination of the mouth and tongue will detect the presence of unusual movements. Poorly fitting dentures may also cause the individual with dementia to make strange mouth movements, which should not be confused with tardive dyskinesia. The best way to prevent this condition is to minimize and regulate the dosage given to patients. Whatever the drug, it should be used sparingly. Drug-free periods or total cessation of the drugs should be considered. Medications do vary in their likelihood of causing tardive dyskinesia, and this should certainly be kept in mind.

Patients who have any blood, kidney, liver, or heart disease, Parkinson's disease, or low blood pressure should not usually take antipsychotics. Individuals on phenothiazines should not be around insecticides or exposed to extreme heat. Antipsychotics should also be used cautiously in patients with glaucoma, epilepsy, ulcers, or problems in passing urine.

It should be clear by now that the use of psychotropic drugs requires the doctor to make complex decisions. Which drug will cause the least harm and provide the best treatment for the right patient? What side effects are most likely to occur? How can they be managed? What alternatives are there to medications, such as exercise, nutrition, or changes in the physical or social environment?

## Antidepressant Medications

### THE COEXISTENCE OF DEPRESSION AND DEMENTIA

Since clinical depression affects thinking, memory, sleep, and appetite and interferes with daily life, the existence of depression in the patient with dementia clearly complicates and worsens the individual's functioning. Depression has been observed in 15 to 20 percent of early dementia victims. However, recognizing depression is often a challenge. Memory-impaired individuals are less able to act and communicate effectively with words. Even early in their disease they may report not that they are sad or depressed but that they feel empty or apathetic. Nothing gives them pleasure, and they simply "don't care" about things. Sometimes apathy and withdrawal—or, conversely, agitation—are symptoms of depression rather than of dementia.

It is important to know that severe depressive symptoms may appear as the result of a disease unrelated to the dementia or the psychological state of the individual, for example, metabolic disorders, such as a thyroid condition, or other physical problems. Depression can also occur as a side effect of drugs used to treat physical disorders, such as certain antihypertensive (high blood pressure) medications.

Since the major objective in the care of the patient is to maintain the highest possible level of functioning, successfully treating the depression can reduce some of the apathy, inattention, and irritability of the patient. One problem, apart from possible side effects of the medication, may be the family's initial enthusiasm that the patient is being "cured." Although this can happen in cases where depression alone causes the dementia, it is not to be confused with a "cure" for Alzheimer's disease or related disorders. Family members still denying the presence of a confirmed Alzheimer's or multi-infarct dementia often grasp at straws and once again go on the emotional roller coaster of optimism, disappointment, and risk, and they develop their own reactive depression.

TREATMENT OF CLINICAL DEPRESSION IN DEMENTIA

Several types of drugs are used to treat major depression in patients with dementia. See Table 2 for a list of the most frequently used antidepressant medications. The most commonly prescribed belong to a group of chemical compounds known as tricyclic antidepressants. Although effective in most instances, tricyclic antidepressants may have adverse side effects, which older patients are likely to show. Therefore, as was discussed earlier, with all drugs lower doses are appropriate. Table 2 identifies the range of therapeutic doses for older patients.

Another class of drugs used to treat severe depressions are known as monoamine oxidase inhibitors. These drugs block the action of a chemical called monoamine oxidase (MAO), which is normally found in the nervous system. MAO acts to maintain a chemical balance in certain parts of the brain by breaking down excess amounts of one of the most abundant neurotransmitters, known as norepinephrine or noradrenaline. One of the major theories of depression holds that depression is caused by the shortage of norepinephrine in key areas of the brain. Whether this shortage is caused by the presence of too much MAO, inadequate production of norepinephrine, or some other factor is not clear. However, since MAO reduces the level of norepinephrine in the brain, a drug which blocks the action of MAO will therefore increase the availability of norepinephrine. The therapeutic result is relief for the depressed patient.

Table 2. COMMON EFFECTIVE ANTIDEPRESSANT MEDICATIONS

| Generic Name | Brand Name | Usual Daily Adult Dosage | Usual Daily Older-Adult Dosage |
|---|---|---|---|
| Amitriptyline | Amitril<br>Elavil<br>Endep<br>SK-Amitriptyline | 100–300 mg | 25–150 mg |
| Desipramine | Norpramin<br>Pertofrane | 100–300 mg | 25–150 mg |
| Doxepin hydrochloride | Adapin<br>Sinequan | 100–300 mg | 25–150 mg |
| Imipramine | Antipress<br>Imavate<br>Janimine<br>Presamine<br>SK-Pramine<br>Tofranil | 100–300 mg | 25–150 mg |
| Maprotiline | Ludiomil | 100–300 mg | 25–150 mg |
| Nortriptyline | Aventyl<br>Pamelor | 50–100 mg | 10–50 mg |
| Protriptyline hydrochloride | Vivactil | 20–60 mg | 5–30 mg |
| Trazodone | Desyrel | 150–400 mg | 50–300 mg |

Several new antidepressant drugs (refer to Table 2), including trazodone, have recently been approved for use in the United States by the Food and Drug Administration (FDA). These drugs seem to act more rapidly, require smaller dosages, and cause fewer side effects than either the tricyclic or the MAO antidepressants. However, since these medications are relatively new, their long-term advantages and disadvantages have not been fully evaluated, particularly not among older persons with dementia.

It is important to emphasize that drugs are not necessary or even appropriate in treating all forms of depression. Alzheimer's patients may have reactive depressions, and here supportive counseling and social interventions are the treatment of choice. Drugs are not! Alzheimer's patients, particularly early in the disorder, may be acutely aware of their losses. They may remember and grieve over the death of relatives when they attend a funeral or feel the loss of friends or pets. It is, of course, always possible that a reactive depression will trigger a more severe depressive disorder in a vulnerable individual. Therefore, grief reactions should be monitored closely.

WHEN TO USE DRUGS

When is it appropriate to use antidepressant medications? They may be effective for the treatment of depressive disorders characterized by a change in mood and the following symptoms:

1. sleep disturbances (either a noticeable increase or decrease in sleep)
2. appetite changes and weight changes (either a significant gain or a loss over a four- to six-week period)
3. loss of energy and complaints of being tired
4. agitated behavior or a marked slowing of behavior
5. loss of interest in pleasurable activities
6. difficulty with concentration and thinking
7. impaired ability to carry out activities of daily living
8. low self-esteem, guilt, and negative feelings about self
9. thoughts of death or suicide
10. persistence of depressive symptoms for several weeks

It is almost never advisable to give the patient more than one drug in a major psychotropic drug class at the same time. This means a person should not receive two or more antidepressant or two or more antipsychotic drugs at once. However, under certain circumstances, it may be appropriate to administer an antipsychotic drug with an antidepressant, such as when the individual with depression also has severe delusions or hallucinations. Here the advice of a psychiatrist or other physician experienced with such medications is valuable.

The choice of a particular antidepressant drug is determined by many factors. The patient may not be able to tolerate a certain medication because of side effects. Some antidepressant drugs will aggravate other physical illnesses or interfere with the action of other medications. As we discussed in the section on antipsychotic medications, the characteristics of the specific drug need to be considered thoughtfully in relation to the patient's problem. For example, some tricyclics have a sedative effect which may be useful for a patient with dementia who is very agitated and has sleep disturbances. These sedative tricyclics would be less helpful for a patient who is apathetic and withdrawn.

DOSAGE

Tricyclics should be given in divided doses or in one dose at bedtime. This reduces the possibility of the patient's developing "postural hypotension," the drop in blood pressure when the patient stands up from a lying or seated position. Postural hypotension may cause falls and injuries, which in turn may require major nursing care. As a general rule, individuals who show clear differences in blood pressure when they change from a sitting to a standing position, even before medications are given, should not be treated with tricyclics.

Once a positive effect is achieved, the dose should be maintained for at least six months. The dose can then be decreased gradually, and if depressive symptoms do not recur, the medication can be fully withdrawn.

SIDE EFFECTS

The different antidepressants have several types of side effects. Some cause sedation, dry mouth, and blurred vision. The tricyclics may also cause tremors and sweating. These occur more often with tricyclics like desipramine, imipramine, and protriptyline. Therefore, these medications may not be the drug of choice for some older patients.

Finally, tricyclic antidepressants may affect heart rate and present a problem for certain patients who also have heart disease. Although no persistent damaging effects of tricyclics on the heart have been reported, a conservative assumption is that the tricyclic antidepressants should not be used within two months after a heart attack or other major disturbance in the heart's functioning. Patients with certain uncontrolled and irregular heart rhythms and those with uncontrolled angina or poorly controlled congestive heart failure should not be on tricyclics.

CAUTIONS AND WARNINGS

In a number of other conditions, tricyclics and other antidepressants either should not be used or should be used cautiously. It is very important that you ask the physician any and all questions you may have concerning the drug effects, dosage, or side effects of these medications.

If MAO inhibitors are used to treat depression in dementia patients, care givers must be careful to follow strict dietary and medical guidelines. These drugs can produce undesirable interactions with certain foods, drugs, and other medications. Mixing MAO inhibitors with any of the substances listed below may cause severe headaches, stiffness in the neck, increased heart rate, and a rise in blood pressure. These restrictions apply while the drug is being taken as well as for a period of ten days after its discontinuation.

Avoid These Foods:

1. all cheese (except cottage cheese, cream cheese, and ricotta cheese), including cheese crackers, cheese sauces, and pizzas
2. liver
3. smoked or pickled fish
4. foods containing brewer's yeast
5. fava beans, broad bean pods
6. fermented sausages

Avoid or Limit These Drinks:

1. red wine
2. beer
3. other alcoholic drinks
4. drinks containing caffeine or chocolate

Avoid or Limit These Medications:

1. over-the-counter cold, cough, decongestant, and allergy items
2. hay fever and sinus medications
3. appetite suppressants
4. pain relievers
5. other psychotropic drugs
6. any prescription medications not first discussed with the doctor

An overdosage of these medications can be dangerous. Symptoms may include confusion, agitation or drowsiness, hallucination, changes in heart rate or heart failures, enlarged pupils of the eyes, convulsions, vomiting, high fever, muscle stiffness, or coma. The individual should always be taken to a hospital emergency room along with the medicine bottle, and the patient's doctor should be contacted immediately.

### OTHER THERAPIES

Drugs may not always reverse the depression. Some patients will not be able to tolerate antidepressants, or they may not respond to treatment, especially as the dementia progresses. In the early and middle stages of dementia, counseling or psychotherapy, maintaining a supportive and stimulating environment, or changing the physical environment should be considered as therapeutic options.

## Antianxiety Medications

### UNDERSTANDING ANXIETY IN DEMENTIA

Anxiety is a normal reaction to certain stressful situations but can become severe enough to be crippling in its own right. The severity of the symptoms and the extent to which they disrupt a person's effectiveness must be taken into consideration in deciding whether the anxiety is a minor psychological upset to be treated by psychological support alone or a serious psychiatric disturbance for which medication is also advised. The truth is that it is sometimes difficult to diagnose anxiety in the patient with dementia. At other times, the irritability, emotional upset, increased activity and wandering, agitation, and fear are easy to recognize.

Nondrug as well as drug interventions may be useful to reduce the anxiety of patients with dementia. A supportive social and physical environment is essential, and the search for activities appropriate to the level of the patient is a constant challenge as the dementia progresses. The loss of mental powers is a legitimate cause for anxiety. This anxiety must be recognized and the patients encouraged to talk about it if they want to and are ready to handle it.

### INDICATIONS FOR USE OF ANTIANXIETY DRUGS

Antianxiety medications may help, but they should not be used routinely or for prolonged periods by anyone. Table 3 summarizes information on a number of common antianxiety drugs also known as tranquilizers. All medications in the table belong to a group of drugs known as benzodiazepines. Meprobamate and other drugs containing barbiturates are not listed in Table 3, because they are not safe medications for older patients. Meprobamate can lead to

Table 3. COMMON EFFECTIVE ANTIANXIETY MEDICATIONS

| Generic Name | Trade Name | Adult Daily Dosage* |
|---|---|---|
| Alprazolam | Xanax | 0.75–4 mg |
| Chlordiazepoxide | Librium | 5–100 mg |
| Clorazepate | Azene Tranxene | 15–60 mg |
| Diazepam | Valium | 2–4 mg |
| Halazepam | Paxipam | 60–160 mg |
| Lorazepam | Ativan | 2–10 mg |
| Oxazepam | Serax | 10–120 mg |
| Prazepam | Centrax | 20–60 mg |

*This is the dosage range for healthy younger adults. Older persons with dementia will usually require less.

physical and psychological dependence. Furthermore, confused patients may kill themselves with an accidental overdose.

The various benzodiazepines listed in the table all relax the major skeletal muscles and also have a direct effect on the brain. Alprazolam (Xanax) and oxazepam (Serax) are probably the best of these drugs, if they are used for *short* periods of time. None of these medications should be used for long periods.

SIDE EFFECTS

The most common side effect of all these drugs is drowsiness, which leaves many dementia patients less able to enjoy daily activities. The benzodiazepines, however, may have additional and serious adverse drug effects: apathy, dry mouth, confusion, depression, slurred speech, nausea, headaches, dizziness, constipation, urinary incontinence, change in heart rhythm, lowered blood pressure, blurred vision, rash and itching, nervousness, water retention, liver dysfunction, and inability to fall asleep. If your relative develops any of the above symptoms, stop the use of the medication and call the doctor.

CAUTIONS AND WARNINGS

Patients taking these medications should avoid smoking, alcohol, other tranquilizers, barbiturates, narcotics, antihistamines, and antidepressants. None of the benzodiazepines should be used if the patient has used one of these compounds in the past and developed an allergic reaction to it. They should also be avoided if the patient has narrow-angle glaucoma, but they may be taken by a patient with open-angle glaucoma.

If patients are not watched, they can overdose on any of these drugs. Symptoms include disorientation, sleepiness, shallow breathing, low blood pressure, lack of response to pain, such as that caused by a pinprick, and coma. Take the patient to a hospital emergency room and bring the bottle.

## Sleep Medications or Sedative-Hypnotics

Sleep problems are common in the patient with dementia, and they often become more upsetting as the dementia progresses. The wakefulness and nighttime wandering of a patient often wear family members out. Indeed, sleep disturbances are among the problems which most frequently cause families to place the patient in a nursing home. Unfortunately, little has been done to study the usefulness and the long-term risks of using sleep medication in patients with dementia.

Two major classes of drugs are commonly used to treat sleep problems—barbiturates and a group of compounds called benzodiazepines. As was indicated earlier, the latter are also employed to deal with anxiety. It is worth emphasizing again that barbiturates are not appropriate for use by older persons, because they are addictive and render sleep problems worse, not better. In some instances, barbiturates can make patients more upset and irritable. Table 4 lists some of the most commonly used sedative-hynotics. Barbiturates are not listed, because they are not recommended.

Benzodiazepines may have some value if used for relatively brief periods, but they are not helpful in the long-term management of sleep problems in dementia patients. The drugs currently available make sleep problems worse when taken over long periods of time. In addition, the use of sleep medication can create psychological problems for members of the family, who may feel emotional conflict about whether or not to provide such medication. Benzodiazepines may initially help the patient sleep (thereby giving the tired spouse the opportunity to sleep). However, they may also cause residual drowsiness and cognitive impairment the next day, thus increasing the burden of care. It is not uncommon to observe family members caught in a vicious cycle of giving the patient sleeping pills "hoping" they will work and developing anger and frustration over the patient's increasing disorientation. Here the family must carefully make a risk-benefit analysis and advise the doctor about its wishes. Most physicians will be glad to work with the family in this complex management task.

As with all classes of drugs, the individual compounds differ in effectiveness. The effects may also vary greatly in different patients. If some drugs have been used for a long time, stopping the use of

Table 4. COMMON EFFECTIVE SEDATIVE-HYPNOTIC MEDICATIONS

| Generic Name | Brand Name | Adult Dose | Drug Interactions |
|---|---|---|---|
| Chloral hydrate | Cohidrate Noctec Oradrate | 500 mg–1 gm at bedtime | Avoid alcohol, barbiturates, and tranquilizers. Anticoagulant drugs may need adjustment. |
| Ethchlorvynol | Placidyl | 500 mg at bedtime | Do not combine with amitriptyline. Avoid alcohol, antihistamines, and other depressant drugs. |
| Flurazepam | Dalmane | 15–30 mg at bedtime | Avoid alcohol, tranquilizers, barbiturates, sleeping pills, narcotics, antihistamines, MAO inhibitors, and other antidepressants. |
| Glutethimide | Doriden Dormtabs | 1 tablet at bedtime | Avoid alcohol, other sleeping pills, and histamines. Anticoagulant drugs may need adjustment. |
| Methaqualone hydrochloride | Mequin Parest Quaalude | up to 400 mg | Avoid alcohol, other sleeping pills, tranquilizers, and other depressants. |
| Temazepam | Restoril | 15–30 mg | Avoid alcohol, other sleeping pills, narcotics, tranquilizers, barbiturates, and antidepressants. |
| Triazolam | Halcion | 0.125–0.5 mg | Avoid alcohol, other sleeping pills, narcotics, tranquilizers, barbiturates, and antidepressants. |

the drug causes sleeplessness, agitation, anxiety, and the need for even higher doses to achieve normal sleep for a few days. This can lead to a spiraling problem. In general we suggest that if medication is used at all for sleep, it should be used only for brief periods, that is, for a few nights and for problems due to a short-term stressful situation. This will prevent the physical or psychological dependence which leads to a spiraling effect in drug use.

Sedative-hypnotics can be dangerous if the patient takes an accidental overdose. In the event this occurs, the patient should be taken to a hospital emergency room along with the medicine bottle.

Behavioral approaches are often the treatment of choice for sleep problems, particularly in the early stages of dementia. Simple strategies such as rising at the same time each morning, eliminating or minimizing afternoon naps, regular vigorous physical exercise, proper nutrition, and a carefully planned active day can go a long way toward improving the patient's sleep pattern. Patients who live through a meaningful and reasonably stimulating day will tire and sleep at night. It is unreasonable to expect that people who are passive all day and encouraged to nap after lunch will use their nighttime for sleep in the same way as others do.

## Cognitive-Acting Medications

A number of medications have been used to treat the symptoms of dementia. Although no current medications can reverse or cure the disease, retardation of the rate of decline may be possible if certain drugs combined with psychosocial interventions are instituted early. The ergot alkaloids, marketed under several brand names—Hydergine, Tri-Ergone, Trigot, Spengine, and Circanol—have been shown to have a minimal effect, especially when used at higher doses in European studies. A few studies in the United States have shown that patients taking ergot alkaloids for a year or more performed at a slightly higher level of functioning than with patients on placebos. Another group of compounds, known as cerebrovasodilators, which improve the blood circulation to the brain, have shown a small positive effect in some patients with multi-infarct dementia.

## General Rules for Drug Use in Dementia

Families and care givers should become knowledgeable enough to judge when drugs are being used appropriately and effectively for the well-being of their loved one. The following principles are important to keep in mind:

1. The doctor should start with low doses and increase gradually, if necessary.
2. A drug should be given only for the patient's benefit, not primarily for that of the family or professional staff.
3. Some drugs have side effects which can make the patient uncomfortable and aggravate the dementia. Refer to the summary in Table 5.
4. Side effects themselves are not necessarily adequate reasons to stop drug treatment. Such side effects may be appropriately managed or be less serious than the initial problem being treated.
5. When the doctor starts your relative on a drug, plans should also be made for withdrawing the drug in the future.
6. A patient's physical condition affects the way a drug acts.
7. The use of over-the-counter medication or alcohol should be avoided unless discussed with the physician.
8. Outdated medicines should be thrown out of the medicine cabinet.
9. Every physician prescribing medication should know of all other medications being taken by the patient.
10. Drugs interact with each other and can cause serious problems.
11. Drugs should always be used in conjunction with psychological, social, and environmental therapies as appropriate.
12. Drugs can hurt the patient if not used appropriately.
13. Drugs may not work at all.

## Clinical Drug Trials

Your doctor may also recommend that you consider enrolling your relative in a clinical drug trial to test the usefulness of an experimental drug to treat the symptoms of dementia. Although this may be a valuable effort, some precautions are in order. Ask questions about

Table 5. COMMON SIDE EFFECTS OF THE FOUR MAJOR CLASSES OF
PSYCHOTROPIC MEDICATIONS

| | Psychotropic Drug Class | | | |
| Side Effect | Anti-Psychotics | Anti-Depressants | Anti-Anxiety | Hypnotics |
|---|:---:|:---:|:---:|:---:|
| Agitation | • | | • | • |
| Bladder problems | • | | • | |
| Blurred vision | • | • | • | • |
| Constipation | • | | • | |
| Dizziness | • | | | |
| Drooling | • | | | |
| Dry mouth | • | • | • | |
| Heart rate change | | • | • | |
| Low blood pressure | • | | • | |
| Postural hypotension | • | | | |
| Sedation | • | • | • | • |
| Slurred speech | | | • | • |
| Stiffness | • | | | |
| Sweating | | • | | |
| Tardive dyskinesia | • | | | |
| Tremors | • | • | | |

the safety of the new compound and about previous research results. Find out whether the study has been approved for scientific merit and ethical use of human subjects by an accredited medical institution. Before signing any consent forms to allow your relative to participate in clinical drug research, make sure you understand the risks of harm to the patient as well as the potential benefits.

Although the probability that any currently available compound will improve learning and memory is extremely low, new compounds may someday be synthesized and tested for safety and efficacy. Clinical drug trials are essential for the testing of new and safe drugs as they are developed and become available. One day we may discover how to treat and ultimately prevent Alzheimer's disease and related disorders. For the moment there exist many strategies for helping the patient cope with and adapt to some of his or her losses. These are discussed in the next four chapters.

# 6

# WAYS
# OF
# CARING

---

"Herman, you really need to start playing tennis again. Look at your stomach. You need it." Sue Ellen, a victim of Alzheimer's disease, spoke these words to her husband as she lay in her hospital bed. As she talked, Herman simply stared at her, then caught himself and replied, "Yes, you're right." And she was. After a few more exchanges Sue Ellen changed the subject. "When do you fly to Rome? Will you take Jamie with you? He so enjoys working with you in the business, and he wants you to be proud of him." Herman gently protested that he, Jamie, and the rest of the family would stay near her until she left the hospital. Sue Ellen sat up in her bed and summoned Herman to move closer. "Please go away. You need a break. I won't die before you return. This disease won't let me die. It's just changing me, but I'll be okay."

FAMILIES and other care givers are often surprised to hear patients voice relevant thoughts and concerns or see them behave appropriately. Sue Ellen Williams had been hospitalized following a fall in which she fractured her hip. The pain and the general stress of being in a hospital had caused her to be even more confused and disoriented much of the time. Sue Ellen's physicians had given her the best medical care, and everyone was optimistic that she would heal and walk again. Even though the doctors were pleasant with Sue Ellen, they said little except hello, how are you feeling, and goodbye. Sue Ellen would often try to ask them questions, but they seemed unable to understand what she said. Indeed, they hardly seemed to listen. However, as the example above shows, her family had just begun to listen.

It is important that Alzheimer's disease not become a stigma. It is a label as well as a disease; when the words are spoken, they can immediately change the way we perceive and act toward the victim. Perhaps one of the most significant barriers to providing good care is our difficulty in recognizing the human qualities of those who have become the diagnosed patients. There is a tendency for everyone, from physicians and other professionals to friends and family members, to act differently around the patients or to avoid dealing with them in a natural way once they are diagnosed. Cognitive deficits, communication difficulties, and strange behaviors make most of us uncomfortable, and we may become angry, sad, and even frightened. These feelings color our abilities to see and react to the "humanity" of the patient. Many patients sense this and withdraw as a result.

It is important to identify and overcome false beliefs and fears about dementia in order to be able to meet the daily challenge of living with a victim of the disease. While Alzheimer's disease involves the slow, irrevocable loss of ability and ultimately even the sense of self, the stereotypical notion that victims of dementia lose overnight the ability to think, write, read, talk, work, or love is a tragic error. Changes do occur, but skills and abilities decline at different rates. In fact, some skills and feelings remain relatively preserved for many years. When changes do occur, they may require that we modify our behavior, but how we change and what we say and do can make the patient function better or worse.

The following letter illustrates how even the most loving care givers may lose their perspective in relation to the patient with dementia.

Dear Sis,

Mom has changed so much in the past several months. She sits in the house most of the day and cries a lot. She talks, or at least strings words together, but they seldom make sense. However, Dad seems to know what she is saying most of the time. I guess it comes from their fifty years together.

Dad would not use the words Alzheimer's disease in front of her. He also would not allow me to talk about Alzheimer's while I was visiting. However, she knows she has a problem. Several times during the day, usually at meals, she asks him, "What's wrong with me?" His reply is always the same: "Your memory is not what it used to be, dear. Don't worry." It took all my strength not to get angry with him. After all he is the one living with her and taking care of her all of the time.

Something happened, however, that convinced me that she understands more than he gives her credit for. Mom and I took a walk together around the orchard while Dad ran some errands. She seemed happy just to be with me. We walked for several hours. Once she stopped to look at a bed of wild flowers that grew by the old woodshed. I bent to pick a small bouquet for her, but she stopped me. I tried to explain that they would look lovely on the kitchen table. She became terribly upset: "Please, no . . . let them live. Don't . . . Cut flowers die slowly—like me."

Sis, I froze when she spoke those words. I looked into her eyes, and she —we—began to cry. We walked back to the house slowly, arm in arm. I knew we—Mom and I—had to have a long talk with Dad.

And talk we did. And for the first time I think they both were honest with each other about Mom's disease. Even though Mom said very little, I think she understood. She and Dad sat together on the couch after I went to bed.

In this letter Alan Hodges shares a story containing one of the most important lessons families must learn in order to cope successfully with the changes dementia imposes on them.

When loved ones have Alzheimer's disease, they are still members of the family, and, despite their dementia, they communicate a great deal about their personal needs and feelings. They do this by the way they act as well as by what they say. However, for them to be understood, those close to the patients need to be open to such communication and relate to the individuals both as patients with deficits and as persons with many human strengths. And who should be more capable of compassion, patience, and understanding than the family? However, the situation is complicated.

Care givers are often unaware of the patient's feelings. This is not because they do not care. Indeed, quite the opposite is true. Family members care so much that they have to develop psychological ways to cope with the intensity of their emotional pain. When they protect themselves from their own feelings, they often block their ability to accurately recognize the feelings of others.

What can the family do to cope successfully with the patient's emotional needs as well as their own? Fortunately, there are well-tested ways of dealing with such needs, and they are a key to living life to the fullest. The first of these techniques involves a reorganizing of family life in ways that make room for the patient. As was discussed in Chapter 4, one of the first goals after the diagnosis is not only to identify appropriate activities and design a structured program for the patient but also to determine what changes need to be made in the family lifestyle to accommodate the patient's needs. This type of planning is a simple and powerful way to reduce stress on the family.

Adjustments in response to the patient's losses do not come easily, even in the healthiest families, and a great deal of emotional energy is expended in dealing with the many changes. Different feelings surface—sadness, anger, guilt, death wishes—and people need to find ways to control them.

Barney Tate lived in a small rural town with his wife of twenty-three years, an Alzheimer's victim. Selma had fractured her hip in a car accident and was confined to a wheelchair. Barney took care of her with the help of their two sons, both of whom lived nearby with their families.

One winter night their younger son, Doug, sat with them by the fire. It was snowing too hard for them to drive home. Doug was a Vietnam War veteran, and he had just finished writing a novel about the war years. He decided to read several chapters to his mother and father. That night Selma sat quietly on the couch, content to be with her family. She insisted, though, that Doug sit by her side on the couch. She even held his arm while he read. It was unusual for Selma to be so attentive. She watched Doug carefully while he read about the night his best friend was killed and about his desire to die and end it all. When Doug finished reading, Selma took the book from his hand. She held it to her forehead and said, "Me too. I want to die."

After Selma fell asleep, Barney and Doug stayed up talking for several hours. For the first time they spoke openly about the awful feelings each had kept private. Both had secretly wished Selma were dead rather than live a meaningless existence. Hearing her death wish had stunned them. That night Selma had taught them a valuable lesson. Part of her was still very much alive, and she was still at the emotional center of the family. And they needed her to be part of the family. Before the Alzheimer's disease had been diagnosed, she had always been the person in the family who settled arguments and helped everyone get what he or she wanted. Strangely enough, through the expression of her own wish in spite of her dementia, Selma had forced her family to deal with their conflicts.

This chapter reviews a number of the more common problems which families may face and some of the techniques that can be useful in solving them. The problems fall into four major categories. The list is not all-inclusive but covers some of the troublesome issues which families and patients have to overcome: (1) cognitive deficits, (2) communication impairments, (3) behavior problems, and (4) maintaining relationships.

## Cognitive Deficits

Cognition refers not only to the ability to learn and remember. Broadly defined, it refers to perceiving, understanding, imagining, willing, thinking, and moving around intelligently in the environment. The mind of the Alzheimer's patient can be thought of as a cognitive sieve, in that various types of information are lost to the individual, who then has less and less capacity to act as an intelligent and accepted participant in the world. Following the diagnosis, families and professionals too often assume that the losses occur immediately and affect all aspects of behavior. Thus, they condemn the patient to a more helpless position than he or she deserves. It is important, therefore, to see that the individual's cognitive strengths and weaknesses are carefully evaluated and that a plan of action to complement them is formulated. Otherwise, chances are high that patients and families will be deprived of important opportunities to enjoy each other and find pleasure in life. One patient told his wife, "The question is not can I talk or think or reason. The question is whether I can suffer. And without you close to me, helping me, I would suffer."

It is important to understand the patients' individuality, even in later stages of dementia—their feelings, beliefs, desires, hopes, and plans. Likewise, it is necessary to provide opportunities for patients to express themselves. Their expressions may not be readily interpretable, but the simple act of setting aside a regular, quiet time for them to talk, however incomprehensible their remarks, seems to fulfill a human need to communicate with a loved one. By listening very carefully to the patients, we can sometimes piece together broken patterns of thoughts or themes to be communicated—pain or discomfort from heat or cold, anger, and hunger. If these feelings and thoughts are not communicated quietly in such a setting, they may be reflected in behavior which will certainly get the attention of care givers. Agitation, aggressiveness, and many troublesome behaviors seen in Alzheimer's victims are not always the result of brain destruction. They may evolve over time in individual patients whose needs are not understood by those around them.

Alison Barnes had been living in a nursing home for more than a year. She was forty-nine, legally blind, a widow, and a victim of Alzheimer's disease. The nursing staff had labeled her as a belligerent, unpleasant woman who was difficult to dress and get out of bed in the morning. Mrs. Barnes yelled at the aides and often struck them. She was frail and therefore unable to hurt people, unless she bit them, which had happened on at least two occasions.

A newly hired nurse's aide assigned to Mrs. Barnes was responsible for making an important discovery that changed the staff's attitude toward Mrs. Barnes. During her first week on the job, the aide would introduce herself by name and chat about the daily news or weather as she raised the blinds, arranged the breakfast tray, and straightened up magazines on the bed table. Then she would sit down close to Mrs. Barnes and ask her how she was feeling, whether she was ready to eat, or whether she wanted to freshen up before breakfast.

For the first two days Mrs. Barnes complained and yelled. However, on the third day she told the aide that she wanted to wash up before eating. After this was done, the aide and Mrs. Barnes talked while she ate her breakfast. Then Mrs. Barnes dressed herself with little assistance and asked to watch the morning news. As the aide prepared to leave, Mrs. Barnes took her hand and spoke slowly,

"Thank you for making me feel real again."

The rest of the staff took their cues from the aide and spent time talking with Mrs. Barnes and learning about her as the woman she once was. They learned to be gentle with her in the morning, talking with her and listening to what she needed to say. Her angry behavior toward the staff had developed out of her frustration and feelings of being ignored.

Although patients often lose their train of thought and are not able to carry out even simple tasks, they are conscious of many things about themselves and their world throughout much of the illness, and they react to changes in their environment. Unfortunately, their difficulty in expressing themselves, and particularly in modulating their feelings, too often isolates them from family and friends.

It is common for many patients in early or middle phases to be angry and privately yearn for a return to their former competence. Frustration mounts when individuals cannot find a way to overcome their losses. One man cried, "I can't live and I can't die. And no one understands how lonely my life is. . . ." Even in later stages patients can express a silent anger by the way they act. Another man, who had dementia for eight years, would walk to the window and raise his fist, almost in defiance, whenever he could not express himself.

Cognitive-training strategies may help improve communication between patients and family members. The results of cognitive testing should also provide a basis for family members to develop realistic expectations for a patient's performance and to find meaningful tasks, however simple, in the family. In order to develop any sort of cognitive-training program, a complete evaluation of cognitive skills is necessary, if available. This may be quite expensive. Is it worth spending hundreds of dollars for a clinical psychologist to do a complete interview and battery of tests? The answer is yes, if the psychologist can use the examination and test results to identify the practical implications of the patients' deficits and strengths. The psychologist can help you understand the patients' awareness of others, their ability to find their way in the home environment, their capacity to plan realistically for the future, to deal with financial matters, and to communicate effectively with the world around them. Knowledge about these and several areas of ability and weaknesses will help you to adjust your expectations for what patients can or cannot do. Patients are able to fill many roles in the family if activities are within their cognitive limits.

Many of the activities which family members report as happy, intimate moments are those when they are doing something together—playing with a child or a pet, sharing a meal, taking a walk, or sitting together reading, listening to music, watching television, or talking. Families successful in keeping the patient at the emotional center of the family are able to find a place or meaningful role for the "relative now patient." Jerome Gardner had cared for his wife, Sarah, for more than seven years after the diagnosis. Even as Sarah declined, Jerome continued to take her camping and fishing in the summer, and during the winter he kept her active in community and church activities:

Sarah is not the woman I married, but she needs me . . . and I still love her. There are times when we are together, and for a second I forget that she has Alzheimer's disease. Several times a week she washes my hair in the kitchen . . . the warm water, the massage, and the intimacy relax me. These are special times when I forget.

Finding appropriate activities beyond quiet intimate involvement is often a challenge, and this is where the results of cognitive testing are especially valuable. Accurate evaluations provide the framework for recommendations about life and work roles for the patient. The son of an Alzheimer's patient told us,

Mom has lived with us fifteen years since Dad died, and she had run the house, since my wife and I both work. Things have been rough since this Alzheimer's started. However, she is still able to do some of the weekly shopping. We try not to stress her. She gets enormous satisfaction if we let her walk to the 7-Eleven to buy a single item once or twice a day. She still feels that we need her.

Dementia can affect concentration, so that individuals stop in the middle of a task or lose track of their thoughts in mid-sentence. Because of these lapses in attention, we cannot depend on the patient to complete an assignment. When attentional and memory lapses occur together, it is difficult to trust the patient to do anything without supervision. But although deficits may make the successful completion of household chores like cooking, cleaning, and shopping impossible, patients often succeed in performing aspects of these tasks. And when they are so impaired that they cannot help, keeping them close by often gives them the security of being part of the hustle and bustle of family life. It is important not to block patients from emotional involvement, even when they are at a loss cognitively.

Social behaviors—the way we act around other people—usually remain fairly well preserved in most patients for long periods. Indeed, it is remarkable that, when losses in memory and attention disrupt many routine behaviors, individuals are still capable of behaving in a socially intelligent way. Many activities with other people remain pleasurable—going to concerts or art museums; sports like tennis, golf, bowling, and cycling; boating, camping, dancing, gardening, and walking. Many patients are so aware of their limitations that they monitor their behavior closely in public surroundings for fear of "giving themselves away." One woman remarked, "I enjoy going on television. My husband and I just tell the interviewers not to ask me hard questions, especially anything to do with numbers. If you ask me things I know—about the disease, ADRDA, my family—I can answer you."

Many steps can be taken to develop a cognitively stimulating and constructive situation at home. The following checklist should help guide family discussions:

1. If you live in a city with a major university or medical center with geriatric specialists, inquire about the existence of a memory clinic.
2. Make a list of all the hobbies and leisure activities which gave your relative pleasure before the diagnosis of Alzheimer's disease. Which ones can he or she still do alone and which of them require assistance? Which ones are dangerous? Is the relative still able to do things with his or her hands, and can someone help while the patient does the actual building, modeling, or planting?
3. List the household chores your relative did and reconsider the division of responsibilities. Investigate the availability of homemaker or chore-worker help when your relative lives alone or if you need assistance. Assign some tasks to the patient.
4. For as long as possible continue social activities which involve

you and the patient with other people—lunch or dinner with friends, picnics, clubs, bowling, golf, tennis, exercise classes, movies, theater, anything you all enjoy.

5. Find acceptable ways to involve the patient in new physical activities—jogging, cycling, or walking.

6. As the dementia progresses, find new ways for the patient to contribute to the household or family activities no matter how simple. Address questions to the patient. Feeling needed is a powerful emotional force.

7. Anticipate changes and discuss ways to deal with them in the future. What will happen when the patient cannot drive safely? (See the next section of this chapter.) What if some household help is necessary? If patients lose their bearings in the home or elsewhere, what should they do? When they have trouble finishing a sentence or forget a word, how might they ask for help?

8. Keep the patient active and mentally stimulated. Many patients still enjoy reading or being read to even though they may forget much of what they read. If the patient cannot read, records, tapes, and "talking books" are available. In many cases you may need to sit with the patient during these activities.

9. Take daily walks with the patient and, when possible, visit different places several times a week—a zoo, a museum, a park, a botanical garden, a shopping center—any place full of sights and sounds. Even when the patient is institutionalized or confined to a wheelchair, try to schedule trips or visits out of the home. Decorate the room with pictures or memorabilia to fit the individual's tastes.

10. When friends or relatives come, introduce them by name and give a clue to their identity. Alert the patient to visitors before they are to arrive; then, when they arrive, say, "Oh, here's your cousin Peter." This may make you uncomfortable at first, particularly when close friends or relatives are involved, but they will usually understand. And while the patient may seem irritated and say, "Of course, I know————," the tactic can be helpful. Frequently, relatives report that after a pleasant evening visit, patients will say something like "Who was that nice young man?" At this point a simple statement will suffice: "Oh, Mother, that was Joe, your favorite grandson."

No amount of cognitive retraining will replace skills and abilities affected by a "failing" brain. However, often unrecognized are those human attributes which make the individual very much a participant, albeit sometimes a passive one, in the family. The challenge is to interact as a family looking for opportunities to enhance the quality of life rather than deal with the patient as someone simply destined to suffer progressive loss and nonexistence. Patience and an awareness of what is lost and what may be corrected are called for.

## Communication Impairments

Patients are capable of higher-order thinking to varying degrees, depending on the individual and the progression of his or her illness. Whatever these abilities are, they are often eclipsed by clear and growing limitations as the dementia progresses. What becomes destructive to the patient's relationships with other people is the inability to articulate thoughts and feelings and to be understood by others. One of the important reasons to have complete psychological studies done early in the illness is to understand the patient's cognitive strengths as well as weaknesses and to develop ways to communicate effectively. These evaluations should be done at regular intervals throughout the course of the dementia to track changes in cognition and adjust communication strategies appropriately. For the family members a certain amount of trial and error will probably occur throughout the illness as they try to communicate.

Alzheimer's disease and other dementias often impair language and speech. However, a variety of other disorders also affect language and speech, as well as other abilities, and these impairments may be treated. More than half of the adults over the age of sixty-five without dementia are estimated to have communication impairments. Communication disorders, if left untreated, will significantly decrease the patients' quality of life as they struggle unsuccessfully to interact with family and friends. Listening, talking, and watching are the primary ways in which people maintain contact with their environment. Every effort should be made to diagnose specific hearing, speech, and language disorders and to treat them to the maximal extent.

Hearing aids and possibly even speech rehabilitation are important for the patient with dementia. Even in otherwise normal people hearing loss causes misunderstandings and arguments and leads to accusations of mumbling or forgetting. Therefore, when the patient has suffered some hearing loss, it can make the dementia seem far worse than it really is. Because the perception of high frequencies is often lost, particularly among older men, certain consonants, especially the silent ones, are not heard well. For example, "thin" may be heard as "sin" and "fat" as "hat." Indeed, entire sentences may be heard incorrectly as a result of hearing problems, but too often the consequent lack of understanding is mistakenly attributed to the dementia. A hearing aid, and in certain instances surgery, will not only improve the patient's understanding but also augment the entire family's enjoyment of one another.

Speech impairments like dysarthria and apraxia are common in dementia. Dysarthria may occur in people who have Alzheimer's disease and in those who have had a stroke. The term "dysarthria" refers to speech that is slurred, slow, and therefore distorted. It is the result of weakness in the nerves and muscles needed to produce speech sounds. Speech therapy can be helpful. The goal in the treatment of dysarthria is to increase the strength and coordination of the muscles used to produce speech.

Unlike persons with dysarthria, those with apraxia are able to produce speech sounds clearly. However, they often say a single sound or word over and over again. Although many are able to produce entire sentences, they speak slowly and with great difficulty. They substitute one sound for another or omit sounds. The speech muscles are not weak in persons with apraxia. The problem results from their inability to consciously use their muscles to make the right sound in a word at the correct time. In some cases speech therapy may be effective. The goal is to increase the individuals' conscious control as they initiate and organize their speech production. When speech becomes too impaired, some patients, depending on the severity of the dementia, may be able to communicate by writing or typing out their messages.

Language problems occur frequently. Patients may have difficulty understanding what certain words mean, or they may not be able to find the correct words to express a thought or identify an object or person. These impairments in language are known as aphasia. Persons with aphasia usually hear speech well but have difficulty finding the correct word for a person, object, or idea. They will speak a sentence smoothly but stop when they cannot remember the word they want to use. In many instances they cannot combine words in the correct order to make a sentence. Depending on the nature of the aphasia, the persons may be able to correctly describe or use the object without remembering its name. They can even make good associations. For example, individuals may lose the ability to say "key" but make motions of turning a key in a lock, or they may repeat "write" for pen and pencil.

Speech therapy has limited effectiveness when aphasia occurs in Alzheimer's disease or related disorders. The therapeutic goals are to help the patient learn cognitive strategies to use remaining language functions to compensate for their losses. It is often possible to teach the individual to ask for the word or to say, "I cannot remember the word I want," or use associated terms. Usually, the most effective technique is to make the patient comfortable in accepting help from others, who will often be able to supply the missing word or words which can be correctly identified by the patient.

Even when specific disorders are not present, patients change their styles of communication as the disease progresses. Although it may seem simplistic, it can be helpful to recognize at least two phases of expression during the course of the illness. The first is seen after the diagnosis is established. Many patients are capable of making themselves understood with a minimum of help. This phase may last for a long time; it is characterized by powerful emotions as well as the desire for active and truthful communication. During this phase the patient can often remain an active participant in family affairs.

During the middle and later stages of the disorder, communication becomes difficult, partly because the individual is less competent cognitively and verbally, and partly because many family members do not have a clear understanding of the patient's remaining strengths. Despite the cognitive impairment, there are strong needs for comfort, intimacy, and assurances of continued involvement. Families should be alert to the messages and to changes in style of communication. In the second phase there is less use of words and more of body language and behavior change to convey the needs of the patient. Verbal and nonverbal acts of care and concern by the family are essential, regardless of the level of dementia. Family members can best help by trying to provide the environment which offers the most comfort and warmth. This is not always easy. When patients lose verbal competence, families tend to talk about the patient less as a person and more as an object, even when patients are sitting in the same room. Professionals who talk to relatives about the patient in the patient's presence share this tendency. Patients should be acknowledged or involved in conversations when they are present. Many, even in severe phases of dementia, seem to understand what is said and may indeed react with signs of agitation and uneasiness.

Even in the later stages of the disease, many patients can convey important needs, and we should be able to deal realistically and supportively with their remarks and behaviors. By responding appropriately to a patient's remarks, families can be helpful both directly, in attempting to fulfill specific needs of the patient, and indirectly, by recognizing that the patient has something important to say. Although almost any topic is likely to surface, there are a number of common subjects. The following examples illustrate only a few of the major issues patients raise, and give general suggestions for how to respond to them.

## 1. "I wish my friends would still come to visit."

It is common for individuals with dementia to feel isolated from others, because they usually are. Many ask whether Alzheimer's disease is contagious, since their friends and relatives seem to shrink from them. Some form of replacement is helpful. Patients can be involved in many social settings, including activities with other patients and families at parties, picnics, and even group meetings. With time, activities with other patients and support groups can become important social events outside the family.

## 2. "I couldn't survive without my family."

Patients often find it easy to talk about their family. Talking with pride about loved ones is something that gives all of us pleasure. What patients really need is the opportunity to be part of their family, to listen, and occasionally to talk while others listen. Many patients have spoken about how lonely they are because they are cut off. They tend to become more dependent on their family and often value expressions of affection and respect as well as statements indicating that they are very much part of the family. They need this security.

### 3. "I want to keep fighting this thing as long as I can."

It is important not only to encourage patients to talk about this topic, which may be a reflection of their anger at having the disorder, but also to praise their courage. We all need encouragement and support from friends and loved ones for our labors, especially when times are difficult. The struggle for survival requires strong positive verbal reinforcement. Since dementia patients have so few rewards or acknowledgments of strength or accomplishment, the family should praise the patients whenever possible. However, this should be done appropriately and realistically, lest the praise become trivialized and lose its value. Praise does not require long or gushy statements. For some achievements this can even be hurtful to the patient. A simple "good" or "nice job" or even "thank you" conveys the message.

### 4. "I don't want help."

This is a very important message. It merits a response. Many older people find it very difficult to ask for help, let alone accept assistance for something as personal and seemingly childish to them as dressing, bathing, and toileting. Less personal tasks like driving a car safely, remembering a name, or shopping for groceries are but a few of the myriad familiar things we do throughout the day and take for granted. Yet, these are precisely the types of things basic to our ability to retain our self-esteem.

Dealing with the issue of "help" is often extremely difficult. In general, there are a few guidelines. Try to let the individuals do things for themselves. When support is needed, avoid using the word "help" as much as possible. Use whatever language is appropriate to communicate effectively, for example, "Let us do this together" or "Can I work with you on this one?" Emphasize that what was once second nature to them is being changed *by the disease*. Simplify the jobs to be done. Analyze whether certain tasks can be subdivided so that only a piece at a time need be done. Learn to accommodate to the short attention span and the memory deficits and to provide organizing cues in the environment. Color codes in the kitchen or bath may make it easier to identify where things belong. It may be helpful to organize the day so that the patient is expected to do the same thing at the same time every day. It often helps to let the patients perform a chore and then later, when they are absent, to complete it or correct mistakes.

## 5. "I know nothing can be done to help me."

Although this theme is expressed in many different ways, it is usually best accepted and not argued with. It is true that there are currently no cures for Alzheimer's disease, but a great deal can be done. However, little is gained by reasoning with the patients, for it often reinforces their dwelling on the negative side. The appropriate response to such comments is a positive statement about anything—the patients' courage, how much the family loves them, or even a comment about a child or grandchild's accomplishment. In essence, change the subject. Later, emphasize that a great deal can be done to help them live as normal a life as possible despite their limitations.

## 6. "I know I'm getting worse." Or "I want to know what will happen. Will I get worse?"

Sometimes it helps to quietly acknowledge that, yes, the patient will get worse, and then affectionately emphasize the importance of living "one day at a time" in the "here and now." Identify the patient's strengths and recent times of enjoyment. Be very specific about the joy of everyday life—food and eating, family outings, any and all activities meaningful to the patient.

Enrolling your relative in a self-help group with other patients can give him or her an important forum to deal with needs to both reject and accept the reality that the dementia will progress. Perhaps acceptance best evolves as we share our thoughts and fears with others who face the same future.

### 7. "I want to stay home as long as I can. I don't want to go into a nursing home."

Many patients say this to their families and others who are caring for them. Institutionalization is a complex issue. It fills some people with anxiety and fear, whereas others find the idea an acceptable and sometimes desirable alternative to a frightening life alone.

For some, talking about going "to a nursing home" is another way of expressing a fear of desertion, often coupled with the fear that this is the ultimate in surrendering to the disease. Going to such a place can be symbolic of giving up the fight to remain independent and an ongoing part of the family.

In order to handle this issue successfully, it is important to know what the statement means to the patient. Often a response like "Don't worry, we'll always care for you" or "We'll keep fighting this together" is the best approach. It probably is best to avoid any promises that you will "never, never, never" use a nursing home as an option, since this is likely to haunt you in the event that institutional placement becomes the best alternative. At such a time the patient may be compatible with the security of an institutional environment while you, as family care giver, are caught up in guilt and intrafamily conflict stemming from remarks made years before.

### 8. "Nothing is wrong with me."

Denial is a common reaction to a difficult reality. It is best not to confront patients, and argue that indeed they are impaired, when they say, "Nothing is wrong." Unless circumstances force the issue, let the patient talk, and gently change the subject, with a remark like "Let's take a walk." Bringing patients together in groups often helps us understand how to deal with their denial. An environment where patients find a "new family" of other people who are living with the same condition sometimes sets the stage for a careful and supportive confrontation with one's own losses. There is safety and solidarity in a group of patients who may not be able to state exactly what is on their minds but who by their presence, composure, or sheer energy speak of their strength to endure.

## 9. "I knew there was something wrong long before the doctors did."

Although some patients deny their illness, most do not. We do not give patients enough credit for the insights they develop into what is happening to them. It is important to give them the opportunity to tell their story. We all know that each of us needs to tell what we have done or what has happened to us. Again, the rule of thumb is to reinforce patients for what they can still do, to bring out the human gifts of hope and solace, and to strengthen the sense that they belong to the family, still have something to contribute, and are loved and valued for their own sake.

Other issues and questions will arise, and the general rule is to give simple and straightforward answers. Impart information when it is wanted and convey a sense of support, love, and commitment. The way we respond to each other's questions and carry on conversations is one of the major ways we create the fabric of human relationships and the home atmosphere. Talking effectively with patients often requires great patience and endurance. One wife commented, "Some days it's like trying to speak Virgil to their Dante. There are also times when we can communicate." It is important to develop confidence in knowing when to respond to the patient's words and when simply to listen, and by doing so convey the love and support we all need.

### How to Handle Disturbing Behavior

Some, but not all, victims of dementia behave in ways that are disruptive and disturbing to those around them. In many instances, the destruction of the brain is causing changes in eating and sleeping patterns, less control of bodily functions, or outbursts of emotions —love, hate, anger, jealousy. Some patients display inappropriate sexual behavior, wander away and get lost, or behave in ways that are improper or offensive without knowing what they are doing.

Whereas some patients become quiet and withdraw from their usual sphere of activities, others become restless and agitated, often pacing relentlessly around the house. Hostility and aggressive behavior become common. Anger is a normal emotion to express in situations in which people or events threaten to harm you and those you love. Patients may experience the same anger we all do when we feel threatened or insulted, but the way they express it may be exaggerated or inappropriate.

One of the most common situations which provoke angry encounters occurs when families stop the patient from driving. The ability to drive requires skills which can become impaired as the dementia progresses. Driving demands sharp hearing and vision, memory for locations, good judgment, quick reaction time, and effective motor skills. Since Alzheimer's disease often impairs individuals' ability to comprehend the full extent of their losses, patients argue that they are competent to drive, and violent arguments erupt when they are challenged. Giving up the car keys is for some a major loss; driving represents freedom to many individuals. Some depend on a car to go virtually anywhere. After a diagnosis of Alzheimer's disease, it is one of the first activities to be questioned, because it affects the safety of others. The more likely an event is to affect other people, the more likely it is to be a focus of concern.

How do you know when it is unsafe for the patient to drive? This is a matter of judgment. There are psychological tests that determine whether an individual has the coordination and other perceptual and memory skills necessary to drive an automobile safely. Having a professional explain the results of the test to you and your relative is an important first step. Your relative may not like what is said, or may not understand, but has at least been involved in the process of making a difficult decision. Give the patient the benefit of the doubt about what he or she can understand.

What happens in the doctor's office and what happens at home are often quite different things. Patients may concede in the office that driving is dangerous. However, at home they may insist on driving, angrily reject any explanation, and often explode in a violent rage over control of the car keys. One woman told us, "Jack wanted the keys, but I refused to give them to him. He grabbed them from me but held my arm tightly. I was terrified. His eyes were filled with such hate. I never saw such hate. Jack was always such a gentle man. He never even raised his voice to me in all the years we were married."

It is important to remember that you are not talking with a rational person about the right to drive, and that arguing only makes the situation worse. Once you make the decision, be firm. Hiding the car keys is probably the most common technique for dealing with the issue of driving. This ploy works well until someone gets into the car with the patient, who then insists on driving. During the period when driving is an upsetting issue—it will fade with time—it may be helpful to have the patient sit in the backseat with someone else to provide distraction. Refusing to drive with the patient if he or she had the keys and insisting on driving control can help, as can the programming of trips when the patient is taking a nap or otherwise distracted.

If driving is dangerous, ask your doctor to write a letter with you to the department of motor vehicles and request that the patient's driver's license be revoked. Involve the patient in discussions about the revocation. As difficult as it may be, give the issue some time to play out. It is painful for patients to accept the multiple losses that come with dementia, and it is legitimate for them to feel anger, bordering on rage. So much is being taken from them. Patients deserves some time and support to work the anger out of their system. Since they may already have problems in expressing themselves, it is often difficult for the family to know how to help the patient. However, most family members do exactly what must be done without really being aware of it. The love and devotion of a caring family often enable it to endure the greatest hardships, with no professional around to tell them what a great job they are doing.

Although the range of disturbing behavioral problems is broad, it is a good idea to learn a few general rules to guide your reactions. As with the problem of driving, these rules involve diverting or distracting the patient, rewarding desirable behaviors, ignoring undesirable behaviors, blowing off steam away from the patient, and using specific techniques to control the environment. Finally, it is important to have a fall-back position for emergencies . . . when individuals may be harmful to themselves or others. If your relative becomes violent, protect yourself. Repeated violent episodes may be grounds for a serious reevaluation of your decision to keep a loved one at home.

DIVERSION

Diversion is often an effective and relatively easy way to eliminate disruptive behaviors, particularly when this involves arguments or an outburst about the car, about leaving the house, or about who you are or the identity of others. Patients with dementia have a relatively short attention span and, as a rule, can be moved to focus on something else without great difficulty. Judy McCormick, the wife of an Alzheimer's victim, was able to calm her husband by saying, "Let's have a cup of coffee, and I'll massage your back." This would often break her husband's angry mood. Care givers will learn rapidly what diversions work best, and they should share this information with others who spend time with the patient.

It is often difficult for care givers to remember to distract the patient. It takes conscious self-discipline and practice to learn to control the natural inclination to argue or try to reckon with him or her. The patient does not look impaired and thus often triggers natural responses which are appropriate for a cognitively intact individual. It is a normal part of daily life to ask questions or have disagreements with others. However, many patients have cognitive deficits that preclude having a rational discussion. They may forget immediately or not comprehend what is said. Some patients have a deficit called perserveration, which means that they dwell on the same ideas, words, movements, or thoughts. Thus, they may continue to ask the same question over and over. This can drive care givers to the limits of frustration if they do not know how to respond appropriately, by distracting the patient with another topic.

## REWARDING DESIRABLE BEHAVIORS AND IGNORING UNDESIRABLE ONES

Praising the patient for successes, spending quiet times together, touching, a hug, or a kiss all give the same message—"I like you. I enjoy your company." It is important to convey warmth and affection. We are, all of us, social beings, and we get satisfaction out of making those close to us happy. For the patients who have so much less to give, the message that they are still giving happiness is a powerful one.

One of our most difficult challenges is the control of our own spontaneous reactions to someone who upsets us. Anger, shouting, or striking out physically are all common responses. What is so difficult to understand is that these reactions often only serve to perpetuate the very behavior we want to eliminate. Years of study have led psychologists to the conclusion that by and large—unless there is some danger involved—ignoring the behavior you want stopped is far more effective than reacting to it. People appreciate any reaction from others. A positive reaction is best, a negative reaction second best, but even second best is more desirable than being ignored. Behavior which is ignored often stops. A technique called operant conditioning systematizes this approach to the changing of specific behaviors. The application of this technique is discussed in the next section.

When patients become repeatedly upset over the same issue, the care giver can often devise an indirect way of calming their underlying fears or frustrations. Olin Wilson dreaded going to bed with his wife. Mona would be fine until he tried to get into the double bed they had shared over three decades. Then she would shout that he was invading her bed. She didn't know who he was and threatened to call the police if he didn't leave. He showed her his driver's license and pictures of their children, to no avail. This happened several times, and Olin became more and more agitated, with the result that Mona grew frightened and even more agitated herself.

Olin finally learned to prevent the situation in an imaginative way. For a few nights he waited for her to calm down and go to sleep before he joined her. A few days later he took out their album of wedding photographs, and he and Mona looked through it before they went to bed. This was a close and quiet time together, and Mona seemed very calm and happy to share her bed with her newly rediscovered husband.

It is common for patients to become angry and frustrated when they are unable to do or say something. Furthermore, they often fear their families will abandon them because they cannot function well. One patient described her situation this way: "I worry that Richard will leave me because I am not perfect anymore. I used to do everything, and now I am no good." Unfortunately, many care givers have not learned how to deal with the patient's fears and anger in a helpful way. In the early stages of dementia it is important to talk with the patient and find ways to work together to compensate for losses. Often it is useful for care givers to convey the message that they accept the losses and still care for and love the patient.

Hans Dyson, whose wife had been diagnosed with dementia for six months, commented,

In the beginning Madge and I were both terribly upset. When she would stop in the middle of a sentence, I tried to help her by supplying the words. She would cry, turn away, or storm out of the room. Madge had always been such a self-sufficient individual. With this Alzheimer's disease she needed help, but she simply could not accept help, even from those she loved.

One morning I found her sitting at the kitchen table crying. There was orange juice in the cereal bowl instead of milk. I placed my arms around her and held her in a long embrace. I told her I needed her more than ever. This Alzheimer's disease did not make me love her less.

### WAYS TO CHANGE BEHAVIOR: OPERANT CONDITIONING

A psychologist or psychiatrist can sometimes help manage patients' incontinence, develop their ability to dress themselves, exercise, and eat properly, and reduce or eliminate their shrieking and screaming. Patients' behavior can be changed by means of the technique of operant conditioning, a type of learning first described by B. F. Skinner. It refers to a strategy in which rewards are given only when the individual performs specific desirable behaviors to increase the likelihood that such behaviors will occur and that undesirable behaviors will stop. For effective operant conditioning the following principle must be obeyed: Ignore undesirable behaviors and pay attention to desirable ones. Attempting to calm patients and paying attention to them when they are behaving inappropriately is "rewarding" their behavior. A smile, a touch, a conversation, or attention should only be given during a period of desirable activity as clear "rewards." As difficult as it may be, leave the room when the patient is behaving inappropriately—is, for example, yelling, throwing food, or cursing.

Rewards or reinforcers do not have to be given to the patient in the form of the care giver's attention or such items as candy, food, and drink or money. The patient's own behavior can be used to change behavior. For example, Jackie Needham, aged eighty, lived in a nursing home but refused to attend any therapeutic or recreational activities. Under the supervision of a psychologist, the nurses observed that she spent several hours of her waking time obsessively cleaning the furniture in her room. Most of her time was spent sitting mutely by the window; none of it was spent with other people or in any ward activities. A special program was designed. Mrs. Needham was allowed to sit by the window only if she attended an exercise class for five minutes in the morning. Over several weeks she began to spend more time in the exercise class and to attend other activities.

Another important example of a positive-reward strategy is "milieu therapy." Milieu programs can be very successful in long-term-care settings. They involve the redesign of the institutional environment, or "milieu," to make it more compatible with the functional abilities of the patient with dementia. Rewards are given to individuals for taking part in specific activities like recreation, maintaining good personal hygiene, exercise, or attendance at group meetings. Establishing a "happy hour" with small glasses of beer, wine, or cider before the dinner hour attracts patients, even dementia patients. One nurse described the changes that took place on her ward: "I could not believe some of the changes. Even Charlie, who has been here for four years and seemed so out of it, began to dress up at four-thirty. He would put on his Sunday sweater and wander into the dayroom at four to wait. I didn't think he could do anything!"

Operant therapies can successfully change behaviors leading to self-injury. These include such actions as the failure to eat or dress and the ingestion of nonfood objects. For example, it was possible to change Adam Thatcher's behavior of refusing to wear clothing by the use of beer as the reinforcer. Mr. Thatcher was given small glasses of beer for wearing additional pieces of clothing for longer periods of time. Eventually, he would stay dressed all day if he had one beer at lunch and one at dinner instead of being given several ounces after staying dressed for a period of time.

Methods of bowel and bladder training have been applied to incontinent patients with mixed success. Incontinence is a multifaceted problem. Operant techniques are particularly effective when incontinence is an "attention-getting" behavior. However, the monitoring of urinary tract infections and drugs prescribed for delirium and the teaching and simplifying of bathroom behaviors must be combined with operant techniques. A watchful eye on the patient will alert the care giver to indications that signal a need to use the bathroom. Being responsive to nonverbal cues often teaches patients to express their need for help instead of urinating or defecating on the spot. The simple act of allowing people to select and buy their own pajamas has been known to reduce incontinence significantly.

It is not always easy to implement contingency-therapy plans, since it often takes time to "extinguish" or eliminate inappropriate and undesirable behavior. These strategies take professional help and time, but they do work.

### PSYCHOSOCIAL THERAPIES

The capacity for changing behavior in patients with dementia depends on many factors—the degree of cognitive loss, personality traits, motivation to perform, and the ability to communicate. When attentional skills are present and reasonably intact in dementia patients during the early and middle stages of the disease, they can be appropriate candidates for certain therapeutic approaches.

Supportive psychotherapy and counseling can be effective for many patients in the earlier phases. More and more clinicians are being trained to deal with the problems these patients endure, including that of adjustment to change and loss. Without appropriate intervention a patient's feelings of dependency and helplessness can hasten the impairment process. Unrecognized and untreated emotional distress can also exacerbate the degree of impairment, even in the patient with serious cognitive difficulties.

Group psychotherapy can also be effective. Groups of patients or patients and family members can successfully confront a range of problems and even help increase the disoriented individual's sense of control over the environment. Groups also seem to facilitate such goals as remotivation, resocialization, and increased activities.

### ENVIRONMENTAL STRATEGIES

Impaired patients are usually capable of handling a number of changes in their environment if they have some choice or control in those changes. Change, especially a change in residence, often causes a stress reaction, but knowledge and a perception of some control over change decreases the amount of stress an impaired patient feels.

Old age for a dementia victim is a period of special vulnerability to a loss of control over the environment. This sense of helplessness has even been implicated in the death of people at home or in nursing homes. One important effect of the operant-conditioning programs discussed earlier is that they not only shape patients' behavior using a system of reinforcements but also give them greater control over what is going to happen to them. This feeling of mastery is itself a very important reward.

A number of therapeutic strategies can be used with the help of professionals to enable patients to cope as successfully as possible. It is important to shape the physical and social environment to support the patient's strengths and to minimize frustrating situations. This means doing such things as simplifying the daily schedule and providing activities consistent with the patient's memory and learning deficits, sensory acuity, and mobility. It is important to deal clearly and directly with those actions that the patient is simply not able to perform. Care givers should express understanding and indicate that these actions are not important. Support for new activities to replace those no longer possible should be expressed.

It is important to work closely with patients not only to determine which actions they can still perform but also to change their expectations of perceived helplessness. Patients can often be trained to use their skills to bring the environment under their control.

Helping impaired patients also requires an understanding of the attributions they make for their failures. Attributions are what individuals identify as the cause of their misfortune. It is important to talk with patients to learn whether they truly understand that they have a brain disease which affects their behavior. If they have unrealistic perceptions about their illness or unrealistic expectations of themselves, these thoughts and feelings neet to be discussed whenever possible.

This brings us to the crucial factor that guides all psychological interventions. There must be an orientation to the individual as a *person*, not as a patient. Only with this respect for an individual with a past and a future will it be possible to maximize the quality of life. Whatever the level of their competence, persons with dementia will respond if they are treated as human beings who are enabled to play an active role in their own care as long as possible.

It is important for care givers to have a well-thought-out fall-back position when emergencies do occur. Is there a physician who can help calm the patient? Can neighbors be available to come if the patient gets violent or tries to run away? Is a son or daughter or his or her spouse available to help? When should you call the police or sheriff? The circumstances will vary, but these emergency measures should be examined and realistically checked out. Knowing what to do in an emergency can help reduce your panic should such an emergency occur; in fact, knowing what to do may enable care givers to solve the problem. Many families have said that just knowing that someone out there was ready to help meant so much to them that they solved the problem themselves. This sort of preparation even has the effect of helping with the decision to keep someone out of a nursing home.

## Maintaining Relationships

Alzheimer's disease challenges the intimate bonds between two human beings. For husbands and wives, though, the love may deepen. A special grace and beauty mark those who have learned to live with the disease and continue to find ways to enjoy each other. For most couples intimacy changes, and, in general, the length of the marriage and the quality of the relationship before the diagnosis say a great deal about how well a couple will deal with the serious challenges of Alzheimer's disease. Long-standing marriages do not suddenly collapse even as the dementia takes its course. Recent marriages, particularly second or third marriages, are more vulnerable and may dissolve if the healthy spouse has not developed a loyalty and commitment toward the patient.

The intimacy of most family relationships is likely to change. Any relative—brother, sister, in-law, daughter, son, grandchild, cousin, or parent—involved with the patient must live with a series of emotional reactions. This reality spreads to other relationships between family members. A daughter or son caring for a mother or father may find that these activities strain the relationship with her or his husband, wife, and children, who come to resent the lack of attention and affection paid to them.

The nature of the relationship with people outside the family is altered. Friendships wither from lack of time given to maintaining them and often disappear. These losses are among the most difficult for the patient and caring family to accept.

Any caring relationship between persons in or out of a marriage is supported by a history of respect, devotion, and commitment to the well-being of one another. Because marriage embodies the most tender bonds of endearment, over time it forges a strong loyalty between people. The shadow of Alzheimer's disease changes the outlook of a couple's retirement years together, but it also provides opportunities for the dearest expressions of love. It hastens, too, what must sooner or later occur in all human relationships—separation and death. Husbands and wives and often other members of the family must work to enjoy each other; in doing so, they will help overcome some of the tragedy of the dementia.

HUSBAND AND WIFE—TILL DEATH DO US PART

Many husbands and wives find the diagnosis a difficult one to accept. For some it becomes a burden of guilt: "I must deserve this for all the bad things I have done." Others see it as a challenge: "We had such a wonderful life together that I should be able to deal with this." For others there is outrage and shock: "Life is cruel. Why did such a wonderful man like my husband get this?"

How do you love someone who begins to change dramatically in front of your eyes and is no longer the person you married? Many family members say that the question never occurs to them and that years of living together have brought them close enough to each other that they can adapt. However, even in the strongest relationships the strain of caring can be significant, especially when opportunities for intimacy are diminished or bizarre behavior is prominent. Many patients may eventually make inappropriate sexual overtures to their spouse, other family members, or friends. One husband exclaimed, "I was shocked. My wife sat out in the lawn chair by the pool—stark naked reading a book!"

Sexuality is an important part of relating to a husband, a wife, or an appropriate partner. Sexuality also has an important impact on the way people feel about themselves. There are many ways to give and receive sexual pleasure, and some couples are able to adjust extremely well to changes in their sexual relationship. They have learned how to engage in a variety of satisfying sexual activities.

Living with Alzheimer's disease challenges the patient and sexual partner to live joyously with one another. Many issues are raised here to help family members at least be able to understand the changing sexuality of the dementia patient and the changes in their personal relationships with the patient. Most of the time sexual difficulties are ignored or not dealt with, because neither partner is comfortable discussing them.

Couples living with Alzheimer's disease face some complex pressures with regard to sexual activity. Unfortunately, most patients and their partners are uncomfortable talking about sex even when they are confronted with a problem. Many individuals are not even comfortable thinking about these issues. They may feel frustrated and upset either because they do not understand what they feel or because they are afraid to talk about their sexual and intimate lives.

Sexual problems should also be reviewed with a doctor or knowledgeable health professional. Although this is a sensitive issue, professionals may help enormously to understand the cause of sexual problems and resolving them. Many such difficulties can be treated successfully. Unfortunately, many physicians neglect to ask questions about sexual problems. Although you may be ill at ease, you should take the lead in bringing these issues up when they are a problem. Once you have begun to talk, the discomfort will often disappear. The cooperation of three people—husband, wife, and professional—is often needed to resolve sexual problems. Sometimes the attitudes and beliefs of an entire family need to be confronted.

Joe Tobias was sixty-seven years old, and he had been diagnosed as having Alzheimer's disease approximately six and one half years earlier. His wife of forty-one years had died on his sixtieth birthday, and within the year he was married again. Six months after his second marriage Joe was diagnosed, and within another six months his second wife had left him. She was unable to cope with the changes in his behavior and the grim future facing the two of them.

Joe's children, five sons and two daughters, formed a close-knit family, and everyone, including their wives, husbands, and children, united to do everything possible to keep Joe at home and happy. And they were able to satisfy all of Joe's needs, save one—his need for a sexual partner.

Furthermore, his sexual needs became an embarrassing problem. Each of the women in the family felt uncomfortable around Joe because of the way he stared at them, obviously fixating on their breasts or legs. Although he never harmed anyone, it was not unusual for him to reach over and fondle someone's arm, hand, neck, shoulder, or other part of the body inappropriately.

The incident that galvanized the family occurred one day when the youngest son stopped at his father's house after lunch and found Joe in bed with a young woman who was a waitress at a local restaurant. A family meeting was called that night (without Joe present), and the consensus was that Dad had to be seen by a doctor who would treat his voracious sexual hunger.

The eldest son, Jason, was elected to escort his father to the doctor. Without referring to the incident, Jason insisted that his father keep an appointment with a "specialist." The doctor told Joe that sexual urges were not normal in a man his age and that, fortunately, treatment was available to cure him. The prescription was for a vitamin E shot once every two to three weeks. The family ushered Joe to the doctor religiously. However, his behavior did not change. Joe would sit in the park and watch the girls, sometimes approaching one of them and asking her to have coffee or lunch with him. And, as the family later discovered, he had been having relations with the housekeeper on a daily basis.

Finally, out of frustration the family sent Joe to visit his youngest daughter, Joanne, who lived in another state. The family members had conferred with each other (including Joanne) and had unanimously decided that it was her turn to take care of her father. Within a week trouble began because Joanne's roommate, a young female artist, was afraid to be around Joe. Even Joanne became alarmed by his "unfatherly hugs and kisses." However, Joanne found professional help.

In the very first meeting, which lasted several hours, Joe described as best he could the distress he felt over his sexual urges. He was aware that his behavior was inappropriate, and he was also aware that his need for sexual relief was powerful. The doctor who ordered regular shots had clearly declared his sexual needs to be abnormal, but Joe was confused. The nurse who gave him the injections was beautiful, and he got an erection every time he received a treatment. Furthermore, although the nurse was aware of his reaction, she did not get angry or indeed say a single word to acknowledge what happened. Once Joe even asked her whether she though that it was abnormal for a man his age to feel romantic and have a relationship with a woman. Her polite answer of "no" made him feel good, but he still remained confused and concerned.

Having received assurances that sexual urges were indeed normal, Mr. Tobias seemed greatly relieved. In fact, he then volunteered that he felt that his behavior toward women was not always appropriate. He very much wanted to talk with someone about what he perceived to be a serious problem—but one that he hoped could be solved.

He had been happily married to a woman who was the center of his life spiritually and sexually. As long as they had been together, they had intercourse at least once or twice a day. One of the reasons he had married so soon after his wife's death was the need to have the intimacy he craved. When his second wife left him, he had clearly lost a socially acceptable partner in his small town. Furthermore, Janice, his second wife, had not deserted him without trying to make the marriage work. She tried hard, and after several sessions with the minister and Joe, the decision she had to make became clear.

Joe's children clearly loved him, but they also made his life difficult. With all of them "caring" for him, he had absolutely no privacy. He felt guilty about having women in his home. He did not want to embarrass his children or make them ashamed of his behavior. But how could he live his life and have the happiness and satisfaction he wanted.

The solution to Mr. Tobias's living situation required the sensitive involvement of the entire family. Many meetings were held to help all of its members identify and understand what their father's needs were relative to their own. It was hard work for everyone. Although his sons and daughters were upset about his sexual needs and behavior, they became more relaxed as they listened to an outsider help them understand how their attitudes and needs had interfered with their father's needs.

With time it was possible to work out an acceptable solution to Mr. Tobias's dilemma. The family members were able to accept the reality that their father wanted and needed a partner. As it became apparent that Mr. Tobias had an affectionate and fulfilling relationship with the housekeeper, the family found the affair acceptable. Mr. Tobias lived another seven years surrounded by his family and the housekeeper-lover, who cared for him until he died.

There exists an extremely sensitive area where husbands and wives report deep feelings of conflict. After a loved one is institutionalized, many individuals describe how their needs for friendships and companionship with the opposite sex cause personal and family distress. Many people are ashamed or embarrassed to be seen together with someone at a restaurant, the theater, a movie, or even on the street for fear of giving rise to hurtful rumors. There is often enormous anxiety about having meaningful affairs or longer-term relationships with a boyfriend or a girlfriend.

Leonard Alexander disclosed his feelings in a group meeting and received support for his desire to ask a friend to spend a weekend with him.

MR. A.:    I love my wife, and she has been the emotional center of my life for thirty years. Nothing will change that. My feelings towards my wife have even intensified in a spiritual sort of way. But I have had to admit to myself that I am interested in women now much more than I used to be.

MRS. J.:   Explain that, will you?

MR. A.:    I was talking to Judy about all the nice women she has introduced me to. When she comes out to the nursing home to visit her husband, she usually brings a friend. It's quite a treat. So when I told her I had an idea about seeing a woman, she encouraged me. I have a friend my age whom I've known for a long time. She was widowed about a year ago, and I thought I would like to invite her for a trip to the islands for a week.

Judy thought it was a great thing to do and encouraged me to ask her. "Lay out the ground rules, split the expenses, and give her a private bedroom. Bring a good book, in case you turn her off that first day, and let things develop slowly."

And frankly, if all I get is some decent companionship, that's fine. But if she wants to seduce me, I don't think I'll protest.

I phoned her up, and she was shocked. But she didn't turn me down. She said she would think about it. I told her to take plenty of time, but if she turned me down, she should have some very good reasons why my proposal was not suitable. So it's going to be rather interesting now to see what she comes out with. I hope it's maybe. I don't want it to be no, but if it's no, that's fine. But you know something—I don't give a damn whether it happens or not now—I feel so good about having asked her. I feel alive again knowing that I can plan a little bit in the future. There were some very hard times when I didn't think I could plan anything. Now I feel that I've ventured a little bit. Yet I haven't abandoned my responsibility or my wife, who, incidentally, I'm probably closer to now than I've ever been before, in a strange sort of way.

I'm starting to take care of my own needs. I feel pretty good about everything.

Someone you trust, whether a family member or a confidant, is often extremely valuable to help you evaluate options in difficult life decisions. There are no easy or right answers, and sometimes the answers are very private. Mr. Alexander did plan the trip with his friend, but he had to postpone the trip a month because he came down with the flu. The illness was fortunate because Mrs. Alexander died the weekend her husband was originally scheduled to be away on his trip.

For many people another relationship outside the marriage is neither a desirable nor an acceptable alternative. Lois Barclay Murphy wrote the moving book *The Home Hospital,* which is not only a practical guide to coping with catastrophic illness in a loved one but also the profound love story of her relationship with her husband, Gardner Murphy, who had Parkinson's disease. The two were devoted to each other, and their ability to sustain and nurture one another is a testament to the human spirit and the bond of love which transcends sexuality. Louis Murphy spoke lovingly of their intimate moments together. They lost no opportunity to hug, kiss, or hold each other, even when Gardner was bedridden and nurses were present. Simply holding hands and being close enough to exchange glances carried the strongest message of love and devotion.

A lifetime of emotional investment between husband and wife often cultivates a depth and style of communication which cannot be undone by Alzheimer's disease. The intensity of the human bond is heightened as couples struggle to live together and care for one another.

Lupe Juarez had been diagnosed as having Alzheimer's disease for eight years. Her husband, Mario, had retired two years before his wife began having noticeable problems. Both Mario and Lupe found great pleasure simply being together, as they had for the past fifty-five years. Most of their time was spent at home, in the garden, shopping, visiting children and grandchildren. During the summer they took to the road in their camper—traveling to new places, fishing, camping, and walking together. The winters were harsh, so they stayed home, quite happy to be together. Meals, family visits, music, and reading were the highlights of the winter days.

Even as Lupe deteriorated, Mario continued to read to her—the paper in the morning at breakfast and novels at night after dinner. Although she could not discuss people, events, or issues as the dementia robbed her of speech, memory, and judgment, she sat next to him on the couch, hand on his knee, listening or perhaps only staring into space. No one knew how much she absorbed, but it was clear that a deep love bound them together.

Mr. Juarez managed well until about two years before his wife's death. His children noticed that he was being more irritable and that he was spending more time at the local tavern. The oldest son called for help, and a meeting with us was arranged. During the interview Mr. Juarez sighed and offered some critical information:

I love my wife more than life itself. It hurts so much to see her wither away. She is like a burning candle which keeps sputtering. I am afraid of the day the flame dies. She and I have been able to help each other live with this thing. But I am getting tired. She is changing a great deal now and is a shell of the person I married. She is becoming a stranger to me even though I know she is my wife, and, strange as it may seem, I love her more than ever.

Now I have to do everything for her. I just wish there was some little thing she could do for me so I would know that the old Lupe is still there. It would help me go on. Please forgive me. It may sound stupid and selfish, but I even miss her washing my hair in the evenings. She gave a wonderful hair massage, and it helped me relax at the end of a long day.

We then met alone with Mr. and Mrs. Juarez and reviewed with them what they planned to do for the next three months. They held hands as Mr. Juarez spoke openly about his drinking. He enjoyed having a few beers in the tavern with his friends. It was a habit of fifty years. We discussed what might be the cause of his excessive drinking, and he began to express his frustrations. He was angry seeing his wife deteriorate. He was also frustrated sexually. Sometimes at night he would make romantic overtures when the time seemed right and she was willing. However, in the middle of foreplay she would change from a responsive woman to a giggling child. Dealing with these abrupt changes was impossible. His wife was still beautiful and attractive in his eyes, but the "child" in bed was someone else. It broke his heart and made him angry beyond words.

The plan we evolved took patience and personal, careful discussions. Mr. Juarez himself suggested that perhaps they should now sleep in separate beds, which would still be kept close together. It was probably not appropriate, at least in this case, to initiate sex with his wife. It took a long time for Mr. Juarez to digest the reality that the Alzheimer's disease was affecting the part of his wife's brain that helped control sexuality and pleasure. He understood this reality intellectually, but emotionally it was difficult to deal with.

We were lucky enough to find something that Lupe could still do for her husband. We encouraged him to reinstate an old tradition —to let his wife wash his hair in the sink several evenings each week. We also suggested that they continue another family tradition—to visit the town diner each Saturday and Sunday morning for breakfast. This was an opportunity to be together and visit other people as they had for so many years.

The strategy was successful. It was a shot in the arm for Mr. Juarez. Hair washing and breakfasts out captured the old intimacy and gave him the emotional strength to continue. Mrs. Juarez died several years later, at home, surrounded by her family and friends. Mr. Juarez never remarried. However, he did have a close woman friend, who had also been close to Lupe. They met several times a week in the diner for breakfast, lunch, or dinner. And together with others friends they took day trips around the area.

After Mr. Juarez died, the children found an attic full of letters as they sorted through their parents' belongings. There were many packages of love letters Mario and Lupe had written to each other. The children were surprised at the sheer volume of letters, because their parents had been separated only during World War II, and the correspondence spanned a lifetime together. Through these letters the children came to appreciate even more what a special partnership their parents had enjoyed.

The memory losses in dementia may, however, weaken the bond between two people. The relationship of marriage partners is a complex one. It is sustained by how events were experienced and resolved in the past, by the sense of perceived loyalty and responsibility, by the degree of emotional (and sometimes financial) investment each holds in the other, and by factors outside the relationship. For example, children, family position, or other social and cultural factors affect the way a couple deal with one another over time. Since Alzheimer's disease is one of the most complex challenges an individual will ever face, it would not do justice to the intricacy of human relationships and experience to try to give simple and easy prescriptions for right and wrong behavior.

SEXUAL DIFFICULTIES IN ALZHEIMER'S DISEASE

Sexual functioning in individuals with Alzheimer's disease and related disorders may be influenced by the physical and emotional effects of the disease. However, there has been little research in this area. Many Alzheimer's patients have difficulty achieving an erection and complain of a loss of potency. Women often report a loss of interest and the inability to achieve organism. Sexual functioning is a major area of concern not only for patients but for their partners as well.

It is important to remember that sexual dysfunction is not unique to patients with Alzheimer's disease. Many happily married people have difficulties at some point in their lives together. In many ways the problems of Alzheimer's patients are not different from those of any other human beings who enjoy physical pleasure, the intimacy of another human being, and the success of giving pleasure to another person. Physical illness, medications, depression, feelings of inadequacy, and many other factors can interfere with sexual prowess and satisfaction. In most instances the condition can be corrected. Since Alzheimer's disease entails the loss of cells in the central nervous system, many parts of the sexual response may be affected. However, many of its victims have been able to overcome their sexual difficulties.

Sexual difficulties in Alzheimer's disease can be divided into five major groups: (1) those resulting from destruction of the brain; (2) those caused by physical illnesses; (3) those that are side effects of medication; (4) those caused by psychological conflicts; and (5) those caused by social pressures and attitudes.

Alzheimer's disease may affect the individual's ability to become aroused sexually. Loss of sexual interest is not the only by-product of Alzheimer's. Increased sexual activity may occur. This hypersexuality may be noticed in many ways, including the heightened desire for sexual intercourse, obvious fondling of one's genitals, masturbation in public or private, and attempts to seduce others.

The short attention span characteristic of the disease also plays a role in sexual activity. Arousal may be short-lived and create frustration in the partner. Childish behavior may emerge, leading to anger and irritability in a spouse who sees the patient as physically intact and, in may instances, no less attractive.

The crucial step is to determine to what extent sexual difficulties are the result of structural change in the nervous system or the consequence of psychological factors like anxiety or clinical depression. Several issues are important here. Individuals must be aware of changes in their own body and be able to share this information with their partner. It is also important for partners to tell each other what they do and do not find pleasurable. However, the Alzheimer's disease often makes this difficult in later stages or when the dementia is more severe. When the impairment is neurological, several devices may be useful to the male. If prosthetic devices are needed, consult a doctor.

When women are having difficulties being aroused or reaching orgasm, they should also seek professional advice. For problems like decreased vaginal lubrication, an appropriate jelly, such as K-Y, may be useful Vaseline is less desirable, because it is not water soluble and often causes vaginal infections.

It helps when sexual partners are able to communicate with one another, but this is precisely the problem in Alzheimer's disease. However, even when the exchange of information is impaired, the healthy spouse can take the initiative. Manual and oral stimulation may become a satisfying sexual outlet or a substitute for intercourse. Not being able to have successful intercourse does not mean that it is no longer possible for an individual to give or receive pleasure.

Husbands and wives have shown the most tender devotion to the other's physical as well as emotional needs. Martin Regan had at the age of seventy-five suffered from Alzheimer's disease for more than seven years. He and his wife, Regina, had weathered the years together surrounded by their two sons and their families. Mr. Regan was hospitalized after a fall in which he broke his hip and also suffered a subdural hematoma. At that time he could recognize his wife and sister as well as his children, but he could not utter more than a few words. Much of the time he seemed disoriented and confused. He needed assistance with bathing and shaving and was incontinent.

Regina's two sons had been urging her to place him in a nursing home. They had become increasingly distressed over her poor health and the strain that caring for him placed on her. Finally, Peter, the older son, and his wife took his mother to lunch to persuade her to put Martin in a nursing home and not take him home again.

As had been predicted, the lunch was a long and tearful one. Mrs. Regan tried desperately to convince her children that her life revolved around her husband and his care. She would not surrender him to a home, because he had made her promise in the early phases that she would never do such a thing. The lunch ended abruptly, but Peter was able to talk his mother into seeing their clergyman. In several sessions with the reverend, she was able to discuss the intensity and richness of her married life—even in her husband's deteriorated state. It had a special intimacy that needed to be preserved for her.

Regina continued to minister to her husband. She described how she often found him in bed, even in the hospital, starting to get an erection. He would hold himself and look distressed. She did the only thing she could. She gave him the relief he needed, and he would fall asleep holding her hand as she sat by the bed.

This section on intimacy may not have been an easy one for everyone to read. Life is very precious, and perhaps nothing is more precious than the shared and private experiences of two people. For some relationships sexuality is a major factor; for others it may have less value. Love is one of the greatest gifts people can give to each other. Sexuality is only one expression of that gift. Intimacy, closeness, familiarity, companionship, and respect are among the other special gifts.

# 7

# CARING
# AT
# HOME

---

WHEN is it best for the patient to be home or in a nursing home or other living arrangement? This is a personal decision for every family.

My friends think that I am a martyr. I feel like both Solomon and Job. Robin has been sick with Alzheimer's disease for less than a year. He has deteriorated very rapidly, and now he just sits much of the day staring out the window. When I talk to him, he may say nothing, smile, or shout nonsense such as "Spitfire! Good! Get them!"

I intend to keep him at home as long as I can. That much I know. The children are pressing me, but I will not let him go.

Robin is company to me. Yes, our life is lopsided, but our love is not. He needs so much care, and as long as I can manage him and me, I will. Robin keeps changing and getting worse a little more each day, but I am still able to understand him. He is not the man he used to be, but he needs certain things—and he needs me.

Each morning and evening we keep an important ritual. He sits at the window watching the birds who visit the feeder in our yard. He is not able to put the food out anymore, but he still enjoys sitting for an hour or often more watching the antics of the squirrels and the birds. He was an avid bird-watcher throughout his life. Now the binoculars, the books, and his sketches are meaningless to him, but the birds still bring him pleasure.

Yesterday a finch flew into the glass door, breaking its neck instantly. I was on the phone with a friend, but I heard the hard knock against the pane. I walked into the living room, saw the bird on the porch, and saw Robin—crying. After checking the bird to make sure it was really dead, I went to the kitchen to find something in which to wrap it. Robin held a brown paper bag while I dropped the bird in. He folded the top down neatly several times and gave it back to me. We buried it in the backyard.

An hour later, I know, he did not remember what happened. But for a few minutes that day I had a glimpse of the gentle man who loved the world of nature. Somewhere deep inside, part of him was still there, but I couldn't hold on to it.


Family members are often correct in the belief that, with assistance and time off, they can take better care of their relative than anyone else can. Familiar faces, sights, smells, and sounds provide valuable reference points for confused adults. Family members know more about the patient and often understand his or her needs and desires more quickly than others.

Many families find a sense of security in being able to supervise a daily routine and in knowing where the patient is at all times. Indeed, care givers often feel comfortable only when they know that the patients are being cared for at home, "where they belong." It is the same feeling as not completely trusting a babysitter with your children. Cognitively impaired individuals respond well to the love and the understanding attention of their family. But successful caring requires devotion, determination, and self-sacrifice on the part of the family.

It is hard to provide for the continuing needs of the patient. Although only minimal assistance may be needed in the beginning, problems become more serious with time. Most families are unprepared for the strain of years of caring, and they are caught in a vise of increasing demands and diminishing resources. This is a burden of love, but the enormity of the demands, the stresses, the isolation, and the uncertainty of the future are difficult to bear. In addition, the erratic sleeping patterns, wandering, clinging behavior, and the physical and time demands of caring are a profound challenge. There are fewer opportunities for rest and little time for personal needs and the many problems that exist in any household.

Care givers must try to be honest with themselves. If the care they are able to provide at home is limited by poor health, financial distress, the need to work, space limitations in the home, or just plain exhaustion, care givers owe it to themselves and the patient to seek help and consider alternatives. Many relatives who have not helped care for the patient may not accept the idea of nursing-home placement, yet they are not able or may not offer to lend a hand with the around-the-clock care. These discussions often make the primary care giver feel angry or guilty. They should be ignored, as difficult as this may be. Only family members caring for the patient's needs on a daily basis know how hard it can be.

Many families find that they can manage home care for years with help from outside sources. Cooperation between various family members in the care of a patient can strengthen ties and bring family members closer together. Young children will have an opportunity to learn the gentleness and love required in the care of a chronically ill older person. Many people, provided they do not have to shoulder the entire burden, find a real beauty in the care of their relative. A helpful book for family care givers is Lois Barclay Murphy's *The Home Hospital: How a Family Can Cope with Catastrophic Illness*. It is a guide to the practical problems of caring for someone at home and a love story sharing the experience of a wife caring for a husband with Parkinson's disease; its theme is universal.

## The Need to Accept Help

One of the pitfalls in providing care to someone very close to us is that we may come to believe that we must do everything ourselves. In many cases there are good reasons for this belief. Care givers may in the past have had experiences with clinics, doctors, and social agencies that gave no help. Over months or years fewer friends call or visit. Even family members may be less available for assistance when needed. Primary care givers may learn to deal with a series of crises in isolation with little help. It is hard to avoid the feeling of being alone in these circumstances.

Some care givers may develop a rigid style of seeing, thinking, and acting. This can be beneficial when care givers reject well-intentioned but ill-advised recommendations to institutionalize the patient as soon as possible. However, in some circumstances blindly opposing any course of action recommended by others, including institutionalization, can be detrimental to all parties. The problem is one of inflexibility and unwillingness to examine and adapt to the circumstances and available resources. Rigid adherence to any pat formula—"Institutionalize in three to six months!" or "Never put into a nursing home!"—paves the way for future difficulties and unhappiness. Such narrow perspectives often prevent people from examining what resources are available in a changing situation, and how the family may find help from a variety of programs for the aged, disabled, and handicapped.

## Resources in the Community

Sometimes there are many sources of help in the community. The ability to find and use these resources ultimately influences the family's ability to keep the patient at home. Although many programs exist, not all medical specialists may be aware of their availability. Even when the doctor knows about their existence, he or she may not refer a patient and family unless a specific question is addressed by the family. Call ADRDA (Appendix 1) or your local Area Agency on Aging (Appendix 3) to find out what services are available in your area and whom to contact for an appointment. Some of them are briefly described below.

*Day health and rehabilitation care:* These programs offer a range of therapeutic, rehabilitative, and support activities, including nursing, rehabilitation, assistance with life activities, social work services, meals, and transportation. They are provided in a protected setting for a portion of a day, one to five days a week.

*Day care:* These day-care programs provide supportive but not rehabilitative services in a protected setting for a portion of the day, one to five days a week. Services may include recreational activities, social work services, a hot meal, transportation, and, occasionally, health services.

*Nutritional programs:* Congregate meal programs feed many older adults as a group in a community center or school. Some communities sponsor home-delivered meals to the frail, homebound aged. One noonday meal is provided, containing one-third of the recommended dietary allowance.

*Home health care:* These are organized programs of nursing, social work, occupational and physical therapy, and other rehabilitation services to individuals in their homes.

*Home health aides:* Home health aides provide personal care to individuals at home under the supervision of a health professional. Aides assist with meal preparation, eating, dressing, bathing, administering medications, as well as light household tasks.

*Homemaker services:* Household assistance is provided by professionally supervised and trained homemakers. Services include shopping, laundry, light cleaning, dressing, preparation of meals, and escort services on medical visits.

*Housekeeping services:* These services usually include cleaning, shopping, laundry, and meal preparation.

*Chore workers:* Chore-worker services include heavy-duty housecleaning, minor home repairs, yard work, and pest control.

*Companionship services:* Companions visit isolated and homebound individuals for conversation, reading, letter writing, and general light errands.

*Respite care services:* Respite care programs provide temporary twenty-four-hour care to give relief to primary care givers. The care may be provided in the person's home, an adult care home, or a nursing home.

*Hospital and surgical supply services:* Supply houses rent or sell medical supplies and equipment like hospital beds, canes, walkers, bath chairs, and oxygen and other equipment.

*Transportation:* Transportation services provide travel by automobile or specialized vans to and from community agencies and services providers.

*Escort services:* These services provide personalized accompaniment to service providers as well as personal assistance.

*Physical therapy:* Physical therapy, or PT, is rehabilitative therapy to maximize mobility. It should be provided by a qualified physical therapist.

*Speech therapy:* Speech therapy is therapy provided by a qualified speech therapist to overcome certain speech and communication problems.

*Occupational therapy:* Occupational therapy, or OT, is restorative therapy to enhance or restore skills necessary for daily living. It should be provided by a qualified occupational therapist.

*Skilled nursing services:* These are nursing services provided in a person's home or in an outpatient or ambulatory-care setting.

*Housing assistance:* Housing-assistance programs exist in some communities to help in the search for suitable housing, in the moving of personal items, and in the finding of emergency shelters.

*Geriatric assessment units and special-care units:* Specialized geriatric units, both inpatient and outpatient, exist in many hospitals and medical centers across the country. They usually provide more-coordinated multidisciplinary services to older patients.

## Finding Help

No matter how educated, experienced, or well-off an individuals is, caring for a relative, especially one who lives far away, is very stressful. How do you find out what services are available when your relative lives alone or in a community far away from you? How do you make proper arrangements? How do you juggle career, family, and responsibilities to the patient? How do you deal with your own distress and frustration?

Throughout the country there is a growing network of health care professionals who offer what are known as case or care management services for a fee. These agencies make referrals for home care attendants, nurses, occupational and physical therapists, homemakers, chore workers, lawyers, financial consultation, and medical and psychiatric specialists. They may also act as your broker, which means that they confer with you about your needs, and then they will arrange for the services you need and take responsibility for monitoring the quality of care.

These care management services can help you when your relative lives far away. For a fee they will find a social worker in any area of the country to assess your relative's needs and arrange for necessary services. In these situations it is important to know that you are getting quality services. Generally, you must rely on your feelings about the responsiveness of the care managers and the quality of the services you have received. Their willingness to spend the necessary time to answer your questions and the actual help they give you are important criteria by which to judge quality.

The major drawback of care management services is their expense. Many people simply cannot afford this type of help, which should be more available than it is. When care management services are unavailable or unaffordable, the family members become the primary managers to coordinate the patient's care. It takes time and the commitment of family members to examine their personal and family resources to decide what can be done.

A local branch of the Alzheimer's Disease and Related Disorders Association (ADRDA) can be a valuable resource, not only as an organization but also through the experiences of individual members who have tried to find help in many different places. They can inform you about what needs to be done and how valuable the help is in relation to the efforts necessary to secure it. In the appendixes we have listed the contact points for chapters of ADRDA (Appendix 1) and for a number of national organizations on aging (Appendix 2).

There are many other organizations for you to consult in the search for services in your community. Every state in the country has a State Agency on Aging, and Appendix 3 provides the address and phone number for every one in the United States. Virtually any major religious group can be an important source of information about available options. For those who are Jewish, interested relatives should call the Jewish Information and Referral Service at 212–753–2288 for referrals to local agencies throughout the United States. Individuals needing Catholic referrals can call the local Catholic Charities Organization in their archdiocese or write the National Conference of Catholic Charities, 1346 Connecticut Avenue, NW, Washington, D.C. 20036. Protestant resources may be located through the individual Protestant denomination. Finally, families can write a letter asking for agencies throughout the country and send it, along with a stamped, self-addressed envelope, to Family Service of America, 44 East 23d Street, New York, NY 10010.

In hospitals the social services department often has a list of community programs, and in many instances the hospital's auxiliary or volunteer group may have on hand published brochures describing these services and giving contacts and phone numbers.

Other sources of help are local colleges and universities. Many schools have gerontology centers or institutes on aging, and their faculty may be familiar with programs in the community. In an increasing number of instances, a university, medical school, or medical center may itself run such programs for training purposes.

The Veterans Administration (and in some states the statewide veterans benefits agency) has been interested in the problems of long-term caring for years. The VA not only has an extensive program of nursing-home care but has also been developing community-based arrangements in certain parts of the country. For qualified veterans this option may be available. Contact the local Veterans Administration office or Veterans Hospital. If that yields nothing, write the Veterans Administration in Washington, D.C., which coordinates these activities (Appendix 2).

One of the great barriers to finding local agencies in your community is that such agencies cannot afford to invest significantly in advertising and promotion. Since most are nonprofit, they tend to devote what resources they have to services and program development, with little in the budget available for outreach to new cases.

## Adapting the Home to the Patient

The environment of the home—size, physical design, furniture arrangements, lighting, decorations, colors, number and configuration of rooms, availability and construction of patios, balconies, and other outside areas—can make living safe or unsafe, comfortable or uncomfortable. As patients become progressively impaired and disabled, homes and apartments can be changed in several basic ways, even when financial resources are limited, to make them more livable. Families can evaluate what may be changed in the home with the following three goals in mind: barrier freedom, safety, and cognitive support.

Barrier freedom is now well recognized. For those persons with physical impairments stemming from accidents or illness, personal devices like wheelchairs or walkers can make an important difference. However, a number of physical barriers can affect the use of those devices. Narrow doorways or high door sills, loose carpets or throw rugs, narrow passageways between furniture, or the placement of breakable objects in or near places which are heavily trafficked can become serious problems. A positive approach to the elimination of barriers, the addition of a number of such features as grab bars in the bath, and the availability of easily accessible showers with stools and easily reached controls can be helpful.

Most Alzheimer's patients do not have physical problems early in their illness. For them other issues are of greater importance. However, as the disease progresses, problems of safety and security need to be addressed. Patients often like to be able to participate in the world by seeing what is going on. Enclosing a porch can serve this purpose, as can allowing patients access to a window. Ensuring that there are adequate safety devices can also help. The value of internal quiet alarms or door locks, including combination locks with four- or five-button codes, should be examined to help contain the patient who is given to wandering.

Different rooms of the house have special problems. The kitchen can be a hazardous place. Gas burners without pilot lights are potential dangers for the patient who turns on the gas but forgets to put a match to the burner. The oven is often mistaken for a refrigerator, with the result that it may be turned on while bags of groceries or unwrapped objects are inside. In general, patients in later stages of the illness should not be in the kitchen unsupervised, even if that means controlling access. The use of fireproof burner pads may help. Putting away electrical appliances or unplugging such devices as toasters, mixers, or food processors can eliminate potential problems.

At least one room in the house should be identified as the patient's own space. A safe room, perhaps with a view, a TV set, a radio, and a source of music, can play a valuable role. It should be a room where the patient can learn to spend time and feel secure. Time spent there with loved ones can often be a foundation for allowing the patient to be alone while the care giver performs chores in other rooms. In places like the bedroom it is helpful to organize objects for daily use. Clothing to be worn that day, eyeglasses or hearing aids, even wallets, should go in a regular place or an appropriate shelf or holder. This routine should be started early.

## The Home Care Checklist

The decision whether to keep the patient at home should be based not only on loyalty and commitment but also on the physical and emotional resources of the primary care giver(s). The following list of general questions is intended as a guide to help you evaluate your continuing capability to keep the patient at home.

### 1. Home Environment: What can you do to make the home safe and comfortable for the patient?

- Is the home large enough that the patient can have his or her own room on the first floor when a separate sleeping area with a bathroom is needed?
- Are there ways to rearrange furniture to make the home less cluttered so that the patient can navigate easily around the house?
- Can you organize the patient's personal belongings so that they are consistently in one place?
- Can you fix up an area outside of the home that is safe and accessible to the patient?
- Is there a place nearby where the patient can walk, jog, or play tennis?
- If there are stairs outside the home, is it necessary and possible to build a ramp?
- In the event that you decide to hire live-in house help, is there adequate living space for that individual?
- Is it feasible for you and the patient to move to special housing for senior citizens?

### 2. Medical Accessibility: Do you have professional help ready in an emergency?

- Is a medical center or hospital nearby?
- Do you have the emergency numbers for the doctor and ambulance service?
- Will your doctor help advise you and visit the home?

*3. Finances: Can you afford to pay for attendants, nurses, and special treatments?*

- Analyze your financial assets and those of the patient.
- Try to estimate the cost of health care—doctors, equipment, procedures—needed each month.
- Talk to an accountant or call the Internal Revenue Service for guidance about what may be deductible on your taxes.
- Investigate your eligibility for home care benefits from Medicare, Medicaid, and health insurance policies (see Chapter 13).
- Keep a weekly budget and each month examine how you are spending your money.

*4. Transportation: Can you drive or do you have transportation for daily needs?*

- Is the home accessible by means of public transportation if and when home attendants and nurses are necessary?
- What transportation can you use in an emergency?
- Have you made contingency plans to keep your home accessible during bad weather and winter storms?
- Are neighbors who can drive close by in the event your car breaks down?

*5. Your Health: Are you realistic about your ability to care for the patient at home?*

- Are you strong enough to help the patient in the bathroom, bath, or shower?
- Can you get away for regular periods of rest and recreation?

*6. Equipment: What do you need to care for someone in your home?*

- Canes, walkers, wheelchairs, and special hospital beds can be rented. Can you arrange the house so that it can accommodate a wheelchair? Is there a place in the home for a hospital bed where the patient will have privacy and still be near family activities?

- What special equipment can you get to help your relative exercise?

*7. Family and Personal Services: Do you have family members who can share the burden or can you afford to hire trained reliable help?*

- Do other family members live close enough to be of assistance?
- Can the family cooperate in making decisions about the patient's care?
- If you are the primary care giver, are you able to share the burden of caring?
- Can you find qualified nurses and home care attendants?
- Can the patient participate in decision making or at least be included in family meetings?
- Have you made neighbors aware of the problem?

*8. General*

- Are you prepared to care for your relative at home even through the final stages of the dementia, when he or she becomes very sick and bedridden?
- Have you investigated the value, availability, quality, and cost of nursing homes? (See Chapter 10.)

In the long run, planning and decision making, based on good information rather than beliefs, enhance the quality of life for everyone. The patient, his or her environment, and your own ability to deal with the inevitable changes are areas about which you need information. There are opportunities for getting help from others, be they community services or health care professionals.

# 8

# COPING
# WITH THE
# STRESS OF
# CARING

CARING for someone with Alzheimer's disease is a task as complicated as any we face. The needs of the patient overshadow everything else, and inevitably the pattern of daily life changes. Since the
dementia usually progresses slowly, the care giver's life is transformed gradually, but the changes can last for years.

Those who have a care-giving role with the Alzheimer's patient
face the constant task of balancing the needs of the patient with
their own needs, and often those of other members of the family.
Tenseness, anger, frustration, guilt, and sadness are normal responses to the strain of living with and caring for any individual with
a prolonged or chronic illness. The constant demands of caring can
and do lead to emotional and physical fatigue. It is easy to feel
overwhelmed and helpless in the situation. A key to coping successfully is to recognize that the care-giver role is impossible and then
to try to do the best you can. Accepting the harsh reality is the first
step.

Most family routines are eventually disrupted when patients become unable to carry out their usual responsibilities. Family mem-

bers report becoming isolated from the mainstream as patients can no longer participate in recreational activities, hobbies, and social engagements which were once pleasurable. Isolation from neighbors and friends leads to feelings of being trapped. As tension increases, family members may quarrel with each other. Financial problems may mount as the expenses of the illness accumulate. Important needs of other family members which require money are frequently postponed.

The behaviors of patients are frustrating to live with, and it is normal to feel irritation and even rage. For example, many patients ask the same questions continually, even when the answer is given over and over. This trivial manifestation of the memory loss of dementia becomes a stressful daily occurrence. Family members, especially spouses, express enormous sadness at the loss of someone in whom they confided and with whom they shared the ups and downs of everyday living. Some family members report being enraged at the dementia itself. One middle-aged man expressed appropriate frustration at his loss: "Why did it have to affect my father? I have been robbed of the chance to be a son and enjoy him."

It is the number and range of problems that often prove to be overwhelming for care givers. Many family members suffer from physical as well as psychological health problems, insomnia, irritability, and physical exhaustion. In order to watch over an individual, it is often necessary to quit a job or at the very least lose time at work. Perhaps the most frequent consequence of the stresses of care giving is depression. In one study 55 percent of the care givers living at home with the patient had a clinical depression. Thus, family members often become unrecognized patients themselves, who as a result of their disability lose the capacity to provide the best care for their loved one and for themselves.

Successful coping involves first identifying your problems and then, most important, recognizing which ones you can do something about and which are beyond anyone's control. Many practical ways to help the patient keep active and feel secure and comfortable are discussed in this book. Friends, self-help groups, and professionals can be enormously helpful. Without outside assistance it is often hard to keep a healthy perspective on the limits of care giving as the dementia progresses. If we lose our objectivity, we can become overwhelmed and sick and cease to be in a position to care for the patient effectively.

The question then is "How do you cope?" or "How do you know if you are coping well or not?" There are several answers. Regardless of how competent, experienced, or sophisticated an individual is, the dementia changes everything, from the most routine daily events to special times like birthdays. There are ways to cope with the stresses, and specific strategies to monitor yourself and determine how well you are doing. These are the focus of this chapter.

## Dealing with Feelings

Emotions are complex. The way we respond emotionally depends on our personality, our mental and physical health, our stage of life, the particular situation we are in, and our previous experience with similar circumstances. The feelings of a care giver are also affected by the nature of the established relationship and style of communication between the care giver and the patient. Although some people will feel little anger toward patients, other will experience a great deal. However, feeling such anger does not mean that you love them less than someone who does not seem to feel it. In fact, for some it is important to feel the anger and then express it in an appropriate way. Furthermore, there are periods in our lives when times are rough and we are simply more vulnerable. The ability to care for anybody when we are hurting and vulnerable is severely compromised.

An especially important determinant of how we feel about the care-giving role lies in the balance between a sense of satisfaction with what you are doing for the patient, and the frustration of caring for someone who is continuing to deteriorate. This equilibrium can be affected by the severity of the dementia, the intimacy of family relationships, and the types of resources and support available to care givers. The pain of watching loved ones in the later stages of dementia, when they become incontinent or cannot eat, or when they develop pneumonia or contractures, is often overhwelming. One woman exclaimed, "I am blinded by my sadness now. My Louie always did for others, and now nobody can do for him. I could handle everything until they put the tube in his stomach. There is nothing but oblivion for him—and me."

It is not always the dramatic, heartbreaking events that upset the emotional balance of care givers. The many years of living with the progressive changes exact a heavy toll. Elmira Jones, the wife of an Alzheimer's patient, told us, "I talk to my pillow each night and cry myself to sleep. Willie still sleeps with me, and I take him every-where—shopping, church, choir, my bridge club, everything. During the day I am okay. It's the nights when I break down. My tears over the past eight years would fill the house."

Personal history plays an important role in the way people adapt or do not adapt. Individuals who have lived through major crises and stressful life events tend to have developed emotional resilience and effective coping skills. Some people simply have adaptive personalities and can handle themselves well in most situations regardless of past history. However, even the most experienced or composed individuals will experience feelings of sadness, anger, frustration, and resentment.

The crucial question is how to deal with the feelings. The answer is complicated. You may have to hide more-negative feelings from the patient, depending on the severity of the dementia. Many patients react strongly to anger, with everything from anxiety to extreme violence. In general, it is wise to protect patients as much as possible from explosive outbursts, noisy arguments among family members, and strong emotions. It is important to judge the patient's ability to respond to expressions of legitimate emotions and when possible to present concerns lovingly and honestly. Some patients can handle feelings reasonably well if they are not too impaired.

However, it is crucial that honest feelings not be bottled up inside you. There are many ways to relieve such pressure. First, look to yourself and try to admit if you are angry, afraid, or upset. Next, do something about it and get the feelings out of your system. Writing letters to family or close friends, telephone conversations, and long discussions with a supportive individual are often helpful. Be open and get it out where you can recognize it.

Pat Conroy wrote several letters each week to her daughter. Even though they spoke often on the telephone, Mrs. Conroy reported that the letters helped her "package her feelings" each day.

My dearest daughter,

I have just finished writing in your father's journal tonight. Jim is asleep now on the couch beside me. Even though he is changing as the Alzheimer's takes its course, he is still the most precious and dearest of beings to me.

I am writing to you now to try and shed my feelings of aloneness and sadness. I know we have done everything possible for Jim, but tonight I feel overwhelmed by my love and my anguish.

Today your father seemed more like himself. He went shopping with me, and we even met friends for lunch at our favorite Italian restaurant. Jim seemed especially happy. He smiled and laughed. Tonight the laughter is a fading memory, but I am fighting to cling to that memory. I need the good times to live through the bad days.

What do you do when frustrations seem to swell uncontrollably? It may not be easy, but try to compose your thoughts. It is helpful to write down exactly what is bothering you. The next step is to do something constructive about it. If you are upset with the patient, talk to someone about it. If your relative is in the early stages, explain to him or her, when possible, what is annoying you. If you are angry with a nurse, aide, or attendant who has committed an error or been lax or careless, be pleasant but firm in your criticisms. You have a responsibility to inform such persons that you expect them to be more sensitive and caring with your relative. If they do not correct their mistake or change their behavior, you may need to dismiss them if they are in your employ. Or if the individual is on the staff of a nursing home, you should report your continued dissatisfaction to one of the administrators.

Dealing with your general anger at the illness is a more complicated matter. If you cannot alleviate your distress at the sad plight of your relative, you may rage with blind fury and only end up physically and mentally exhausted. However, there are ways to lessen the frustrations of living with dementia. It is important to learn how to do these two things:

First, focus on ways to enjoy as many activities as possible, with and without the patient. Al Rogers cared for his wife over fifteen years: "Jill and I went everywhere together for many years. Even though she could do very little, she seemed content just to be near me. Indeed, she seemed happiest when surrounded by her entire family." Lorraine Thomas remembered the two years she cared for her husband: "Roger went downhill so fast. It was hard to accept that he wasn't my husband anymore. I did everything I could to care for him, but I had to get out of the house every day to rejuvenate myself. I had to do things I enjoyed, or I would have gone crazy."

Second, cultivate a philosophy of "living one day at a time." One way to cope with catastrophic events of all kinds—war, natural disasters, terminal illness—is to live day by day, focusing your energy on survival. June Anatole said it this way:

Bart has been dead two years, but I still think of him every day. I remember the five years of hope and suffering. Yes, we had both. For most of our married life, Bart would get out of bed each morning, extend his hand to me, and say, "Come on Mama, we have another day ahead of us. Let's not waste it." It was a simple ritual in our lives, but it was the way I loved to start my day.

I remember the awful loneliness I felt the morning Bart forgot our ritual. It was about a year after the doctor had told us that Bart had Alzheimer's disease. He simply got out of bed, went into the bathroom, and called out to me that he wanted breakfast. I remember how afraid I was. This Alzheimer's problem was getting worse, and Bart was changing.

The days took on a special meaning after that. It wasn't easy, but we changed roles. I was the one who got up first and extended my hand, "Pop, it's time to spend another day together."

Bart lived another four years; no, not years, more than 1,400 days. And each day carries a special memory for me. I know we did everything we could.

People handle their emotions in many different ways during the long months and years of caring. Some individuals are able to deal quietly with the sorrow and sense of loss, while others enlist the active support of friends and family. The capacity of family members to care and cope are often profound testaments to the love individuals feel for each other.

Samuel Jackson took care of his wife, Nadia, for eighteen years with the support of his daughter and two sons. Their daughter had never married and continued to live with them, which proved to be enormously helpful during the long period Nadia had been ill. Sam cared for Nadia tenderly morning and night, day after day. They continued to go out and do many things together. Around the house Nadia was on the move constantly. When she tired Sam out, he would ask her to sit on the couch so that he could lay his head on her lap to rest. No matter how agitated or active Nadia was throughout the entire course of her dementia, she would sit quietly stroking his hair while he rested. If anyone walked in, she would raise her finger to her lips: "Shh! Sam is sleeping!"

The bonds between people are of many types. Not all relationships are characterized by such devotion, but that does not mean that other people do not love as well or as much. Many good and stable relationships are hard-pressed by the demands of caring. Indeed there are many situations in which family members should, in the best interests of everyone involved, find a nursing home for the patient. Caring is hard work, physically and emotionally. Amanda Potter finally let her son make the arrangements for her husband, Albert, to go into a nursing home. She simply wasn't physically strong enough to care for her husband after he was bedridden, and she could no longer afford home help. Amanda told her son, "Your father and I lived through the concentration camps, but I never expected another Holocaust! I love your father, and I am powerless to protect him from this."

## Who Takes Care of the Care Giver?

The primary care giver, usually the spouse, may find it very hard to accept the reality that Alzheimer's disease or a related disorder cannot be managed without help. Over the years of living together, husbands and wives develop unique patterns of caring for each other's needs and desires. Indeed, what makes entire families special is the way different members relate to one another with various degrees of loyalty, obligation, and commitment. Families are often able to meet many of the complex personal and social needs of their members. However, Alzheimer's disease is akin to a major catastrophe—to a natural disaster. Responding to it requires a lot of individual effort, but it cannot be handled alone. Other people are necessary, and by working together and sharing responsibilities, you and they can do a great deal. You will find it easier to cope if you let yourself accept help when you need it.

The availability of a people support system is one of the most important resources anyone can have. It is common for a husband or wife to feel he or she can do everything necessary to care for the patient. However, even though a spouse may have the yeoman's job, it is important, even lifesaving, to share the responsibility of caring.

Children, grandchildren, brothers, sisters, in-laws, friends, neighbors, and other important individuals can provide much needed assistance if you will let them.

Hugo and Alicia Prado had been married forty years and had raised five children. Two daughters, Anne and Jean-Marie, had started their own families and lived within ten miles of their parents. The eldest son, Jacques, who was divorced, also lived in the same town and ran his father's business. The other two sons were still single and lived in other states: George was in law school, and Bryan worked for an insurance company.

Hugo had been diagnosed as having Alzheimer's disease a year and a half earlier. Indeed, it was on their fortieth wedding anniversary that Alicia knew she could no longer delay taking her husband to a doctor. Their five children threw a surprise party, at which Hugo, in making a toast, stunned everyone by wishing his wife happy birthday!

Mrs. Prado reminisced about the past several years:

My family has been my anchor. I would not have been able to handle myself without them. There were so many days when I felt completely lost and helpless. The pain welled up inside me, and I . . . I wanted to die. The children surrounded me and gave me the strength to face Hugo's illness. There is no greater agony than to see the one you love obliterated, and without the kids I would have fallen apart.

It is also important to find ways to get away from care-giving responsibilities on a regular basis. However, this goes against natural instincts and desires. Ordinarily, someone caring for another looks for ways for them to be together, but the toll that dementia extracts is a high one. Even people with normal routines need vacations and breaks during the day and week. Alzheimer's disease and related disorders are extremely demanding, and if care givers are not able to refresh themselves, there is a danger that their energies will be depleted and that they will have less to give.

## Depression: A Danger for Care Givers

Depression is not a rare condition in care givers, and sometimes it can become quite serious. If clinical depression goes unrecognized and untreated, it can worsen and can indeed become deadly. It is a complex emotion, spanning the continuum from normal and appropriate feelings of sadness and despair to any one of several major clinical disorders. The first question is how to recognize when you are in danger of becoming seriously depressed; the next is what to do about it.

In order to develop some insight, it may be helpful to examine the many faces of depression. All of us have felt despondent, gloomy, despairing, helpless, and hopeless at some time in our life. Sadness is a normal and appropriate response to an illness. Death, the anniversary of a loved one's death, a financial loss, a personal failure, or any one of many life stresses can cause such feelings. Sometimes we get the blues when we have been working too hard and are simply overtired.

Living with and caring for a relative with dementia can bring on great sadness. Some of the emotions become overwhelming, and help for those feelings is warranted. Unfortunately, depression is not always easy to recognize and diagnose. There are many different symptoms to look for. Some of them are psychological and others are physical. You do not have to look and feel consciously sad to have a clinical depression, and this is one of the most difficult things for nonprofessionals to understand.

Problems with memory and with concentration are often characteristics of depression. Many care givers complain that they have a memory problem. It is common to hear, "I must be getting demented myself. I cannot seem to remember things any better than my husband." Depression contributes to slower thinking, feelings of confusion, and real memory losses. Making the simplest decisions becomes difficult. One husband described his situation:

I sat in my office and worried. I could not get any work done. I would read a report and would reread the same paragraphs over again. At the end of the day, I knew I had accomplished nothing. I had paced around the office, shuffled piles of paper, and stared at the walls. I felt impotent—psychologically impotent.

Depression can also be a psychological state often characterized as the blahs—your zest for life is gone, you feel low and empty. You may also think about your life and feel guilty about all the mistakes you have made. In a clinical depression people often dislike themselves and feel like failures. They may see themselves as incompetent and unworthy—unworthy, even, of the time and help of a professional.

The depressed person is often pessimistic and convinced that things can only get worse. The future seems bleak and hopeless to them. Their feelings of oppression are so strong that others become depressed from being around them. Depressed people may also talk and act more slowly. The answers to even simple questions may be accompanied by long sighs.

Pain is a prominent symptom of depression. The presence of depression in a care giver may exaggerate the pain of arthritis and other chronic illnesses. Indeed, the combination of emotional distress and physical illness may in the long run seriously disable the care giver and compromise the quality of care he or she can render.

Depression shows itself in bodily functions. Not only is it visible in one's face and posture, but other changes occur. The sleep cycle is altered. Although falling asleep may be relatively unchanged, people who are depressed often awaken in the early hours of the morning and cannot fall asleep again. This condition is also known as terminal insomnia—that is, insomnia at the end of the sleep cycle. Sometimes people stay in bed and sleep many hours. When awake, they complain of being tired all of the time. Appetite changes. Most people lose their appetite, eat far less than usual, and lose weight. Others eat more and gain weight. Constipation also occurs as a result of depression.

Be on the alert for the signs of serious depression, and if and when you see them, seek help. You are doing yourself and the patient an important favor. If something is wrong, the longer the depression lasts, the harder it is to treat. Often a friend or relative first suggests to the care giver that he or she should see someone. Try not to be angry or defensive if persons you trust say that they are worried about you and that perhaps you need help. It is often sound advice. At least give yourself the benefit of a checkup.

Untreated depression may affect the way a care giver reacts to the patient. Although it is a sensitive issue, it should be discussed openly. Husbands, wives, children, or whoever the primary care givers are may become so angry or depressed that they neglect or physically abuse the patient. Seemingly uncontrollable emotions and actions impair the care giver's thinking and ability to care for the patient. However, these conditions can be treated. Sadly, neglect and abuse of a patient do not usually come to anybody's attention until the patient is hospitalized and medical staff become suspicious of the patient's injuries and circumstances.

Hope Conti had been married to her husband, William, for over forty years. William had been diagnosed as having Alzheimer's disease at the age of sixty-four. Eight years into the Alzheimer's disease, Hope hired a home care attendant to help with bathing, dressing, feeding, and light cleaning around the house. She and her husband continued to do as much as his strength permitted. Each day they would drive somewhere for lunch and later take a walk or go shopping. During the summer they drove to the country with the attendant every weekend; there she and her husband would hike in the woods, swim in the pool, and go boating on the lake. William enjoyed the exercise and seemed to continue to take pride in his athletic prowess.

One afternoon while William was napping, the home care attendant announced that she was quitting. She accused Mrs. Conti of beating her husband. There were large bruises on Mr. Conti's chest, shoulders, and arms. Mrs. Conti was horrified at the accusation, and angrily told the woman to leave.

The next weekend the Conti's drove to the mountains for a weekend with friends. Sunday afternoon Mr. Conti lost his balance and struck his head on the rocks. With the help of her friends and of a local ranger, Hope was able to get her husband to the car. They drove to the local hospital, where Mr. Conti was admitted.

Mr. Conti was hospitalized five days before being transferred to a university hospital in his hometown. He stayed there another three weeks before being sent home. He had sustained a subdural hematoma, but he also was anemic, malnourished, and had a urinary-tract infection.

Mrs. Conti's daughter Carol had successfully persuaded her mother to talk with one of the doctors at the hospital. During the interview Mrs. Conti described her firm desire to take her husband home and not place him in an institution, as everyone on the hospital team had recommended. Staff and family were united in their concern about Mrs. Conti's health and her continued ability to care for her husband. She had lost twenty pounds in the past month, was waking up every morning at five, and even admitted to having thoughts of wanting to die. She also conceded that she was extremely frustrated with her husband and that she sometimes wanted to hit him when she couldn't understand what he wanted or needed. In the intimacy of the conversation, she gradually admitted her shame and embarrassment that she had struck her husband on a few occasions. The few turned out to be many.

The doctors conferred with Carol to share their concern that Mrs. Conti had been abusing her husband. For his own safety Mr. Conti needed to be institutionalized. And just as important, Mrs. Conti was suffering from a severe depression and needed help.

Placing Mr. Conti in a nursing home could be a temporary placement until Mrs. Conti felt well enough to assume his care again. Depending on how she felt after her depression was treated, she might also decide that institutionalization was an acceptable solution. Caring for William, as much as she deeply loved him, had become an overwhelming task for Hope. The physical exertion of turning him in bed, helping him to the toilet or with his bath, even with home help, was akin to an olympic decathlon for Mrs. Conti, who herself had multiple health problems.

Mrs. Conti responded to the antidepressant treatment. She retained a deep regret and shame over her behavior, and her family also had difficulty accepting what they perceived as her cruelty. However, after several family sessions they were able to understand how the situation had become so toxic. They also saw ways to help one another prevent such a problem from recurring. The entire family was enormously relieved to understand the cause of Mrs. Conti's actions and was prepared to support her in the future.

## Dealing with Ambivalence toward the Patient

The very nature of dementia causes ambivalent or confused emotional reactions in care givers. If we are unsure about an individual's competence and safety, we find ourselves vacillating between wanting to help patients maintain independence and forcing them to accept our help. It is emotionally confusing to live with individuals who look to us like the human beings we knew yet who lose the capacity to carry out the simplest actions. Everyday situations may generate powerful mixed feelings of love and anger, tenderness and rejection. The need to come to grips with these ambivalent feelings is extremely important. The consequences of not recognizing them are inevitably reflected in unnecessary anguish and a poorer quality of caring.

Alexander Frishman lived at home with his wife, Betty, who had been diagnosed as having dementia two years earlier. He explained how he tried to maintain a normal life:

Betty tries to do many things around the house—set the table, wash the dishes, dust the furniture, and little things like that. She is always eager to help, but she gets confused and doesn't finish anything. That's what gets me so upset. I get so frustrated sometimes that I want to lash out. For example, she will get the silverware out of the drawer, walk to the table, pick up the napkins, and walk back to the drawer with both silverware and napkins. I know that the Alzheimer's is causing her to act this way, but little things like this happen every day. She seems so normal in many ways, but it's like only half of her mind is working.

Coping successfully with the stress of caring requires improved insight into our own behavior. However, it is often difficult to recognize what we are doing wrong unless someone points it out to us. Mr. Frishman responded to the advice of his daughter to take Betty for a psychological evaluation. After the testing was completed, the psychologist met with the entire family. He identified the types of tasks Betty could do and gave the family explicit instructions on how to respond when she made mistakes. Alexander Frishman was upset about Betty's confused behavior, and his anger and frustration actually made Betty anxious and tense. When she insisted on doing the smallest task, Alex would often become so frustrated that he would shout, "Go ahead and do it if you can." This would only aggravate the situation. Alex eventually learned to deal with his own anxiety about her mistakes. Even if Betty would stand for twenty minutes fumbling with the silverware, she was not hurting anyone. Indeed, she seemed to be happy to be doing something, even though it made no sense to anyone else.

There are many constructive ways to deal with ambivalence, but usually this can be done only with help. Unfortunately, many people are afraid to seek help, and the results can be dangerous to the patient or the family. Mrs. Grace Arrow became increasingly frustrated about attempts to keep her husband, Ronald, in bed at night. After retiring, he would get up and walk into the kitchen eight or ten times, try to remove his pajamas bottoms, and hold them over the stove burners. On several nights he turned the burners on, igniting his pajamas. This routine went on for several weeks before Mrs. Arrow, becoming increasingly agitated, took her husband back to the doctor. The visit was precipitated when Mr. Arrow screamed at his wife and struck her in the face while she was trying to prevent him from repeating this dangerous activity.

Everyone was baffled by his ritualistic behavior, and Mrs. Arrow was weary from lack of sleep. She was legitimately upset and angry not only because she was tired but also because she did not understand her husband's unusual actions. They had been married over fifty years, and she had prided herself on her ability to care for her husband's needs. During the daytime he seemed quite content. However, his "craziness" and violence at night were devastating because Ronald had never raised his voice to her in all the years they had been married. She loved him deeply but could not understand the action of this man, who seemed to be someone else. She was so upset about her feelings of anger and guilt that she endured Ronald's behavior—as dangerous as it was—until his blow appeared to snap her out of her conflict and led her to seek help.

It was possible to make sense of his actions. It was the middle of winter, and to conserve fuel and money Mrs. Arrow kept the thermostat at sixty-six degrees. This had been their custom for as long as they had lived in the Northeast. Since it was possible that Mr. Arrow was trying to communicate that he was cold, the doctor suggested an experiment. Raise the thermostat to seventy degrees and observe whether there was any change in his behavior. The very first night, Mr. Arrow slept soundly and did not get out of bed except to go to the bathroom.

It is often difficult for spouses and other family members to reconcile their ambivalence toward a loved one. Furthermore, patients themselves are capable of experiencing ambivalent feelings. Mrs. Abigail Truman lived with her husband, Dale, aged sixty-nine, who had been diagnosed as having Alzheimer's disease more than three years earlier. This was the second marriage for Mrs. Truman and the third for her husband. They were a handsome couple, who enjoyed each other's company and were devoted to one another's happiness. The marriage had lasted twenty-two years, and although they had no children, Dale's three daughters from his second marriage were devoted to both of them.

The oldest daughter, Mary Jane, became deeply concerned about a growing depression in both parents. Her father had begun to deteriorate. His memory was worsening, and he napped more often during the day. It required three or more hours for her stepmother to get him out of bed, dress him, and feed him in the morning. Dale claimed he was too tired and simply did not want to leave his bed.

Mrs. Truman was a strong, beautiful woman determined to keep her husband active. Having become distressed by his inability to rise in the morning, she was increasingly frustrated and tired. Once he was out of bed and dressed, she kept him active in the afternoon and evenings. The ceaseless hours of caring, however, were taking their toll on her, and with time she found herself averting her husband's romantic advances. He, in turn, became irritable and began to withdraw from her. Dale ate and slept more and began to put on excess weight.

It was at this point that Mary Jane invited her parents to visit with them for a few weeks. She also persuaded them to see a specialist in Alzheimer's disease to see whether anything might be done for Mr. Truman.

Several discussions with Mr. and Mrs. Truman, together and separately, were revealing. It was clear that the marriage of twenty-two years was a solid one and that despite the dementia there were several areas of mutual pleasure—eating, shopping, collecting stamps, and building miniature furniture. Both were gourmet cooks, and although Dale could no longer cook, he could still enjoy his wife's special meals. Although both had also enjoyed stamp collections and miniature furniture, these hobbies had been among the first pleasures to be dropped as expenses mounted. Finally, it was clear that sexual relations were extremely important to both of them.

The couple were approaching a crisis during the visit to their daughter's home. They had not had relations in the past month. Mrs. Truman cried frequently but was unable to confide in her daughter, and both she and her husband were trying to act as if nothing were wrong.

Mr. Truman was greatly distressed about what he perceived as his wife's rejection and withdrawal. He knew that the Alzheimer's disease was progressive, and his greatest fear was that his wife would reject him and abandon him as the disease destroyed him. He described how his wife refused to discuss the future with him. She would hide articles on dementia, and she even tried to keep him from watching a television special on the topic. He knew that his future was a grim one, but he also wanted dearly to talk with his family and help prepare them emotionally. He was becoming increasingly angry that his wife would not cooperate. He felt excluded, and he was also afraid that the disease would rob him of his senses before he could complete his preparation.

His wife's sexual withdrawal was the ultimate rejection. He was ashamed that the Alzheimer's had deprived him not only of his dignity but also of the woman he loved. He wanted to die and often said so to his wife.

Mrs. Truman was deeply troubled by her husband's wish to die. In fact, she was so overwhelmed by the situation that she felt she would soon be on the verge of a breakdown. She was adamant that her husband must not know about the final stages of Alzheimer's disease, and it took time to convince her that he already knew. Indeed, the two of them had been so busy protecting each other that neither had any sense of the other's real thoughts or feelings.

Mrs. Truman understood the possible effect of her sexual withdrawal. She loved Dale but was exhausted from the long hours. She had no energy and was depressed and angry. She did not know how to deal with her confused feelings of love and anger and sadness.

After several meetings it was possible to help Mr. and Mrs. Truman communicate with one another and to understand how this situation had evolved. Mr. Truman was enormously relieved that his wife was not rejecting or leaving him. And at first Mrs. Truman found her husband's fears unbelievable. As his loneliness became clearer to her and as the two began to see how each was torn by ambivalence, it became easier to plan the future together. Mr. Truman responded well to antidepressant medications, and both he and his wife participated in several therapy sessions. Eventually, they reestablished their former intimacy and trust.

## Maintaining Balance in the Family

Changes in the patient threaten everyone's ability to sustain a rewarding and loving relationship. At some point in the course of the disorder, patients may no longer understand what is happening around them or be able to share experiences with the family. Some patients become so belligerent and unpleasant that it is easy to see why even close relatives and friends become resentful and upset. Even when families understand that brain damage is causing the irritating, unreasonable, or violent behavior in a loved one, it is still difficult for them to tolerate the upsetting behavior. Feelings of hurt, anger, and frustration may become so unbearable that family members isolate themselves from friends. In some families this isolation only further increases the emotional turmoil and leads to a premature decision to institutionalize the patient. Other families may refuse to institutionalize their relative regardless of the disruption in the family.

Even families which have coped well for years may find they need help as the dementia worsens. Alice Chen and her husband, Frank, accompanied Alice's mother, Mei, and father, Hong, to see a physician. Hong was seventy-two and had been diagnosed as having Alzheimer's disease approximately six years earlier. The entire family was involved in the decision as to whether Hong should be moved to a nursing home. Mei and Hong had three other daughters (and sons-in-law) who could not be present for the meeting, because they either lived too far away or because work responsibilities prevented their attendance. However, all of them had reached the consensus that if their mother could not accept the help of a home care attendant, then perhaps it was time to think about an institution.

Over the past years the children had become more concerned about their parents. Their father had changed very gradually through the first five years, but in the past year he had begun to deteriorate more rapidly. Mr. Chen required more help with dressing, feeding, and other personal activities. Mrs. Chen managed well for a while, but she gradually became overwhelmed, as his nightly wanderings interrupted her ability to rest.

Family and close friends would visit and offer to schedule time to be with Hong and give her the opportunity to get away, sleep, sew, and resume her volunteer work at the local hospital. Mrs. Chen had been very active raising funds for her church. Even while her husband was sick, at least until the last six months, she had been on the phone and at meetings night and day to raise money. Mrs. Chen, however, refused help, and took great pride in caring for Hong by herself.

At the same time Mrs. Chen refused help she also placed her daughters in a double bind. She called them daily to ask them to visit her and keep her company, but then she withdrew and even asked them not to visit. She was a proud woman and embarrassed by her husband's behavior. He would shout obscenities, undress himself, or pace restlessly around the house throughout the day. It was the children's concern with this situation that precipitated a visit to us for professional assistance. They could not deal with repeated cries for help followed by rejection.

Mrs. Chen submitted to the children's demands to have a home care attendant. However, as might be expected, she had great difficulty surrendering the responsibilities of caring to anyone else. Mrs. Chen refused to leave her husband alone with the attendant, Bertha, and insisted on helping with every single task. Even though Bertha was a well-trained, bright, and sensitive individual who understood Mrs. Chen's feelings, she was becoming increasingly frustrated. Mrs. Chen was not just stubborn in her determination to care for her husband; she interfered with everything and was unfairly critical of everything Bertha attempted. Mrs. Chen would ask Bertha to feed her husband and in the middle of lunch would take over the feeding and criticize Bertha without cause. She would ask Bertha to bathe her husband and within minutes send her away, accusing her of being too rough. Or she would ask Bertha to accompany Mr. Chen on a walk, only to change her mind and insist that the two of them must help him to prevent him from falling.

In desperation Bertha called the oldest daughter, Lois, to plead for their intervention, or she would have to quit. She could not do her job with Mrs. Chen's interference. Bertha understood Mrs. Chen's suffering but sensed that Mrs. Chen was in a serious emotional state and needed help.

With great difficulty the children persuaded Mrs. Chen to see a counselor. After Mrs. Chen was treated successfully for a severe depression, the entire family agreed to several family therapy sessions to develop a plan for working together to care for Mr. Chen. Even though Mrs. Chen felt better, she resumed her old pattern of demanding and rejecting help from her family. This became one of several important family problems to be resolved.

Mrs. Chen described how she had cared for both of her parents when she was only a teenager. She nursed her mother for three years and her father for five years before they both died. Her brothers and sisters were all younger, and that left her with the burden of supporting the family and physically ministering to her parents. In the course of several discussions, Mrs. Chen's children learned a part of their mother's history that was new to them. They began to understand the basis for her double-bind behavior in regard to care giving.

Mrs. Chen was also able to relive painful memories and share her frustration that she had had no help in caring for her parents. She even believed that had she been able to do more, her parents might have lived. She wanted her children to care for their father (and her) with the same intense devotion she had rendered to her parents. At the same time she sheltered them the same way she had protected her own brothers and sisters. She was the oldest, and therefore it was her responsibility to do what needed to be done. This, too, was part of her culture. In the context of family discussions, Mrs. Chen and her family were able to understand each other better; they learned to collaborate in such a way as to share in the decisions and in the hands-on caring of Mr. Chen.

When families are in trouble, they can benefit a great deal from meeting together (if necessary with professionals) to discuss the needs, hurts, and rights of various family members, including those of the patient. Negotiations may unearth the various problems of all family members involved and lead to a plan of action to balance needs and responsibilities. Furthermore, as was evident in the foregoing description of the Chens, family interventions can bring to the surface those intergenerational and cultural issues which help explain an individual's behavior.

Continuous family negotiations are needed to help everyone decide what must be done to balance the needs of various family members with those of the patient. Since the patient is changing, however slowly, the delicate balance of family relationships is threatened, and family members must reevaluate what they are doing. Some family members may not be able to cope well, and if it is not possible to restore equilibrium in the family system, it is likely that some of its members, including the patient, will suffer. When serious conflicts between family members exist, a patient's care may be seriously jeopardized.

Sue Ellen Grant was seventy-seven years old and a widow. She had lived alone in her apartment for more than ten years since the death of her husband. According to her family she never seemed to recover from his death, and over the years she socially isolated herself from everyone, including her family. Mrs. Grant had three married sons, all of whom lived far away from her. The youngest, Teddy, was stationed in Europe. Richard, the oldest, was a minister whose parish was several hundred miles away, and although Todd lived the closest, he was still more than a two-hour drive away. Teddy had joined the armed forces at an early age and was estranged from his brothers. However, each month he sent his mother short letters with a check. Todd was a successful banker who had little time for his family, and it was Todd's wife who called Mrs. Grant several times a week. Richard was very attached to his mother. He called her daily and visited at least once a month with his family. In the last year he had noticed that she had some mild memory problems and often forgot what she was saying or repeated stories over and over.

Several events caused Richard to become greatly distressed. His mother called him several times with complaints that her landlord was trying to poison her and that men in dark hoods entered her home at night. Richard visited her to investigate, and it was clear that she was very paranoid and needed help. There was rotten food in the refrigerator, piles of newspapers were stacked throughout the house, and she was very forgetful.

When Richard tried to arrange to have his mother see a doctor, Todd objected violently, insisting that she was only old and a little eccentric, just as she had been for her entire life. When Richard argued that she was quite sick and that Todd should see for himself, Todd did visit, and promptly took his mother home with him. However, within three days Mrs. Grant was back in her apartment, and Todd was more insistent than ever that nothing was wrong with her.

Mrs. Grant immediately began to call Richard at all hours of the day and night. She was afraid to be alone because her neighbors were plotting to kidnap her or poison her with gas. Once she claimed to have been raped by several of the hooded men. Sometimes she would call in the middle of the night, thinking it was morning.

Richard contacted several doctors and with their assistance persuaded his mother to check into the hospital for a complete examination. Although Todd objected, the rest of the family, including his
own wife, insisted that she get help. Mrs. Grant's paranoia was
successfully treated, and she even seemed to enjoy the experience of
being in the hospital. However, the results of the medical, neurological, psychiatric, and psychological evaluations all suggested Alzheimer's disease. She had serious memory deficits and would not be
able to live safely in her home.

The medical team insisted that Richard, Todd, and their wives
meet together with them to discuss discharge options. Todd domi-
nated the discussion. He was angry throughout the conference,
insisting that his mother had been taken to the hospital against her
will, that she was old enough to be a little senile, and there was no
good reason for her to need any additional medical help. He refused
to talk directly with his brother and would speak only with his wife.

The meeting concluded with everyone tired and angry, except for
Mrs. Grant, who was present for part of the conference. She felt that
she was ready to go home and live by herself as before. She admitted
to being a little afraid but thought all would be well once she was
settled in her apartment. Todd insisted that he would take his
mother home with him for a few weeks and then find another
apartment for her close to them. Richard protested vigorously, but
he was exhausted from caring for his mother as well as from his
demanding duties at the parish. He and his wife had also suffered
a major tragedy. Their eighteen-year-old son had been killed in a car
accident two months earlier.

Within a week of discharge, Mrs. Grant was again alone in her
home, calling Richard day and night. She was confused and paranoid. Richard began to search for alternative housing arrangements
for his mother, since it was clear she could not live alone. Todd called
Richard several times, accusing Richard of trying to take his mother
away from him. The bitterness of Todd's sibling rivalry tortured
Richard. He wanted to help his mother, and he was angered and
hurt by Todd's lack of cooperation and angry assaults, which
impeded all of his efforts.

On the same day Richard had completed arrangements for his
mother to move into a health-related facility, Todd "kidnapped"

her. He told the family that he had taken her away to care for her, but he would not tell anyone, not even his own wife, of her whereabouts. Richard called a close friend of his brother to use whatever influence he had with Todd to bring him to the discussion table. The talks began but broke off many times over a period of a month, before the "mediator" asked to remove himself from the emotional deadlock.

Richard made the difficult decision to call the police. Todd was forced to divulge his mother's location. The police found her locked in Todd's country home, malnourished and extremely confused. Todd had hired someone to look after her, but the attendant had visited her only once a day to bring food. Mrs. Grant was hospitalized, her physical health was restored, and she moved into a nursing home near Richard. Richard refused to press charges against his brother.

Family dynamics are extremely complex. Powerful loyalties bind family members together, and although many of these forces are nurturing, others are destructive. Mrs. Grant's son Todd interfered with her care, despite his perception that he was helping her. If circumstances had been different, Richard might have been able to work around Todd. However, in this situation Todd's denial of the reality of his mother's problem, coupled with his own psychopathology, created trouble.

This sad family saga is clearly an extreme example of how an older parent with Alzheimer's disease further unbalances the complex relationships among family members. Unless significant disruption exists in a family, regular meetings are an effective way to minimize family conflict, to anticipate future problems, and to develop alternative solutions in order to care effectively for the patient. The process of developing contingency plans is one of the most effective means of minimizing stress. It also provides opportunities for family members to examine how they can best cooperate with each other in various situations.

In preparing for family meetings, each member would do well to prepare a list of issues, as is done in labor-management negotiations. Identify the important issues, write down the steps needed for a solution, and specify exactly what you will do and what you expect others to contribute. Clearly, this analogy is a limited one because of the special nature of family commitments, but the approach has real merit as a way of discussing problems and solutions. If you become deadlocked, bring in a mediator, who can be a trusted friend, a clergyman, or a health professional. Mediators can help identify the loyalties and obligations people feel toward each other and get family members to deal with each other's needs. Some conflict is normal in this process. The discovery and ventilation of angry feelings is healthy and paves the way for constructive actions to help correct the situation.

Talking about feelings and difficulties associated with caring may sometimes be done productively with the patient present. Great caution needs to be exercised to avoid the mistake of blaming the patient. When the focus of the meeting is planning, however, it is valuable to have the patient share in the experience.

## The Effects of Dementia on Children

Young children and adolescents may find it extremely difficult to accept that a parent or grandparent has dementia. They may not understand the strange behavior of someone they love and admire even when they are aware that something is wrong, and for some the explanation that the behavior is due to an illness seems to have no meaning. They may withdraw from friends and family or become angry and rebellious. Children vary in the way they cope, and many factors are important—the child's age, the number of other children in the family, the closeness of the relationship between the child and the patient, the culture the child lives in, and the availability of other family members. Some children assume the role of a care giver in the household, whereas others are unable to deal with a "changed" parent and become more childlike in dealing with the healthy parent. Occasionally, young children and even teenagers who cannot understand what they interpret as a loss of interest or of love by a patient may act out, becoming demanding and rebellious, or show violent outbursts, and generally misbehave at home and school. Clearly, these behaviors create even more stress in the family.

Some children seem unaware of their parent's suffering or seem to adapt to it. Others become preoccupied with worries about parental loss or about the possibility that they will become sick like their mother or father. Dr. James Turner was a young, respected surgeon in his late thirties whose father, uncles, and grandfather had each developed Alzheimer's disease sometime between the ages of sixty and sixty-five. He was married and the father of a three-year-old girl, Beth. Both he and his wife, Ann, talked openly with each other (and once in a while consulted their clergyman) about the possibility that he would someday get the disease. Both were actively involved in the care of Jim's father, and everyone, including their young daughter, frequently visited the nursing home.

Jim had two wisdom teeth extracted and spent several days at home recovering from the oral surgery. The first afternoon, Beth crawled next to him on the couch and asked, "Daddy, is this the beginning? Are you starting to get Grandpa's disease? . . . I have a toothache too. Will I lose my memory before I have a chance to grow up?"

There are several guidelines for dealing with younger children. First, it is important to involve children at a level appropriate to their ability to understand and participate in family activities. In the earlier phase of dementia and when the patient is not aggressive or violent, the presence of infant grandchildren can bring laughter and smiles. For the most part young children should not be kept away from the patient. Hiding a relative with dementia only makes the person and situation more difficult for a child to understand. Even two- and three-year-old children are able to sense their parents' anxieties and fears. Children learn many of their fears from others. Involve them with you and the patient, and let them see and feel your comfort. Whenever possible find time to be alone with your children. Talk simply and directly. Provide opportunities for them to be around the patient and to do even simple tasks like carrying food and drink or playing in the same room with the patient.

Children often give us valuable insights into our own attitudes and behaviors. Sometimes another person, usually an outsider, is necessary to help us see accurately what is actually happening. Robert Blanc, a fifty-two-year-old retired mechanic, had been diagnosed as having Alzheimer's disease more than three years earlier. His wife, Louise, and two daughters, Cindy and Marjorie, had been doing well until Mr. Blanc started to become more agitated and combative. The younger daughter, Cindy, aged seventeen, whom everyone reported to be a great deal like her father, had a rebellious relationship with her father prior to the diagnosis. Following his diagnosis Cindy withdrew from everyone and became sullen. The arguments with her father intensified, and within six months Cindy angrily moved out of the house. She refused to confide in her sister or her mother. She spoke of her father as an arrogant, stubborn, unfair person, and the anger spilled out into all of her relationships, with girlfriends at school as well as with her boyfriend.

One of the teachers at the high school finally called Mrs. Blanc to arrange a meeting. Irene Dalton had been Cindy's student adviser and teacher. Mrs. Dalton had also been Cindy's hockey coach for several years and had become a special person in Cindy's life. In the course of the meeting, Irene relayed what Cindy had confided to her over the past several months.

Cindy was angry not only with her father but with her mother as well. She resented the fact that no one had told her about the seriousness of her father's memory problems or the many doctor appointments which led to the diagnosis. Her response to her anger was to cut the family out of her life. The only person she had been able to talk to for any length of time was her father, and now she was so blinded by her anger that she could not accept his illness. Instead of dealing effectively with her hurt, she lashed out against all of her family. She rejected her family because she felt that they had rejected her. She also had deep feelings of rejection by her father because he was not the father she knew. He was there and not there at the same time.

Irene recommended that Louise take a brief weekend trip with both her daughters. She thought that the lack of communication between them could be repaired. The relationship between Cindy and her father could also be improved but would probably be handled best with some professional help.

## Guidelines for Families to Evaluate Coping Skills

Is there a healthy family response to caring? Yes, the healthy family is one that is able to cope with change. Is there one right way to cope with change? No. There are no easy prescriptions, and there is no prototype for the healthy family. There are many different ways to successfully respond to the challenge of caring for a relative with dementia. Families differ in numerous ways, and the history of what happens to every person within and across generations affects how each responds as an individual and as a member of the family.

There are several questions family members can ask themselves to evaluate their coping skills as a family unit. Asking questions and searching for answers helps care givers adapt to the challenge of caring.

1. What was the patient like before the disease? Was he or she open and sharing with the family or aloof? Did he or she have close friends or keep counsel only to themselves? Did he or she express anger or happiness easily, or was he or she emotionally controlled? Family expectations for the patient's behavior must be consistent with the individual's previous personality style. There are no "gold standards" for how a patient should behave throughout the course of the illness.

2. Who is providing most of the care—husband or wife, children, brothers or sisters, in-laws, or perhaps a parent? Is there a natural leader in the family to whom everyone looks to for decision making? Do several members of the family share the burden of caring? If one person such as a spouse, dominates the caring, does he or she know how to ask for help or let others help? Solving problems together and sharing the burden of caring is a continuing challenge to the family.

3. How did the patient relate to other members of the family prior to the diagnosis? If relationships were ruptured or if conflict was prominent, is it feasible to repair the relationships before the patient deteriorates, or is it better to leave things alone? If the patient was married several times, is it possible for the different families to relate to each other, if only around the care of the patient?

4. If the patient is married, is the relationship a stable one? If long-standing disruptive marital conflict preceded the diagnosis, it will probably continue or worsen. What steps, if any, can children or other family members take to ensure the safety and care of the patient and still respect the autonomy of the couple? Is professional help useful?

5. How close do family members live to the patient or to the patient and spouse? What plans can be made to allow distant family members to participate in caring? If geographically close relatives feel overburdened, what steps can be taken to remedy imbalances or perceived imbalances?

6. How well are different family members accepting the diagnosis? Does anyone need professional help?

7. Does anyone else in the immediate family suffer from a major physical or emotional illness? When several people are sick the family's emotional and financial resources are strained. It is not uncommon for family members to feel that a child with leukemia, an adult with multiple sclerosis, or a younger paraplegic relative is "more deserving" of family resources. Families often face difficult decisions which need to be made carefully, and often with help.

8. Are there any recent life crises affecting other members in the family? Did someone die, lose a job, get married and move away, or go to jail? Many major as well as minor unpleasant life events can disrupt families. The family's ability to deal both with the stresses of everyday life and with major crises potentially jeopardizes the balance of care for the patient.

9. How well-informed is everyone in the family about dementia and the problems of caring?

10. How well do family members cooperate with each other to solve problems around the patient's care? It is sometimes useful to get outside help to improve the communication patterns among family members. It is often possible to find solutions to a problem if individuals are able to avoid conflicts of style and personality. Sometimes the way people talk interferes with the message. Anxiety, anger, and other emotions often color a conversation and precipitate unnecessary arguments.

11. Do family members take responsibility for what they do and say, or do they blame others? When things go wrong, it is easy to say it is the other person's fault. In family meetings focusing on the patient's problems, try to examine your own actions honestly.

12. Do family members listen to one another and are they sensitive to each other? Do people speak for one another rather than let the other individuals speak for themselves? Do family members let patient speak up or do they "bury" the patient? It is important to give patients time to talk. It often takes them longer to make a response, and this may be difficult to do in a group where people tend to interact quickly with one another. Remember,

patients often experience the world differently. Their world may be slower, less coherent, and less organized.

13. Have financial matters been addressed? Unless these issues are being solved, anxiety about money may color discussions about everything else. This is not unusual. Throughout the lives of most people, financial transactions have been known to cause many domestic arguments.

14. Are there irresolvable conflicts in the family? If so, seek help. Families are complex systems, and it is not legitimate to expect to change an entire family. However, it is realistic to focus the family on the needs of the patient as a member of the family.

Changes do not occur immediately. It takes time to work on problems, and when solutions are identified, implementing them also takes time. The cruel reality of dementia allows time to live and to fight for meaning and happiness.

# 9

# REHABILITATION: A FOCUS ON FUNCTION

---

"YOU have a beautiful chapel. Will you let me visit sometime?" Shirley Everitt, a victim of Alzheimer's disease, spoke those words as she and her attendant, Henrik, took their morning walk. Before Henrik could answer, Shirley darted into the dark room, walked to the front row, and sat down. He followed and sat down next to her. Shirley turned and whispered quietly, "Follow those trees up the hill to the stone wall and push open the gate. You will see my house in front of you."

Henrik placed his hand on hers and replied, "I don't think we will find your house there. But we are in a house now . . . a house of God, the chapel. Do you want to stay here awhile?" Shirley nodded and said, "I wonder if we have gone out of our minds. I want to go home, but I can't find it. This place looks familiar. But there is no chandelier, no fountain, no furniture. I will sit here and wait for it to change. We can read this book."

Henrik opened a prayer book and gave it to her. Shirley sat holding the book for several minutes. She then stood and circled the room as if looking for something. She touched each of the colored glass windows and said, "This glass will have to be replaced. I want new ones. We have to keep this place in shape. This house is messy, and people will be here soon. We can't have people see it this way."

Henrik agreed with her. She was right. The chapel was in a state of disarray, and the windows were dirty. The two of them spent about an hour cleaning things up. They stacked the prayer books, moved tables and chairs, and even dusted the altar. When they were finished, Shirley wanted to sit down again. "The windows are still dirty," she said, "but you'll do that later, Henrik, won't you? I like my house. You may call me at my house anytime now."

As long as Shirley could walk or be pushed in a wheelchair, Henrik would take her to the chapel regularly. On some days she enjoyed simple cleaning tasks, but most of the time she seemed happy to spend time there—sometimes it was minutes, sometimes hours. Although Shirley deteriorated quickly and became increasingly confused and unable to express herself clearly, Henrik could understand her needs most of the time, keep her occupied, and make her comfortable. Up until the last few months of her life, when Shirley was confined to bed, the chapel retained its special meaning.

During her last months Henrik arranged for students from a nearby divinity school to visit Shirley regularly. Several of the young men even set up a small altar in her room. After that, other nursing-home residents would gather in her room when the priests visited to pray or talk. Even though Shirley was dying, she was continually surrounded by the people who cared for her.

Several weeks before her death a young priest was playing his guitar in her room. More than twenty residents and staff spilled out of her room into the hall listening. After an hour the priest finally placed his guitar in its case. As he bent over Shirley's bed to say good-bye, she reached for his hand and kissed it. Only the priest and Henrik could see the tears in her eyes. Even though Alzheimer's disease had rendered her frail, helpless, and unable to speak, Shirley Everitt could still communicate with others.

Shirley Everitt and others like her are evidence that dementia is not a hopeless condition for which nothing can be done. Patients are human beings—first, last, and always. They usually live for years with the disease, and those are long and difficult years. The challenge during that time is to maximize an individual's ability to function at the highest possible level.

Rehabilitation is an important concept in the care of dementia victims. It is both a philosophy and a technology. As a philosophy, rehabilitation is the way we think about people's problems and make decisions about what we do or do not do to increase their ability to function. For example, if a dementia patient develops a disease of the hip the response may be a wheelchair and institutionalization after hospitalization rather than orthopedic surgery and physical rehabilitation, with walking as a reasonable goal. Surgical decisions should be made on the basis of information about a person's physical health and orthopedic status, as well as the severity of the dementia. However, the presence of dementia per se should not be a deterrent to appropriate treatment. When a child, young adult, or middle-age person sustains a disability, parents and family as well as doctors are usually aggressive in finding ways to reduce the degree of handicap. This usually includes some form of rehabilitation. Unfortunately, a diagnosis of dementia often leads to professional nihilism toward the patient—an attitude of "Why do anything? The patient has Alzheimer's disease."

Intellectual decline should not by itself be a barrier to rehabilitation. Cognitively impaired older persons deserve to be treated as people. Patients often develop a number of such disabling conditions and disorders as arthritis, osteoporosis, immobilization, fractures, incontinence, and infections. It is important to do everything possible to rehabilitate the patient and restore function when possible. What you learn here, from other medical sources (see reference list at the end of this book), and from your doctor will, we hope, not only help you maintain your relative's comfort and mobility but also lessen the need for hospitalization or premature institutionalization.

Even when patients are living in a nursing home, a great deal can be done to keep them mobile and active. Although many nursing homes have active rehabilitation programs for residents, family members should become vigorous advocates for the patient. They have an important responsibility to work with nursing-home staff, and they often need to be aggressive with administrators and other staff. Being aggressive here means taking time to meet with various professionals, asking questions about realistic expectations for a program of care, including rehabilitation, and teaching staff what you would like them to know about your relative—what he or she was like before the dementia. Help them see the human side of the patient and let them know your expectations.

The first week after Rachel Breton had moved her husband, Jean, into the nursing home, she made appointments with everyone on the staff—all the administrators, the nurses and nurse's aides, and the director of social services as well as the social workers assigned to her husband, the medical director, the dietician, and the recreational, occupational, and rehabilitation therapists. She wanted them to know a little about him as the man she had lived with, not just the frail, angry, agitated figure who had been wasted by Alzheimer's disease for the past seven years.

She began each talk the same way.

I know you are terribly busy. I will only stay a short while. Here I have a few photographs of Jean taken at different times in his life. He was born in 1893 to a poor Parisian family. His father died when he was fourteen, and in 1909 he moved his mother and his four brothers and sisters to the United States. He worked very hard to support them.

"We met in 1915 and were married within the year. We had no children and have spent the past sixty years together. He was a good man and spent his life helping others.

"I know his condition is getting worse, but I want him to be as comfortable and happy as possible. He can still walk, and he enjoys other people when he is not in one of his angry moods. I know some ways to control that. He needs to have regular exercise every day. I do not want him to be in a wheelchair. What will you do to help him live out the rest of his days? I wish I could keep him at home. Since that is impossible, I will do what I can to help you here.

The staff members were receptive to Mrs. Breton's questions and desire to help with her husband. She was pleasant yet persistent. She wanted to know what could be done as well as what she could do. Needless to say, there were times when staff felt Mrs. Breton was making unrealistic demands on them; likewise, there were situations in which she was legitimately upset with his care. She was an aggressive, loving advocate for her husband, just as she had been throughout their life.

Not all nursing homes have administrators and staff as receptive to family involvement as the last example indicates. There are many reasons for this, but whatever the reason, families have the right to see that a relative is receiving optimal care. Do not let staff brush you aside. The director of volunteer services, a clergyman, or a patient advocate can be valuable informants to help you understand and deal with the personalities in a nursing home. Remember that staff may not always be the obstacles. Your own anger, sadness, or guilt may be so great as to interfere with your ability to deal with other people. Even when your message is legitimate—"I want the proper therapy for my relative"—it may not be heard if the staff react to your anger. These emotions are natural reactions in care givers who have moved someone into an institution, but it is futile to take your anger out on those who could be your allies.

Families and professionals have an important responsibility to work together as a team. Goals need to be established and plans implemented to keep patients healthy, active, and comfortable. The mandate for everyone involved with patients is to have a realistic set of expectations based on assessments of the patients' physical cognitive and emotional status. It is also important to understand the personality of the patients. Who were they? What were their accomplishments in life? What were they like before the dementia? Knowing the person behind the mask of dementia is often the first step to successful rehabilitation. "Rehab" embodies the principle that the individual has a distinctive personality with specific physical and emotional needs and the potential to restore functioning.

## Identifying and Stabilizing Treatable Disabilities

When is it realistic to attempt to restore physical, mental, and social functioning? How are decisions made to help dementia victims overcome their disabilities to the full extent possible? Before answering these questions, we will do well first to identify different treatable problem areas: (1) chronic diseases, (2) conditions that reduce mobility, (3) psychiatric illness accompanying the dementia, (4) social rehabilitation, and (5) rehabilitation of life skills.

Very specific rehabilitation goals in each of these areas can be defined if the patient is evaluated properly. Family members should search carefully for the right team of people to help them. Rehabilitation is a necessary process throughout the course of dementia.

When the patient is living at home, it takes time and effort to find health professionals unless a good home care agency is available. As was discussed earlier, rehabilitation specialists are available in most nursing homes. In addition to rehabilitation specialists, the people to look for include physicians who specialize in chronic conditions, psychologists, nurses, social workers, physical and occupational therapists, audiologists, speech therapists, podiatrists, and, where available, dance therapists and exercise specialists.

## Recognizing and Stabilizing Chronic Conditions

If your relative has one of the chronic conditions briefly discussed below, ask the doctors about treatment strategies. Families that want to learn more can consult the references in the back of this book or search out reading materials in medical libraries.

### OSTEOARTHRITIS

Osteoarthritis is a condition in which the cartilage of the joints degenerates and inflammatory reactions occur in the surrounding tissue. Physical therapy combined with anti-inflammatory drugs is often an effective means of improving mobility and easing pain.

### RHEUMATOID ARTHRITIS

Rheumatoid arthritis may occur suddenly, with severe inflammation in the joints, or it may progress for years and gradually incapacitate the individual. Anti-inflammatory medications are the treatment of choice. Question your doctor carefully about anti-inflammatory therapy and especially about the side effects of these medications. Enteric-coated salicylate drugs like diclofenac sodium and ibuprofen are often effective and have few side effects. Naproxen is another drug which has been shown to reduce inflammation. Small doses of steroids may be effective when the objective is to keep the patient comfortable in later stages of the illness.

All anti-inflammatory drugs should be given with food. The patient should be monitored very carefully, because side effects are very common in the aged and because patients with dementia living at home may take them more frequently than is safe for them.

## PAIN

Rheumatoid disease, osteoporosis, and many other conditions are all painful. Treating pain in patients with dementia requires careful observation of the patients. Often we do not know how much pain they experience, because of language and cognitive losses. Poor memory tends to prevent them from describing the onset of symptoms.

Drugs should be used carefully, with the smallest dose to achieve pain relief with the fewest side effects. When the patient is in constant or extreme pain, drugs should be given on a regular schedule. This may sound simple, but in the best hospitals and nursing homes the need to care for many patients or staff shortages may disrupt these simple routines.

Morphine and addictive medications should be avoided whenever possible. However, in the later stages of dementia, near the end of the patient's life, the use of these agents should be considered. They may provide comfort for whatever limited time remains. Since we know so little about the world of late-stage patients, because of their inability to communicate, regular physical examinations and careful monitoring are essential.

## MUSCULOSKELETAL DISORDERS

Osteoporosis, progressive bone loss, causes significant disability, especially when there is a history of fractures of the spine, hips, arms, and legs. The most important treatment is to keep the individual active. Walking as much as possible is important. Bed rest leads not only to more immobility but also to more bone loss.

Consult your physician about other forms of treatment. Calcium supplements and Vitamin D, when prescribed by the doctor, may be useful. Three eight-ounce glasses of milk contain the daily requirement of 1.5 grams of calcium. Milk substitutes are available for patients who are allergic to the lactose in milk. The use of estrogens and sodium fluoride must be carefully justified by your doctor.

MULTIPLE CHRONIC DISEASES

The older patient with dementia often has several different disabling conditions. Diabetes, heart disease, resppiratory disease, and many other disorders are severe problems by themselves; when they exist together in the same person, especially in the very old impaired patient, they may be profoundly disabling and painful. How do we understand impaired patients' needs when they are withdrawn, agitated, or violent, when they talk and act as if in another world? How do we measure their discomfort? Severely demented patients who are living their last years in the nursing home pose an enormous and complex challenge to staff members and family. A thorough knowledge of patients' medical conditions, the potential for pain, and astute observation of their behavior are crucial. Family members can make a considerable difference by working closely with professionals to monitor the patient.

SURGERY

When is corrective orthopedic surgery helpful to the older dementia patient? This is an important and difficult question. Family members should get several medical opinions when patients have peripheral vascular disease, soft-tissue contractures, or a wide variety of other anatomical impairments. Dementia patients should not be denied appropriate corrective surgery and therapies. However, the decision for surgery requires a careful evaluation of medical risks as well as the potential benefit to the patient.

## Maximizing Mobility in Frail Dementia Patients

Although keeping patients active is relatively easy in earlier stages of dementia, keeping them active and mobile in later phases becomes more difficult. But physical activity in later stages is vital. Bed and chair rest and prolonged immobility usually lead to even more immobilization. Rehabilitation efforts should focus on walking, where possible, and appropriate exercises to limber up stiff limbs.

There are many profound disabling consequences when even the frail older patient is not kept active within the safe limits of their condition. Read the list below carefully and ask your doctor what is being done to ensure that your relative is being cared for in ways that protect him or her from these disabling conditions:

- loss of muscle tone and strength
- stiffness and contractures
- accelerated osteoporosis
- thrombosis in arteries or veins
- pressure sores, known as decubiti
- dehydration and malnutrition
- urinary-tract infections, incontinence, urinary retention
- constipation, impaction, incontinence
- chest infections

Although there are limits on what can be done to mobilize the patient as the dementia progresses, families should discuss these issues with health professionals to feel confident that appropriate decisions are being made to care for their relative's comfort and well-being.

DEHYDRATION

Many dementia patients do not have an adequate intake of liquids. At the very minimum six to eight glasses of liquids are required daily. Dehydration causes fatigue, apathy, constipation, and abdominal discomfort because the concentrated urine irritates the bladder.

INCONTINENCE

There are many different causes of incontinence, but in most instances it can be prevented. During aging, the bladder becomes smaller and more insensitive to stretching. The result is that the urge to empty the bladder comes when the bladder is almost full. In men, prostate problems may cause retention of urine with "overflow incontinence." In women, constipation may block the bladder, so that urine leaks past the blockage point when the pressure has increased sufficiently.

The more immobilized the patient, the greater the risk of incontinence. Simply being in a bed with guard rails, restraints, and anything that causes immobility increases the risk. The absence of a commode near the bed may make it impossible for the individual to go to the bathroom.

In many cases getting the patient to the bathroom regularly will prevent incontinence. In more cognitively impaired patients it may be necessary to schedule trips to the bathroom every two hours and be watchful for warning signs. Although language is impaired, patients may reach for their belt or groin and look distressed.

When the incontinence cannot be controlled, diapering the patient respectfully becomes necessary. An indwelling catheter is hardly ever recommended, because infections are inevitable and lead to other problems. Catheters are necessary only when the patient has significant skin sores or when there are other strong medical reasons.

A thorough continence diagnostic evaluation is important because there are so many possible causes of incontinence. Make sure the doctors conduct a thorough history and physical examination, including laboratory analysis of a urine specimen, if "bladder training" does not work. If the cause of the incontinence is still unknown, a series of urodynamic tests can determine how well the urinary system is functioning. This may also include cystoscopy, a procedure for directly observing the bladder. These procedures are uncomfortable, involve the risks of repeated catheterization, and are expensive. They may or may not be practical and beneficial with the dementia patient. Caring for the patient requires continual decisions about what helps and what hurts.

CONSTIPATION AND IMPACTION

Adequate fluids and fiber are needed to prevent fecal incontinence. Eating bran with cereals, drinking at least six to eight glasses of fluid, and getting adequate exercise will usually maintain regular, comfortable bowel movements. Sometimes it is necessary to use stool softeners when patients have a history of constipation.

Untreated constipation leads to fecal impaction—hard feces that block the rectum. This not only is a serious physical problem but also tends to be associated with very agitated behavior. A rectal examination is necessary to diagnose the problem; once it is discovered, the bowels must be cleaned.

## PRESSURE SORES

Pressure sores, or decubiti, can be prevented by turning bedridden patients every two hours and using special mattresses to keep pressure from reducing local circulation. Pressure sores start as red irritated areas with reduced blood circulation and proceed to become ulcers , which may spread deep and wide. They are extremely painful and may take months to control and heal.

Bedridden dementia patients are vulnerable especially if they are frail and malnourished. Individuals at risk should be examined daily. The key to prevention is early recognition of red skin areas.

## THROMBOSIS

Confinement to bed impedes the return of blood from the legs to the heart. In normal circumstances the blood is moved through the veins by one-way valves in the vessels and by the movement of the leg muscles. Thrombophlebitis occurs when a clot forms, most commonly in the legs or pelvic area. If a clot breaks off, is passed through the circulation, and is caught in the lungs, this condition is called pulmonary embolism. Nothing may happen, or the patient may die suddenly. These individuals are at high risk for chest infections. If pulmonary embolism persists, the patient may develop progressive breathing problems.

Activity and adequate intake of fluids will often prevent thrombosis. When patients with dementia have had hip surgery, low doses of heparin—an anticoagulant, or blood-thinning agent—may be helpful for certain patients. Discuss this with the doctor. Even in severely impaired patients massage and passive range-of-motion exercises help ward off circulation problems. Automated massage devices are expensive but effective in patients at high risk for embolism.

## POOR NUTRITION

Malnutrition is a common problem for the frail older person with dementia because many eat improperly. Dietary consultation is a crucial aspect of patient rehabilitation. Wounds do not heal, teeth and gums decay, weakness and apathy result. This is an area in which families can educate themselves by consulting the references at the end of this book. In nursing homes and hospitals, do not hesitate to be gently aggressive with the dietary department.

## CARDIOVASCULAR DISEASE

Diet and exercise are important factors in the reduction of vascular disease even in the older cognitively impaired patient. When individuals have high blood pressure, it should be controlled and monitored carefully. Spend time with the doctors to understand the impact of different vascular diseases on the dementia. Ask them to explain to you what is being done when congestive heart failure, arteriosclerotic heart disease, high blood pressure, arrhythmias, diabetes, and other conditions are present in the patient.

## ORAL HYGIENE

Regular dental care is essential, as are regular brushing, adequate hydration, and a nutritious, balanced diet. Eating is one of the great pleasures of life for many people. Rotting teeth and sore gums make eating difficult, unpleasant, and often painful.

## FOOT CARE

A good podiatrist will help prevent many foot problems. It is difficult to walk when feet are swollen and cracked, toenails are long and thick, and fungal infections are present. Regular care is needed, as well as properly fitting shoes.

## INFECTIONS

Patients with advanced dementia appear to be extremely vulnerable to infections. Regular, thorough physical examinations and immunization are important. Pneumonia and influenza vaccines should be given each year. Also check to see that the patient is current with diphtheria and tetanus shots.

Urinary-tract infections can be prevented by appropriate exercise, adequate intake of fluids, and avoidance of catheterization. Frail dementia patients are at high risk for pneumonia, a common cause of death. Mobilizing the patient as much as possible, proper hydration, and chest therapy go a long way toward helping prevent pneumonia.

FALLS

Keeping patients mobile and active carries the risk that they will fall. However, in many instances the consequences of not moving around may be more serious than the degree of risk from falling. Falling is an issue that must be considered carefully; when the risk is high for certain patients, careful management with appropriate exercise patterns is important.

Many factors increase the likelihood that patients will fall. Work with the doctor and other professionals to evaluate the following problems:

· poor vision
· loss of peripheral vision
· poor night vision
· unstable walk and swaying
· coordination problems
· muscular stiffness
· osteoporosis
· postural hypotension (dizziness caused when people stand up quickly)

The larger the number of problem areas in the above list, the higher the risk of falling. However, a few practical environmental alterations can be made to help the patient compensate for some problem areas. Canes, walkers, and wall handrails help patients get around. Low tables and chairs and uneven floors are hazardous. Carpeting and throw rugs should be secured. Chairs should be solid, with arms but no rollers that bear the weight of a person sitting down or standing up.

Certain conditions seem to cause repeated falls. These include irregular heart rhythm, epilepsy, cerebrovascular disease, heart failure, and diseases causing dizziness or vertigo. A number of medications may cause dizziness, increasing the likelihood of falls. Dementia patients deserve regular "falls evaluations" by the internist, psychiatrist, and neurologist to determine their vulnerability, so that care givers can plan accordingly.

## Recognizing and Treating Psychiatric Disturbances

See Chapter 5, which discusses the recognition and treatment of psychiatric conditions that may coexist with the dementia—depression, anxiety, paranoia, and sleep disorders.

## Social Rehabilitation

Family, friends, and acquaintances, social and professional contacts, co-workers, and other people around us are an important part of our lives. One of the greatest challenges to everyone involved with the patient is to keep the patient socially engaged. Since other people affect our feelings about ourself, our life satisfaction, and even our health, working with the patient's social network is often an effective means of reinforcing feelings of independence and self-worth. Friends help us believe in ourselves when we see ourselves as less valuable. Other people are thus important resources for rehabilitating the patient's motivation to continue to live and feel wanted.

Scientists have long known that social ties have a profound impact on physical and mental health, but they do not know exactly how they do so. One theory is that social relationships give people a feeling of support that, in turn, leads to a sense of control which is important for health. Another theory suggests that people important in our lives help us stay healthy and force us to seek medical help when we need it. Still other scientists propose that support from our family and friends helps us adapt to stress and that this in turn prevents illness.

## Occupational Therapy and Rehabilitation of Life Skills

Occupational therapy is a profession in which registered occupational therapists teach patients skills necessary for the activities of daily living. During the course of dementia, individuals gradually develop more difficulties in taking care of themselves, in doing what each of us does every day—we dress, bathe, eat, go to the toilet, groom ourselves, get around, work, and play.

Although cognitive losses affect many things the patient tries to do, occupational therapists can help the family and patient understand what the limitations imposed by the dementia are and what can be remedied. Occupational therapists help patients learn to use strategies and techniques to compensate for losses. Many stroke patients have lost function in parts of their body and have cognitive losses as well.

Special attention should be paid to ensure that patients are doing the appropriate exercises to strengthen muscles and restore maximum function. It is common even with patients who have access to good medical care to find that they are not doing what they should to rehabilitate themselves.

Occupational therapists examine social and physical barriers in the home or institutional environment which impede the individuals' ability to do for themselves. Family members may insist on dressing patients because it seems simpler, when patients can in fact do much of it themselves if some accommodations are made. In later stages of the dementia, if patients are confined to a wheelchair, the clothes rack in the closet may be too high for them to reach. Shorter racks can be built or purchased. If motor dexterity or hand impairments make buttoning difficult, pullover clothes should be substituted or Velcro fasteners used. Families need to understand when memory losses are the problem and when other problems inhibit patients from helping themselves.

Many patients in long-term-care institutions have coexisting problems like Parkinson's disease or other physical diseases which further reduce functional abilities. Many specialized devices are available. Eating utensils and cups come in many different sizes, weights, and shapes. A weighted spoon may help patients who have hand tremors eat by themselves. Spoons with long handles are useful when a patient's arm range is restricted. Although many types of specialized equipment are available, much of it is expensive and should be purchased only after a thorough professional evaluation of the patient's limitation and assets.

Patients may also need special equipment in order to participate in leisure-time activities. Devices are available that enable individuals with a paralyzed arm to hold playing cards or books. There are ways to help people write letters, knit, crochet, build furniture, and do many other tasks.

## The Courage to Live

Much of what occupies daily life is very ordinary and task oriented —shutting off the alarm clock, getting out of bed, walking to the bathroom, bathing, preparing coffee and breakfast, turning on the TV or radio for the morning news, and so forth. It is difficult to imagine not being able to hold a fork or spoon and to move it to our mouth, not being able to swallow juice from a straw, or not being able to move our own body out of bed and to the bathroom.

The losses of dementia tear the family fabric. However, the family can triumph over dementia if everything has been done to prevent physical deterioration, to rehabilitate patients as much as possible, and to keep them active. Even the most impaired patients can be active if the tasks are simple enough. Seeing and smelling flowers, watching people and traffic on the street, watching children play ball, walking through a park, sitting on a dock watching boats, walking along a beach collecting shells, drinking a beer or a glass or wine, listening to music, or having a photograph taken—all these things and many more can be done to stimulate life.

One patient's husband brought a mocha cake and a bottle of champagne to the nursing home for his wife's eighty-fifth birthday. Elmira Jones had been a victim of Alzheimer's disease for thirteen years and was now confined to a wheelchair or bed for most of the day. She did not speak except for incoherent sentences or an occasional yes or no. Mrs. Jones enjoyed the cake but refused the champagne. However, when her husband and the staff raised their glasses to toast her, she smiled and clutched her glass. After the party Mrs. Jones quietly watched her aide clean the room, but she cried out when the aide went to throw the champagne bottle in the wastebasket. The aide heard her and placed the magnum on the window where she could see it. Even after her husband left that day, Mrs. Jones would not let go of her glass. How many of us have saved matches from a restaurant, a wine label or bottle, or pressed flowers to remember a special occasion. Simple pleasures are often available even to the most impaired.

## The Future

With research advances, we can hope, there will come more techniques and devices to help rehabilitate patients and help them cope with losses and live life to its fullest. Rehabilitation research is a focus of many federal agencies and institutes. Write to the National Institute of Handicapped Research (NIHR), the National Institute on Aging (NIA), the National Center for Health Care Technology, the U.S. Department of Transportation, and the U.S. Department of Housing and Urban Development for information they may have about new procedures, devices, and equipment to help Alzheimer's patients (see Appendix 2).

It is hoped that technology from computers to robots will someday be available to meet a portion of the needs of the aged who are cognitively impaired. Several rehabilitation research centers across the country are attempting to develop devices to improve mobility and communication and compensate for sensory and motor losses in the disabled, including patients with Alzheimer's disease and related disorders. In the future, robots may carry out home tasks by voice command and help patients communicate their needs more effectively. Currently, telephones with computer memories can help patients place phone calls; eventually, other memory computer aids may be invented.

The challenge to the family is to search for information and trained help to rehabilitate the patient. Several books listed in the back of this volume are valuable references containing helpful ideas for families that do not have easy access to health professionals. Rehabilitation is a philosophy and a set of strategies and techniques to maintain the self, even when the disease disabling the individual leads to the loss of self.

# 10

# CHOOSING A NURSING HOME IF THE TIME COMES

---

I will never forget the day we brought Dad to the manor. He slept later than usual, and he refused breakfast. Dad and Mom stayed in their bedroom with the door closed for more than an hour. The rest of us waited in the kitchen. It was a strange morning. This was the first time all of us kids had been together at home except for Christmas and Thanksgiving holidays, and even then one of us was often missing.

Sitting around the table together stirred childhood ghosts and memories. Mickey, Joe, Ellen, and I each felt transformed to our childhood selves. We also felt inadequate and scared of the task ahead of us that day. How could the four of us move Dad from the home in which he had raised us and take him to a strange place—a nursing home? We felt guilty and nervous.

Mickey was the oldest, and she finally stood up and walked to the window. With her back turned to all of us she spoke slowly and solemnly: "I feel empty inside. There is no justice in a world where we must move those who gave us life into a house of death."

EACH year thousands of families make the difficult decision to place someone they love in a nursing home. It is often a heartbreaking and painful decision. Unfortunately, in most instances institutionalization is seen as a tragic defeat rather than as a natural transition to the best possible care for someone with dementia. Mickey's lament reflects the overwhelming grief of a daughter grappling with what were irreconcilable feelings. Her guilt and that of the rest of the family was real and unavoidable. Mr. Ascot needed a nursing home, yet they abhorred surrendering him. It was a cruel defeat for them to have to cast him out of his home. Even though they had done everything possible to meet his needs over nine years, he had deteriorated considerably and required constant nursing care. Mrs. Ascot was eighty-six and frail herself. Each of the children lived in a different state, and to transport Mr. Ascot in his present condition would be difficult and uncomfortable for him. Moving would also take Mrs. Ascot away from her friends and the home she loved dearly.

Institutionalization is agonizing for many reasons. First, it is a major life change which disrupts the fabric of relationships woven over many years of being together and depending on one another. Second, moving to a nursing home is not a natural part of the family life cycle. Whereas people anticipate going to school, getting jobs, leaving their parents' home, marrying, having children, and going through many other life transitions, moving to a nursing home is not something people plan for their later life. Third, institutionalization confuses the bonds of loyalty, commitment, justice, and kinship between children and parents, brothers and sisters, husbands and wives. Placing a parent in a nursing home, under the care of others, arouses guilt in children who once were the beneficiaries of parental investment for many years.

One woman cried, "How can I live with myself if I cast off my mother in her old age? She and Dad did so much over the past seventy years. Mom never abandoned us kids—how can we abandon her?" Fortunately, her own son answered her:

You are not casting her off, Mom. That is what you may think that you are doing. I wish there was some way I could help you understand how I see what is happening. You will never stop loving Nana. None of us will. And you do not love her less by moving her to a home. You are spending every minute of the day with Nana, and it is taking its toll. You must care for yourself as much as you care for her.

Several important messages lie in this man's response to his own mother. Caring for persons with dementia does not mean that their needs must dominate the lives of family care givers. As was discussed in Chapter 8, optimal caring is achieved with a balance between the needs of the patient and family members. Dementia requires a long-term emotional investment, and the well-being of many people is important. Family members are interdependent on each other. It is absurd to think that the price a wife should pay to care for a cognitively impaired husband is her own poor health, impoverishment, and perhaps death! It is also wrong to think that the bond between a child and parent can be repaid by total devotion between an adult child and parent to the exclusion of everyone else in the family.

Making the decision to institutionalize a relative is difficult for all the reasons stated. However, there is another important factor. Nursing homes have become emotionally loaded symbols. Many individuals see them as houses of death or warehouses for the sick and dying, and the thought of moving a family member into one often ranges from unacceptable to repulsive.

Nursing homes were created as a societal response to a need. Although they are a less-than-ideal solution to the problem of caring for the increasing numbers of frail older persons with dementia, or with any other disorder that impairs individuals' ability to care for themselves, nursing homes have their place in the continuum of care. The quality of care many such facilities provide may be much better than what families can offer at home.

At present, nursing-home beds are more common alternatives in most communities than day care, home care, respite care, or other long-term-care service options. As will be discussed in Chapter 13, our current policies for financing health care encourage institutionalization rather than other options.

## Searching for the Right Facility

Once the decision is made, it is important to invest time searching for the right facility. After their admission most patients are likely to remain in the nursing home for months or years. Therefore, selecting the right place is almost as important as choosing one's own home. Unfortunately, most people postpone the decision and prefer not to think about it until the last possible moment. The problem then is that the family has to decide in a time of crisis, when it is under intense pressure and must act quickly. Many new and different problems emerge.

First, in most places nursing-home beds are not easily available when needed, and some facilities have waiting lists months long. As a result families may have to accept the first bed available. There is also little time to prepare the patient for the move, since beds which become available may have to be filled "immediately," at least according to the hospital discharge planner or nursing-home admission worker. The tragedy is that decisions are thus made precipitously, and patients are often placed in inappropriate or inadequate facilities.

Second, nursing-home care is expensive. People may live in a nursing home for several years, and the cost of the average stay in a long-term-care facility may be $75 to $100 or more per day. Therefore, costs of $30,000 a year or higher are not rare. As will be discussed in Chapter 13, it is important to know that Medicare, which pays most hospital costs for older Americans, does not pay for nursing-home care except in rare instances. Most of the costs for nursing homes are a private matter unless (or until) the patient's and the family's resources are reduced to such a level that they are eligible for state financial aid through Medicaid. Each state has different financial requirements for Medicaid eligibility, but all states have a "means test," which requires that the patient must be "medically indigent" to qualify. The specific financial levels—how poor you have to be—vary from state to state, and many states are changing their eligibility criteria as they try to meet the rising costs of long-term care. This shifts even more of the burden onto the family. Even with these additional problems, however, the main question remains, How does one choose a suitable nursing home?

## Types of Facilities

Nursing homes in the United States fall into several categories— those run for profit and three types not run for profit. There are

18,000 nursing homes across the country, 14,000 of which are non-profit. The latter are run either by a branch of government, by a religious organization, or by a nonprofit philanthropic organization or foundation. Of the for-profit, or proprietary, nursing homes, a substantial number are owned and operated as chains and managed by employees of larger corporate groups. Nonprofit and religious groups may also own and operate a group of facilities in an effort to reduce operating costs through larger-scale purchasing.

It is worth remembering that long-term-care institutions are a profit-making business for some and that the quality of their product —caring—may be tempered by the profitability factor on the one hand and the marketing strategy on the other. This does not necessarily mean that facilities run for profit are worse or better than those in the not-for-profit sector. Large chains may have more capital to invest in the physical plant and more efficient operations and programs. On the other hand, the corporation, individual managers, and regions may be driven more by the fiscal "bottom line" than by their role as service providers. Not-for-profit facilities also have financial incentives and may minimize or reduce the quality of programs to meet fiscal constraints, the needs of the local sponsoring group, legislated budget cuts, and bureaucratic controls.

What the Alzheimer's family must know is that although long-term-care facilities are among the most regulated enterprises in the country there are significant differences in the quality of care found in individual homes. The old adage "Let the buyer beware!" must certainly be applied to the choice of a nursing home at the present time. Some are outstanding caring settings, while others leave much to be desired.

## How to Locate a Good Nursing Home

The first step is to identify a selection of facilities in a location relatively convenient to you. Your physician may know of some fine nursing home, and it is a good idea to inquire whether he or she has an ownership interest in these facilities. If so and if you are satisfied with your doctor's care, ask him or her to personally guide you through the facility. Ministers, especially hospital chaplains, may be knowledgeable about facilities where they have visited patients or facilities which are related to their church. It is also helpful to contact the state health or welfare department to obtain a list of nursing homes licensed by the state, names of administrators, and the level of care offered in each facility. Hospital discharge planners and social workers are also excellent sources of information. It is then up to you to find out as much as you can about specific nursing homes using as many sources as possible:

- other patients and their relatives
- your rabbi, priest, or minister, who may have parishioners in these facilities
- your family physician
- friends
- local chapters of the American Association of Retired Persons or the National Council of Senior Citizens (see Appendix 2)
- your Area Agency on Aging
- other nursing homes
- ombudsman nursing-home organizations
- National Citizens Coalition for Nursing Home Reform (see Appendix 2)
- local chapters of the Alzheimer's Disease and Related Disorders Association

Directories of nursing homes may also be obtained from state nursing-home associations, which usually have their offices in the state capital. Every state also has affiliates of the American Association of Homes for the Aged, representing nonprofit or church-sponsored homes. The American Health Care Association, which has its national office in Washington, D.C., represents for-profit homes (refer to Appendix 2).

## Guidelines for Determining the Quality of Long-Term Care

Once you have identified one or more facilities, what should you look for to assure that the institution is a suitable environment for your relative? There are at least eleven areas to examine closely in your investigation of nursing-home options. Each is discussed briefly in the remainder of this chapter.

- philosophy and conduct of ownership and management
- quality of professional staff and management of patient care
- range of activities and programs
- patient participation and involvement
- resident/staff relationships
- physical plant and housekeeping
- food services
- physical design and accessibility
- community ties
- professional affiliations
- cost

The next important step is to call and visit the nursing homes you have selected. It is a good sign if you are welcome to visit them at any time. You may see the real flavor of the home if you time your visit to occur during the change of shifts, between seven and eight in the morning (when breakfast is served), between eleven and one (when lunch is served), or at night. The more open the facility, the better, usually, the care.

## Ownership and Philosophy of Management

Does the ownership have a philosophy of care? You may be assured that places are run with a specific orientation in mind, and that orientation, whether expressed or left unsaid, should be clear to you. If you cannot get the senior administrator or intake worker to articulate the facility's approach, you may have to get it indirectly, by interviewing patients, families, or other staff. If this is the case, think twice.

There are several questions to keep in mind. Is the point of view of the staff similar to yours with respect to the use of medications, the sedation of agitated patients, resident participation in the nursing-home community, the care of the dying, the role of staff, family involvement, and other aspects of care? Is there a special ward for patients with dementia? Are less deteriorated patients integrated with other patients? The more satisfied you become initially, the easier it will be for you in the months and years to come. Having once settled your relative in a nursing home, you should avoid moving him or her to another. The longer patients reside in a home, the more disturbing any move is likely to be for them. Therefore, choose carefully and deliberately.

- Interview the administrator. Ask to see the nursing-home license and the administrator's license. In most instances they are required to be posted by law. Is the administrator the owner? What is his or her educational and employment history? Does he or she have any other business interests? Is the administration on the premises? Is it easily reached during normal working hours, on weekends, and in emergencies?
- Inquire about the number of nurses—full-time and part-time. Who is the nursing director? Take down the names and check them against the nursing registry in your state.
- Make sure there is an R.N. in charge of all three shifts of nurses.
- Since most employees are nurse's aides, find out whether the home provides in-service training for aides.
- Check to see that only licensed personnel set up and give medications.
- Discuss whether R.N.'s really spend most of the time with patients or on administrative work.
- Ask how much nurse's aides are paid and how many there are. Do they know what to do in an emergency? What is the turnover rate?
- Inquire whether patients may bring personal furniture and belongings.
- Do the administrators seem to know patients and their families?
- Do they spend time on the floors, or do they seem aloof from the resident population?
- What is the ratio of personnel to patients? Nursing homes should have roughly the same number of employees as patients.
- If you are shown cards on a time clock as evidence of the number of employees, check to see how many are either blank or for part-time employees.
- Ask the administrator how many full-time and part-time therapists are available. Good homes provide speech therapy, occupational therapy, and physical therapy. Write down the names of these employees and check their credentials with the appropriate professional associations.

## Professional Staff and Care Management

The quality of professional staff is not always easy to judge without your spending time getting to know them. As a minimum, however, you can judge the credentials of the medical and nursing directors and of the chief of social services. Along with the administrator, they set the professional climate of caring, and you should try to meet with them and learn as much as you can about them. The following questions may be helpful:

- Is the medical director the house doctor who treats patients who have no personal physician, or does he or she care for all the residents? Most nursing homes expect the patients' personal physician to continue to care for them in the home.
- Will your physician continue to provide care in the nursing home?
- Are medical specialists available?
- Are psychiatrists with expertise in geriatrics and the special problems of residents in long-term care available?
- Are there any specialists connected with the nursing home who are interested in patients with Alzheimer's disease and related dementias?
- Who is responsible in an emergency?
- What procedures are followed when a patient is admitted to the nursing home?
- Are all patients given a complete medical and psychiatric examination on admission?
- Does the home have the services of a dentist or podiatrist, and how often do they visit the facility?
- How many incontinent or nonambulatory patients does the home have? The way these patients are treated often tells you a great deal.
- Do the patients have bedsores?
- Are they left sitting in their own waste? Turn down a few made-up beds and look for stains or worse.
- Are many patients restrained? If so, how long are they restrained? Are they sitting in adult high chairs? Is there a physician's note to justify restraints?
- Do patients look sedated, or attentive and happy? Are their feet

swollen from constant sitting? Is there evidence that they get exercise? Can they walk on the grounds?

- Check the nursing stations. Narcotics should be kept in special locked areas within the locked medications room.
- Can the nurse see down the corridors from the nursing station?
- Do the drugs appear to be kept in a neat fashion? Beware of boxes full of drugs on the floor.
- Do over-the-counter medications have prescription labels on them? Are drugs all supplied by the same pharmacy? Patients may have the right to retain their own pharmacy. Check on this. Denial of this right often leads to inflated prices.
- What agreements does the nursing home have with nearby hospitals if the patient becomes acutely ill?
- Are there trained, caring social workers available to help patients and families?

## Activities and Programs

Just as activities are the backbone of family life at home, so should programs and activities be available for nursing-home residents. Games, social engagements, clubs, organizations, musical events, classes and lectures, and crafts and hobbies are only a few of the innumerable opportunities people have to enjoy the company of others. Not only should there be a wide variety of programs; options should be meaningful and available to even the most impaired residents.

- Is there an activities director?
- What activities are available? How are they conducted, and how are they received by patients?
- Is there evidence that activities actually take place?
- Do patients have a wide choice of activities?
- Are the activities and programs appropriate to the cultural background and previous experiences of the residents?
- Are there religious services?
- Are there efforts to involve patients who are withdrawn and uninterested in activities?
- Are volunteers available to help patients? Talk to volunteers and find out how they feel about the home.

- Are there special programs for patients with dementia?
- Are there physical exercise programs for the severely disabled?
- Are there appropriate activities for men as well as women?
- Are there trips away from the hospital?
- Are there activities where residents can be of service or help to others? Older adults can often give a great deal of emotional support to children, especially to those who are mentally retarded or physically handicapped.
- Are family members encouraged to participate in activities?

## Patients' Rights and Daily Life

The challenge of long-term-care institutions is to provide a home-like environment along with a range of health services to a chronically ill population. People have many needs—for privacy, accomplishment, independence, self-identify, and self-determination. Unfortunately, institutions can be dehumanizing environments. It takes administrative leadership and a compassionate staff to create an environment that is pleasurable, comfortable, and stimulating for the people who must live there.

- Become familiar with the Patients' Bill of Rights set forth by the Department of Health, Education, and Welfare in 1974. Copies should be available in the nursing home.
- Are there combined patient-staff meetings?
- Observe staff and patients together. Do people seem particularly sad, angry, or irritable? Is morale high?
- Observe how patients are treated by staff (from housekeepers to administrators).
- Is there kindness and respect?
- How do staff respond to requests for help?
- Can patients come and go as they please?
- Can patients have pets?
- Are rooms personalized?
- Do patients have any areas for privacy?
- Can husbands and wives share a room?
- Are patients clean?
- Do patients seem happy?

- What opportunities do patients have for decision making? What choices do they have?
- Is there a residents' council or some other mechanism for involving patients in decision making? Do they meet with the staff on a regular basis?
- Are certain patients segregated?
- Do privately paying patients receive the same food as patients on Medicaid?
- Talk with a few patients. What is their feeling about their "home"?
- Do staff members involve residents in their own care?
- Do staff members encourage patients to be dependent, or do they encourage them to make certain decisions for themselves?
- Into what kinds of decisions do residents have some input?
- How stable are staff positions? Is there a high turnover rate?
- Do staff seem to enjoy their work or do you sense a lack of satisfaction and lack of involvement with patients?
- Does each resident have a primary helper or designated staff member? Even though team care is important, patients or residents relate most to people, not to a team.
- Do you feel that the staff work together for the benefit of the patient?

## Physical Design

The physical and architectural design is important. The environment should meet the personal needs of the patient as well as foster efficiency of operation. Pleasant, supportive surroundings may be one of the most significant factors to maintain or enhance the comfort of even severely impaired patients.

- Is the lobby attractive? Do patients use it? Do staff use it?
- Are there windows in patients' rooms?
- Is lighting adequate?
- Are there areas for socializing?
- Is there a separate dining room on each floor? Is it attractive?
- Does the physical design allow enough space for the patient?
- Are patients overcrowded?
- Are beds comfortable?

- Is there a call system at every bed? Does it work?
- Are there grab bars and call buttons in bathrooms and showers?
- Are there reading lights for patients' beds?
- Are there sprinklers/fire extinguishers in patient's rooms? Are exists clearly marked?
- Is there carpeting? Is it fireproof?
- When was the last fire safety inspection?
- Are exits clearly marked? Are ramps available?
- Are stairways enclosed? Are doors shut?
- When was the last fire drill? How often are they held?
- Is there enough space for a reasonable number of personal belongings?
- Are there opportunities for personal touches—pictures, personal desks, chairs, chests, or bureaus?
- Does the decor make you feel comfortable?
- Are there spacious activity rooms or dayrooms on each floor?
- Is there a library or quiet room or chapel?
- Are patients lined up in hallways? Are some patients isolated in the corridors or hallways?
- Are colors pleasant and bright?
- Are rooms and areas clearly marked (with color codes or large signs)?
- Are the grounds spacious and attractive? Can patients with walkers or wheelchairs get outdoors easily?
- Is there a closed outdoor area where patients with dementia may use the corridors?
- What is your general impression of the place?

## Housekeeping

The cleanliness and attractiveness of the institution have a powerful effect on morale.

- Is the home well kept?
- Is the home comfortable?
- Are there stains on floors or odors (urine, feces)?
- What is the condition of patients' rooms?
- Are there noticeable odors?
- Is there fresh water at the bedside?

- Is the heating and cooling system effective? Do patients seem comfortable? Ideally, thermostats should be set between 71° and 76°F year round.
- Are burned-out bulbs replaced?
- Does the facility cut back on heat or turn off air conditioners at night?
- Check more than one floor. Sicker patients are usually kept on separate floors.
- Is a barber or hairdresser available?

## Food Services

Our quality of life depends on many physical and environmental factors—the comfort of our home, financial security, family and friends, good times, and good food and drink. Invest time inspecting the kitchen area, visit during mealtime hours, and even ask to taste the food. Eating is not only a biological necessity; it is one of life's greatest pleasures.

- Is the kitchen clean? Examine floors, stoves, refrigerator, storage areas.
- Is there evidence of roaches, ants, or rodents?
- Does the home have an extermination service?
- Evaluate the cleanliness of people preparing food. Do they care for patients as well as prepare food?
- Have all kitchen employees had tests for infectious diseases?
- How is garbage disposed of?
- Check the alley where garbage is stored.
- Does the home have a dietitian or nutritionist? Who makes up the menu?
- Does the food served conform to what is written on the menu?
- Are therapeutic diets followed? Examine special-diet meals to make sure.
- Is food appetizing? Is it adequate in quantity and quality?
- Are warm things served warm and cold things cold?
- How many meals are served each day? At what time? Do they allow time for patients to eat? May people have seconds? Are snacks served between meals and at bedtime?

- May patients have beer or wine or other alcoholic beverages?
- Who feeds those who cannot feed themselves?

## Community Ties

Nursing homes should be part of the local community. The home should not only be physically attractive but also be seen by the local residents as a desirable place.

- Do children in the community volunteer in the home?
- Do local organizations such as the Lions Club or the Rotary hold their meetings in the auditorium?
- Do the police stop by to visit or eat in the institution's cafeteria?
- Do older people who live in the neighborhood volunteer?
- Do staff members live in the neighborhood?

## Professional Affiliations

Many nursing homes have affiliations with university medical centers or community hospitals. In larger cities they may be fortunate to have ties with large medical centers with specialists in geriatrics and Alzheimer's disease.

- Does the institution have student volunteers from local high schools, schools of podiatry, nursing, and physician's assistants?
- Is there a formal affiliation with a medical center, medical school, nursing school or other professional training programs?
- Have residents in the nursing home participated in research projects conducted by scientists or professors from neighboring colleges or universities?

## Cost of Nursing-Home Care

Ask specific questions about the cost of care provided in the different institutions you visit and compare prices. Establish in detail exactly what you would be paying for each month—room, board, laundry, therapies, drugs, and miscellaneous expenses.

- Contact the local Social Security office to learn about Medicare. Medicare pays only for certain skilled nursing care following hospitalization. Eligibility is strict and limited.
- Contact the local welfare office to learn about Medicaid. Medicaid is a state and federal program, and eligibility varies from state to state. Medicaid is given to people with limited assets.

Last, but by no means least, what is the attitude of the facility toward you and the patient? Will the staff work with you to get a careful history of the patient and try to understand what is important for a high quality of life for the patient? Do they wish to know key dates in the patient's life, such as wedding anniversary or children's birthdates? Is visiting encouraged? Are you expected to participate in any of the institution's programs? Does the institution itself have long-range plans?

In sum, our advice is that you get to know everything you can about the place and its people. If you do not feel good about a facility, try another place. Remember, it is best to plan ahead for placement. Waiting for a final crisis to occur before you decide may deny you the options you need. Excellent facilities exist, but most are full and take time to process new applications. Many will also have their own rules about patients with dementia. Some will accept only those who are bedridden; some will want to admit only those patients who are more intact so that they have the capacity to adapt to the facility.

Remember, too, that once the patient is admitted you will still be a part of the caring process, and you should feel comfortable in your new role. Adaptation to the institution is not always easy. It may even be easier for the patient than for the guilty relative. Sometimes the guilt surrounding institutionalization is so strong that the decision is made much later than it should have been, and after the patient is admitted, the guilt keeps spouse, children, and other members of the family away since they cannot face the new setting.

## Preparing the Patient and Making the Move

When possible, talk with the patient about moving into a nursing home, or allow him or her to sit in on family meetings when the topic is being discussed. Even when it is clear that the person is severely impaired, in most cases the simple act of being present in relevant discussions often reinforces the patient's importance as a person in the family.

Include all family members in the decision-making process. Even when you are the patient's husband or wife you do not have to do it all.

Carol Reiss had cared for her mother, Patricia Brown, for almost eight years. Mrs. Brown's husband died two years after she had been diagnosed as having dementia, but she had continued to live in the duplex next to her daughter. Carol was able to cook and clean for her mother and to check on her several times during the day, and every day Mrs. Brown joined her daughter's family for supper and the rest of the evening.

This arrangement had worked well until Mrs. Brown began to wander around the neighborhood, sometimes half-dressed. Although their friends were watchful and often gently guided Mrs. Brown back to her home, it was becoming evident that the family would have to consider moving her into a nursing home. Carol could not spend time with her mother during the day. She was divorced and had to work to support herself and her two teenage children.

For the next six months Carol hired a young woman to stay with her mother during the days. Mrs. Brown continued to deteriorate physically as well as mentally, and the young home attendant found the job too demanding. After hiring and firing several more attendants, Carol reached the conclusion that a nursing home would be a safer place for her mother.

Many phone calls later, Carol selected six places to visit. After making the rounds, she eliminated four of them. One was particularly appealing, and she decided that her mother should see it with her.

One evening after cooking a special supper for her mother, Carol and her two daughters, Bess and Evi, sat with her and spoke directly and quietly about looking at a few nursing homes together. Mrs. Brown listened carefully for several minutes before breaking in: "Carol . . . I'm not sure it's a good idea. But . . . we can visit if you like."

The four of them—Mrs. Brown, Carol, Bess, and Evi—visited two nursing homes in their town. The two girls felt it was important to do this with their grandmother to emphasize how important she was to them. For each trip Carol and the girls took the full day off. After visiting the home, they all had lunch and later went shopping.

Mrs. Brown moved easily into the nursing home they chose together. It was Carol, Bess, and Evi who felt upset, sad, and guilty. They had arranged to move Mrs. Brown on a Monday morning so that the family could have a special weekend together. Carol invited close family members and special friends together for a party. Mrs. Brown enjoyed the festivities and the company of those she loved.

The gathering was so successful that Carol almost changed her mind. During the day her mother seemed happy even though she was unable to say very much. However, the nights reinforced the importance of following through on their decision. Mrs. Brown would not sleep, wandered about the house, and even went outdoors several times to roam the streets. Carol had not slept well for months, and she could no longer bear the worry. She was exhausted, and she reached the painful decision that she could no longer keep her mother safe and comfortable at home.

The day of the move went smoothly. Their family and friends had agreed to accompany Carol and her mother. Carol later admitted she needed the moral support more than her mother did. All pitched in to help in many different ways. They agreed on an intensive visiting pattern for the first month so that she would have a few visitors each day rather than everyone at the same time. Carol and other members of the family worked out plans in many areas—to decorate Mrs. Brown's room and take her out for lunch, short shopping trips, or just for a walk.

As Carol and the girls saw how well Mrs. Brown adapted to her new home, they were able to relax and feel less guilty. Indeed, with time they were able to reflect on recent events and feel very good about everything they had done. Mrs. Brown lived another three years and remained an integral part of her family until she died.

Not every patient and family make the transition so easily. The key factors appear to be the amount of emotional preparation for the move, the insight of family members that they have done everything possible within their financial and human limits, and the availability of acceptable nursing homes.

It is important to recognize when home care ceases to be a viable alternative. Financial matters often make home care impossible. Especially in cases involving other dependents, the main care giver may find some form of employment necessary for the family's financial security. Bringing home a paycheck while carrying the burden of responsibility for a relative with Alzheimer's disease can be too taxing for the most dedicated and energetic of care givers.

Sometimes it is simply not possible to keep a relative at home if the apartment is too small or if other family members have serious health problems. Even families that care for their relatives at home for years often eventually decide that, for one reason or another, the care the patient is receiving at home is simply not as good as nursing-home care would be.

In many cases care givers are unable to handle the patient because of his or her violent or unmanageable behavior. Care givers may be powerless to handle a patient who is bigger than they are, especially if the patient becomes violent or insists on wandering out of the house and into dangerous situations. One woman with severe arthritis, who used a walker to do what needed to be done to care for her husband, tolerated being knocked down by her husband until she was so incapacitated that she could not stand up after an assault. Often a whole family will become tyrannized by a violent patient. Nursing homes are advisable in situations like this, not only for the protection of the family but for that of the patient as well.

As this chapter has indicated, there are positive steps you can take when the issue of nursing-home placement becomes a real one. Institutionalization is not a defeat. It is often an important and realistic choice in caring.

The following interview is with Helen Lucho, the sixty-five-year-old wife of a dementia patient. She describes how she coped with her husband and the events surrounding his institutionalization. Her feelings, actions, and thoughts capture much of what we have reviewed in this chapter. Her doctor tries to help her to continue to cope adaptively with the future.

DR.: I understand your husband just moved into a nursing home.

MRS. L.: Yes, in January of this year.

DR.: How was that for you? And how are you doing now?

MRS. L.: Well, it's upset me, to say the least. He was in the hospital three months before he went into a nursing home, and in that time I think I learned to adjust a little.

DR.: So you had some time to get used to the idea.

MRS. L.:  Yes, I did, but to have him picked up and taken in—it is the hardest thing I ever did in my life.

DR.:  It sounds painful. What led up to this decision?

MRS. L.:  He changed a great deal over the past two years. He became very abusive and struck out at me. And for two years I put up with it. He knew something was happening, and he begged me not to leave him. I told him I would not leave him—that I would take care of him as long as I could. But I couldn't stand much more abuse. Just before he went into the nursing home, I had a feeling I needed help soon or I would fall apart. I went to the medical center, and they helped me.

In January I had him committed. I hate to use the word "committed." Louis is not in his right mind, and this is pretty hard to cope with. At least, I find it so. I know that it isn't his fault, and I love the man.

DR.:  It's very painful for you to see all this happening. You were saying it's hard to cope. What kinds of adjustments have you had to make?

MRS. L.:  I have had to make all the financial decisions in the last two years. Before the illness he wouldn't let me do anything, and that was fine with me. Gradually I took over, but I had to do it carefully. I would give him a choice: "Do you want me to write a check for the rent, or do you want to do it?" He would accept that. But I have had to do everything because there is no one else. We don't have a family.

DR.:  So you have really been alone trying to struggle with these changes.

MRS. L.:  Yes, making decisions that I hope are right. I really had no choice when it came down to it. I do have some good friends, and they kept telling me that I should do something before he hurts me badly.

DR.:  What was it like for you to hear that?

MRS. L.:  I knew they were right, but I was going to put up with it as long as I could.

DR.:  Do you find yourself feeling guilty about anything?

MRS. L:  At first I did, but then I remembered how he would take a swing at me when we were alone. I put up with it as long as I could, and I don't feel guilty about that part. I feel I did the best I could.

DR.:  It sounds like you have done exactly what you needed to do. Is there anything that bothers you now?

MRS. L.:  Yes, financial problems. It's expensive to keep Louis in a nursing home, and I am worried about what might happen to me. I'm not getting any younger. Do I spend all my money on him? And what do I do then? This would go on for years, even after I run out of money. This is a community state—do I spend his half and save mine for me? I may end up in a nursing home.

DR.: Did you have any financial advisers?

MRS. L.: Well, I did go to the bank to see about a living trust. If something happened to me, he would be taken care of.

DR.: Have most of the nursing-home issues been resolved?

MRS. L.: Well, he's settled down now. He's not happy, but he's there. And I feel as good as I can about it. I feel it's the best for him.

# 11

# DEATH
# AND
# DYING

ALZHEIMER'S disease is a terminal disease. It is incurable. However, in many instances patients and families are so distressed by its immediate impact on their lives that only after some time do they grapple with their legitimate anxiety and fear about the future and the eventual death of the patient. Patients are often the first to bring the subject up. It is important not to overreact to the patient's talk about deterioration and death. The fears and sadness of each individual family member often impair communication and lead everyone to withhold information from one another, including the patient. Often we hear, "If I let him find out too much about Alzheimer's disease, I know he will kill himself." Unfortunately, families often shrink from discussions with loved ones about deterioration and death, precisely at the time when they need to talk as an affirmation of caring and life.

Mrs. Proto, the wife of a professor with Alzheimer's disease shared a story with us:

One afternoon I came home to find my husband in our library looking at an art book. He was staring at Chagall's *Gate to the Cemetery*. When I walked into the room, he showed me the picture and asked when he would join that community of graves. He seemed peaceful, but I was scared. I turned and walked out of the room upset and angry that he should suffer such a cruel disease. I cried in our bedroom for several minutes; I didn't want him to see me cry. As I sat alone, I realized it was wrong of me to walk away and not respond to his question. I returned to the library ready to talk about death. He was still sitting in the chair with the book closed. I asked him to show me the Chagall picture. He didn't remember the right picture or the book. He asked to go outside for a walk. I felt confused and angry and, even more, sad that I had lost my chance to communicate with him.

This experience and many others were extremely painful for Mrs. Proto. She spoke at great length about how difficult it was to talk with her husband when he wanted to share important issues with her. She felt out of synchronization with him and was frustrated with his periods of confusion. At times she also thought that he might actually kill himself if she allowed him to talk about death.

Mrs. Proto's predicament is one that many families experience. Although it is natural to avoid the issue of death, each family member involved in the patient's care must face it sooner or later. However difficult it may be, beginning to face a relative's death is necessary to be able to live and work effectively with him or her. Eventually, Mrs. Proto decided she could convey to her husband her own feelings about death. She did not share her husband's view that death is a continuation of life under more just conditions. She felt that death, specifically his death, was a cruel waste. She communicated this to her husband by showing him a picture of another work which she thought reflected death destroying their lives together even before he actually died. She described her condition as a restless peace. Although she was taking good care of her husband, her feelings were confused by the two deaths—the psychological and the physical.

Family members need to cope with the emotional dilemma presented by the two types of death—the physical death and "the death of self," which precedes the physical death by many years. The deterioration and death of a relative from Alzheimer's disease is experienced differently by every family. Many factors contribute to the way family members feel and act as the dementia progresses: the personality of different individuals, the history of relationships between family members, the ability of people to communicate with the patient, the speed with which the illness progresses, and the quickness with which physical death occurs.

Many victims of Alzheimer's disease die emotionally and spiritually alone. Even the most loving relatives may inadvertently isolate the patient psychologically and socially. Patients need to feel needed and be treated like responsible human beings even though they have dementia. The unspoken attitudes and behavior of family, friends, and professionals influence how the person with dementia feels and responds. One patient told us he felt like someone wandering by himself along the lonely seashore. He knew that everyone in his family loved him, but they did not know what the disease meant to him. He wanted his wife to understand how much it hurt him not to be able to care for her and meet her needs: "What makes me so upset is not that I have no one to share my burden. It is that I have only my own burden to bear. I am only a shadow of my former self." Mr. Boyle was finally able to communicate his sadness to his wife and family before the dementia robbed him of his ability to express his feelings. After he died, his wife told us she felt that his death had been a good one and that she had been able to help him retain his sense of identity to the end. She considered herself blessed to have had a husband whose love for her had transcended the dementia.

The challenge for the family is a difficult one. The ongoing psychological death of the patient causes profound grief, and the grieving is very much like the reaction to terminal illness, but with one major difference. The patient appears healthy, looks very much like as he or she used to look, and is likely to be alive for many months or years in this peculiar state of physical health and psychological decline. It is not easy to deal with the invisible changes that alter behavior and mood and destroy the husband, wife, patient, or friend whom one has known for years.

Grieving is healthy, but with it there emerges a subtle, inevitable change in the way we relate to the person for whom we grieve. This change involves getting closer to him or her initially and then developing a degree of emotional distance. Although we may actually do more for the patient as he or she becomes more dependent, we also begin to regard the patient as the shell of someone we once knew —much as we treasure an object we inherited for its power to evoke memories of another time. It is hard to say that this distancing process is wrong. The greatest danger of distancing is that the patient becomes an object—a flesh-and-blood container holding memories and deep emotional ties to the past but with no real function or humanity in the present. Although emotional separation is helpful in dealing with our psychological pain, it affects our ability to try to relate to the patient and to keep him or her as involved as possible.

The following two principles are important guides to interactions with an individual with dementia.

1. *Do not let emotional ties die too far ahead of the patient.* The changes in dementia are gradual. It is important to engage the individual in meaningful activities consistent with his or her cognitive and behavioral limitations. Nurture the hope to enjoy today and tomorrow for as long as it is possible.
2. *Treat your relative like a human being, with a role and an identity, not like a patient.* Share information as you see him or her ready to receive it. Do not minimize the seriousness of the disease, but do not overreact. Goethe wrote, "If we take people as they are, we make them worse. If we treat them as if they are what they ought to be, we might help them to become what they are capable of becoming."

## Suicide

Alzheimer's disease patients speak frequently of the desire to be dead rather than enter a nursing home or be bedridden and incontinent. In this situation, family members and close friends often become disturbed and fearful that the patient may actually commit suicide. Yet, there is no evidence that individuals with dementia attempt suicide or take their lives more frequently than do other persons. Occasionally, the fear of suicide may be legitimate, but most of the time it is unjustified.

Why is suicide not more prominent in patients with Alzheimer's disease and related disorders? We do not know the answer to this question. Indeed, we still do not know enough about the social and psychological nature of suicide in the general population, where it ranks among the first ten causes of death in the United States. Data are simply nonexistent for dementia victims. We can speculate, however, that the very nature of Alzheimer's disease limits the individual's ability to think about and carry out such an action in much the same way that it impairs other abilities in the later stages of the illness. In a number of instances patients with dementia have overdosed in a confusional state. This appears to be accidental, however. It is important to keep medications out of reach of patients when they can no longer manage their own drugs. Several patients have gone into deep coma and died after consuming too many pills, in all likelihood unaware of what they were doing.

Accidental death or apparent suicide are painful experiences when they occur because so many questions are left unanswered. Professional help, if available, is often vital in dealing with many of the complex psychological and family reactions of the survivors. These are times when it is necessary not only to grieve but also to come to grips with the uncertainty of what really happened. Did my wife, my husband, my friend, really take his or her own life? In the absence of a genuine suicide note, this question often lingers.

The following letter was written by an eighty-year-old widow whose husband had dementia for more than ten years. Thomas Bucht was not actually diagnosed until shortly before his death. Although his wife, Erma, knew that something was wrong, she was afraid to ask for help. For years Mr. Bucht went from doctor to doctor, receiving numerous medications, but the dementia went unrecognized. It was only after an episode during which Mr. Bucht beat her unconscious that Mrs. Bucht telephoned her family for help.

As the events unfolded, it became clear that Mr. Bucht had deteriorated greatly over the last eight months. Mrs. Bucht had struggled to deal with his "craziness" alone and as a result became physically and emotionally exhausted. Mr. Bucht was diagnosed as having Alzheimer's disease after a two-week hospitalization and was then discharged home with twenty-four-hour nursing coverage. Mrs. Bucht sustained a heart attack shortly after her husband was hospitalized. She never saw him again. A week after he left the hospital, he overdosed in a confusional state and died.

Mrs. Bucht recovered with time, and during the year following her husband's death she wrote a series of letters to her doctor. The excerpt below is from one of those letters.

Dear Doctor,

I am writing to let you know that I am doing as well as can be expected. My family is wonderful, and I have some good friends. But I miss Tom, and I think of him all the time. It has been nine months. I still think I might have saved him if I had been home.

You have always told me not to blame myself for his death. I understand that Tom did not really commit suicide, but if I had been home he might not have been so unhappy. I might have kept him from taking all those pills. I know the night nurse was watching him all the time. She heard him get up from bed and go into the bathroom that night. She heard tap water running and opened the door to find Tom swallowing the sleeping pills. He smiled at her and said, "Darling, please get my breakfast. I am late for the office." Poor Tom, he was so sick for many years. His brain was not working right.

I have talked to my pillow all these years. I did not know what else to do. Tom would take so many pills. He took two for his heart, something for his sugar, pills for his nerves, and then there were the sleeping pills. Tom was forever taking pills. There were pills hidden all over the house. He went to so many doctors, and they all gave him pills, pills, pills.

Tom slept all day except for meals. And then at night—the nights were terrible. Tom would kiss me and say it was the last kiss he would ever give me because he was going to die. Each night I would sit in the chair fully dressed, wrapped in a blanket waiting for something to happen. If Tom began to have problems, I wanted to be ready to take him to the hospital. For more than a year I waited for something to happen.

Tom could be so cruel sometimes. I knew he did not know what he was doing. He would scream at me, and once, no, more than that, he struck me. I finally had to call my son one weekend because Tom hit me so hard I could not get up again. I must have passed out and been unconscious for more than an hour. When I came to I could not walk. My leg was broken, and my hand was throbbing. And more than that, my heart was breaking.

Now that Tom is dead, I think back and try to remember the good times. But it is hard to erase those last years. The doctors should not have given him all those pills. They were not helping him. He was a sick man, and they should have figured out what was wrong. I also made things worse—I think I hurt us both. I hid it from the family and worse still, I tried to hide it from myself. I made myself sick, and if I had asked for help earlier, maybe he would still be alive today.

Sometimes I wonder if he killed himself because he thought I had left him. He was my husband for fifty-nine years. But the last ten years he was not himself. Forgive me for sounding this way. You and the other doctors have all told me that Tom did not know what he was doing when he took all those pills. His brain disease affected the mind. He was confused. He was not himself.

With time and the continued support of family and friends, Mrs. Bucht recovered her strength and a sense of the future. She was fortunate to have an attentive family and many friends, mostly widows, who surrounded her during the months following Tom's death. Her family was surprised at the numbers of other widows who always seemed to be present. This network helped Mrs. Bucht deal with her deep feelings of loss. And as time went by she moved on with her life. Mrs. Bucht was able to deal with her grief in a healthy way, and she also reached a point when she could review her past objectively. Although she accepted the results of the psychological autopsy, which indicated that her husband did not commit suicide, she still admitted that there was some doubt in her mind but she could live with it. She had to live with it.

A psychological autopsy is the process whereby a group of professionals examine all the available evidence to determine the likelihood that a suspicious death was a genuine suicide. When the results of this deliberation are communicated to the family, they can provide the information needed to deal with the uncertainty about the cause of death. Since many professionals may take part in the psychological autopsy, the outcome reflects a reasonably authoritative opinion. After the decision is made, the family may need to hear the professional analysis several times. The accidental death or apparent suicide disrupts the normal grief process because the notion of suicide may be almost incomprehensible, as Mrs. Brucht expressed in her letter.

If you are concerned about your relative's "suicidal" behavior or death wishes, seek professional help. Research suggests the following danger signals:

1. Someone with a history of a suicide attempt or serious gesture (prior to the diagnosis of dementia) may be at heightened risk. People who have attempted suicide are more likely to attempt it again.
2. Individuals with a diagnosis of depression have a higher rate of suicide. The presence of a significant depression should not be

ignored in anyone. Depression is a treatable disease even in patients with dementia.

3. A history of mental hospitalization of other family members is more common in groups of people who have committed suicide, particularly if depression, in any of its forms, was diagnosed.

## Facing the Terminal Stages of Alzheimer's Disease

Living with a dementia victim in the later stages of the disease is a struggle for everyone. It is a more intense experience of what families have been engaged in since the diagnosis. It is not unusual during this period to wish the patient a speedy and painless death rather than to see the ongoing destruction of his or her human dignity.

These wishes stem from deep feelings for the patient as well as from notions of how we ourselves would like to end our lives, yet they provoke upset and guilt. Death would clearly be a release not only for many patients but for the family as well. This then becomes the basis for an internal crisis—"How could I want my husband to die! I am so selfish." Death then comes not only as a release but often generates pain-provoking guilt and self-doubt.

The emotional turmoil around the patient's decline is extraordinary. The physical presence of the person evokes thoughts and feelings which bind the patient to the family at the same time as the individual's suffering makes us wish him or her dead. The following excerpt from a letter expresses the impulses we often hear from families.

Dear Sis,

We visited Mom and Dad again today. Just as old leaves struggle hard to hold onto the vine in a strong winter wind, Dad is fighting not to die. He doesn't want to give up, but I wish he wouldn't fight anymore. I wish he would die. Sometimes I find myself thinking about ways to end his suffering.

Last week when Mom was in the hospital, we stayed with Dad. It's rough! He has really gone downhill this winter. He paces up and down all day long, and he doesn't sleep at night. It's impossible to get any rest with him wandering around the house. I don't know how Mom puts up with this.

We did find a solution to at least get him to sleep for a few hours. A hot bath at night relaxed him, and once we got him into bed he would sleep three or four hours. One night I found myself staring at the open-face heater by the tub. I know what I felt—lonely and scared. I wanted to place the heater on the edge of the tub. If he accidentally pulled the heater into the water, then it would be God's will . . . and I almost did it!

The desire to see the patient die is a confusing feeling. Yet, it is natural to have these feelings. It is also natural for thoughts of death to be accompanied by guilt. Alzheimer's disease is painful for everyone, and one of the reactions to pain and hurt is to run away from or attempt to eliminate the cause of the pain. As a result, some family members shy away or limit time spent with the patient. As the letter expressed, some people even have the impulse to act in a way that increases the risk of an "accidental" death. Living with a loved one exacts an enormous emotional toll because you not only see and feel the suffering of the patient but also have your own reactions to contend with. The desire for the death of a patient evolves naturally from the desire to end the irreversible suffering of another human being and sometimes—when you identify yourself with the patient—from the fear of being a burden to others. These feelings may emerge soon after the diagnosis or only after a period of time has passed and the losses and changes seem to have become almost bearable.

It is important to acknowledge death wishes and talk about them with family, friends, or clergymen. The process of sharing these difficult thoughts often shows us that we are not sick or cruel—that others also feel helpless and hopeless in the face of Alzheimer's disease. Many people would rather see death come soon than watch progressive suffering. If these unspoken wishes are not expressed to someone, they can build up and become more and more troublesome and difficult to manage.

The strong feelings we all have about dying and death often bring family members into direct conflict with one another. In the turmoil seemingly forgotten emotions tend to be confused with present feelings toward the patient. Adult children may be upset and torn between the desire to care for a dying parent and anger toward the person who was never a "good" mother or father to them. Old rivalries between children or between children and parents reemerge, and the patient's death becomes the new battleground for old playroom feuds. Raw emotions which everyone had considered long buried emerge again.

The family may be torn apart, just at a time when collaboration is essential. Sensitive decisions are needed about the patient's comfort and well-being, family needs, legacies, the sharing of the deceased's possessions, funeral arrangements, autopsy, and even the use of the patient's brain for research. At best these can tax even the strongest family. Part of dying "a good death" is that family members (and the patient, as long as it is congnitively possible) derive comfort knowing that they acted together to do what they could, and, as much as possible, helped one another. When families work as a unit and do what is right for all concerned, they can face the end with a greater sense of peace. If conflicts are disruptive, families may need a counselor to help them understand their responses or even to serve as referee to mediate the problem.

## Death with Dignity

Family members have described the long process of watching a loved one die with Alzheimer's disease as a "living funeral." Inevitably, physical death becomes a reality. The moment of death is often painful despite the years of mourning and adjustment during the course of the dementia. With Alzheimer's disease and related disorders the grieving process begins well before death, and while this "anticipatory grieving" helps family members deal with their emotions, it does not entirely alleviate the pain of the final loss. The period following death is difficult even though families often feel a sense of relief that the agony is over, both for them and for the patient.

Whether death occurs in a nursing home, a hospital, or at home, only a few families are prepared for it. A number of decisions suddenly must be made about funeral arrangements, including costs, the acceptability or desirability of an autopsy, notification of family and friends, and rearrangement of other commitments.

Modern medical technology has also created new ethical dilemmas for family members and for medical care givers even before death occurs regarding decisions to use life-support systems and emergency cardiac-resuscitation measures. Victims of dementia may undergo many medical crises or prolonged suffering before they die, and most die in a hospital.

The following interview with Geraldine Mason was conducted five months after the death of her husband, James. He had suffered from what was probably a multi-infarct dementia for seven years. The ethical challenges are evident in her description of the last seven days. For many patients the painful dilemmas may last months or years.

A week before my husband died—he died on a Wednesday—we took him to the doctor because he had great difficulty breathing. The doctor said it was bronchitis and prescribed some medicine, but it didn't help. In fact, he became worse.

By Saturday he was so much worse that I took him to the hospital. The doctors checked him and confirmed that it was bronchitis. They told me he would be fine, but I wanted him to stay in the hospital. I was certain he had pneumonia. What bothers me is the way they treated him or, more accurately, did not treat him. They really did not treat him as a human being. Nor did they examine him carefully, as I found out later. They did not understand that he did not comprehend their questions.

The next day, Sunday, was horrible. He woke up about ten in the morning. He slept sitting in a cuddle sack in the couch because he was unable to breathe lying down. When we tried to help him off the couch, we noticed his lips and fingernails turning blue. We took him to the bedroom and sat him on the bed. I kneeled in front of him and looked into his eyes. And then he collapsed on top of me.

I screamed to my daughter, "Call 911!" All I remember thinking was, "Don't die, James. Please don't die!" My daughter gave him artificial respiration until the medic team arrived. One medic ordered me to leave the room until they got him talking. I tried to tell them he would not talk as they pushed me out of the bedroom. I screamed, "He has Alzheimer's disease and does not communicate well with people—especially strangers."

Two medics worked on him for about ten minutes. Finally, one gentlemen came out and asked me several questions, something about medications and James's swollen feet. They told me that my husband was in heart failure and had been for several weeks. I was shocked! We had seen two doctors in the last two weeks, and nobody said anything about heart failure!

The medics continued to work on him for a long time. Finally, one of them told us James was breathing again, but that he had suffered a massive coronary. If they were not able to get the heart started within another twenty minutes they would call the coroner. I remember pleading with them not to stop.

They finally got the heart started again and took him to the hospital. The doctor there talked to us. He was very kind. He wanted to know if James had another coronary, did we want resuscitation and life support. The entire family were there, including several friends, and we all agreed, "No." The doctor explained that the coronary was so severe that there was probably very little brain functioning. James was living off machines. We instructed the doctor not to resuscitate him if he had another coronary.

That was Sunday.

On Monday, things were the same. The doctor told us that he wanted someone to check James's brain waves. He also asked us if we wanted the life-support system removed if there were no brain waves. I told Dr. P. that if my husband was not going to be conscious on his own, I did not want the life-maintenance system. James had always thought it was terrible for instruments to be put on people who would probably never recover.

And that was the case. I guess there were no brain waves. He passed away Wednesday afternoon.


Mrs. Mason's story touches on many issues. She and her family were able to make decisions together which reflected the wishes of her husband. The physician at the hospital shared information and alternatives with them. He gave them information and asked them what they wanted him to do.

These are not easy decisions for families, nor indeed are they for professionals. Death with dignity is a humane goal—particularly when life as we know it seems absent from a human body which is functioning marginally and then only because it is attached to machines by wires and tubes. Caring for the dying person, however, confronts the clinician with ethical dilemmas. Physicians are committed to keeping people alive and to the principle "Do no harm." It may be a painful internal struggle to adhere to this mandate and also respond to the need to relieve human suffering. Active euthanasia is unacceptable medical practice and can be considered murder. Passive euthanasia, the withholding of medical procedures or drugs in order to allow someone to die "when there is irrefutable evidence that biological death is imminent," is sanctioned by many, including church leaders, but these decisions are for the patient and/or the responsible family to make, not the physician alone.

Families have the right to expect guidance and information from the doctor. Families should seek out someone who will be regularly available to them to provide information, advice, and opinions about the alternatives available. If it is at all possible, these discussions should take place during the early phases of the disease, when the patient may be able to discuss issues and let relatives know his or her desires. It is helpful if the patient's thoughts and feelings can be made as explicit as possible to provide guidelines for family action when the time comes. If the patient cannot or will not participate, it may be desirable for the family to be guided by a trained professional who can listen and answer questions about the rights of patients, family rights, the position of physicians, and the rulings of the legal system.

## After Death

After the patient's death, the spouse and remaining family are likely to change their pattern of living. During this period of adaptation, the family will continue to feel great sadness. Usually, a spouse has the most difficult time finding a new personal identity. Grieving takes time, and months may pass before the worst part is over.

The following interview with Ollie Richards, a middle-aged woman, took place approximately eighteen months after her husband's death. She and Albert had been married twenty-six years and had raised three children. Mr. Richards had been diagnosed as having Alzheimer's disease at the age of fifty-two, after perhaps a year of disturbing symptoms. He deteriorated quickly and died at the age of fifty-three. Mrs. Richards kept him at home, involving him as much as possible with friends and family up until the end.

DR.:     How did Albert die?

MRS. R.: He just died one night after I had put him to bed. He had been incontinent, and I had him in Pampers. I changed him after dinner, put him to bed and kissed him. He was perspiring like crazy, but I thought he was upset about wetting his pants since we had company. Three other couples had come for dinner that night. They were in the living room when he died. I was preparing tea. I went into Albert's room to see if he was still awake and wanted a cup. When I walked into the room, he wasn't with us anymore.

DR.: What did you do?

MRS. R.: The first thing I did was to tell one of my friends, "Albert is sleeping. I can't waken him."

DR.: Did you know he was dead then?

MRS. R.: In the back of my mind I think I did. But his eyes were open and his hands were behind his head, just as he normally slept. My friend went in, came back, and said he could not waken him either. At that point we called the doctor.

DR.: And how long did it take before the doctor arrived?

MRS. R.: We never reached the doctor. We called Medic I. I had had a nurse out to the house the Friday before he died. I called the hospital to say that Albert had not bathed himself for three weeks, nor would he let me do anything for him. They sent a visiting nurse out on Friday, and the nurse said to me, "Should your husband aspirate"—and I really didn't know the meaning of the word "aspirate"—"call Medic I immediately, but tell them he is a terminal patient and not to use any life-support equipment on him."

DR.: What did you do when they arrived?

MRS. R.: I told them I didn't want any support equipment used on him. They said they would just test to see if there was a heartbeat, which, of course, there wasn't. From there the police came and next the funeral home. I also called a good friend who came right over and helped me.

DR.: Did you know what to do when Albert died?

MRS. R.: Yes, I did. I had made a list of priorities.

DR.: When did you make that list?

MRS. R.: The day before he died. After I spoke with the visiting nurse, she really brought it home to me that maybe he might die. Up to that time Albert had been very weak. He couldn't get out of the chair or the bed. I had to lift him, drag him to the bedroom, and put him on the bed. He was very weak. But I never—I don't think I ever thought he was going to die.

DR.: How did you feel when you knew he was dead?

MRS. R.: Relieved . . . for him. Because I think he went through hell. Albert had not been able to hold a conversation with me for a year. It was like talking to a child. He would just smile or grin. Every time I tried to make conversation, he would just say "seven four seven" or "spitfire." Airplanes were his life. So I never ever got to talk to Albert in that last year.

DR.: During your marriage did you and he ever discuss what to do when one of you died?

MRS. R.:   Yes, we wanted to be cremated. We never wasted our money. We did not feel the lavish funeral was the thing for us. We would spend our money whilst we were living.

DR.:   After Albert was diagnosed, did you and he ever have a conversation about his death, at least when it was possible to communicate?

MRS. R.:   Albert never accepted the fact he had Alzheimer's. He never admitted he was going to die. Albert was a perfectionist. Immediately after the diagnosis he wanted to go back to England. He thought if he could go back to his earlier days he would recover and be fine. He never admitted he was sick. The only time we discussed it, I just said, "Well, we'll work it out together." He simply answered, "Okay." We never really talked about it.

DR.:   Were your children home when their father died?

MRS. R.:   No.

DR.:   Were your children helpful to you during the year that you were caring for him?

MRS. R.:   My youngest one was very supportive. She was eighteen at the time. She would take Albert out for a drive or walk with him, at least when he was able to walk. I also have a middle daughter —Albert transferred all his aggressions to her, so she moved out about a month before he died. She is the one that is having the hardest time accepting Albert's death. I think she feels bad about leaving when she should have stayed home.

DR.:   Have you talked about that since—

MRS. R.:   To her? Yes. But she doesn't open up very much either. We are very reserved people. We don't discuss our feelings too much.

DR.:   So, after Albert died you didn't spend too much time discussing your feelings?

MRS. R.:   No, no. Because we have all accepted what is. There is nothing we can do to change it, so we must go on from there.

DR.:   How did you go on from there? What plans did you make?

MRS. R.:   I didn't make any plans. I tended to drift.

DR.:   Were your children and friends around you during the period after Albert died?

MRS. R.:   Yes. But I am a self-sufficient person. I don't need—I don't want a lot of sympathy. I never have wanted sympathy. I needed support, yes, and most of my friends were very helpful. But the children were very good. In fact too good. They smothered me. They were always telling me what I should do and what I should not do. I told them to get on with their lives because that's the way we wanted it. And they have adjusted quite well.

DR.: What changes do you face now?

MRS. R.: I am engaged to be married now. My husband and I were friends with one couple for more than twenty-five years. Peter's wife died of cancer two months before Albert died. We just gravitated together and have gone on from there.... And it's marvelous.

DR.: When did you get engaged?

MRS. R.: New Year's Day. About a year after Albert's death. I'm excited now. Things go on, you know. It's no good looking back. You can't look back.

DR.: How do the children feel about your getting married again?

MRS. R.: They're pleased because it makes me happy. I'm more relaxed with them, and I don't worry about their lives as much. But they're not too keen on the choice. But then I don't think they ever would be.

DR.: But you're happy about the choice!

MRS. R.: I'm happy, yes. And I think it's a relief for them to know they don't have to worry about me. They can go on with their own lives.

DR.: And you?

MRS. R.: Oh, I'm very pleased. I'm relieved for Albert that he died when he did. I'm relieved for me that I didn't have to go through the experience of finding a nursing home. Everything just worked out beautifully, it really did. He went quickly. By and large, as I look back—the longer he's gone . . . you know, you look back and think. I have a few guilt feelings wishing that I hadn't been so . . . I was mean to him sometimes. He needed constant attention and care. He would follow me around, and I would hide in the closet just to get away from him for five minutes. And I wished I hadn't done that, but you can't change what was. I did the best I could. I pray he is at peace now.

Grief differs from person to person, family to family, and culture to culture. Complex emotions are expressed—sadness, anger, hurt, guilt—and many thoughts and feelings erupt. It is painful to lose someone we love. It is also difficult to lose a spouse or parent when the relationship has been strained, ambivalent, or disrupted. The nature of the relationship we cultivate with someone throughout life greatly influences the way we react when he or she dies.

Getting on with the future does not mean that the sense of loss disappears. Death does not erase the impact of one human life on another. The memories of a relationship will always exist at some level. Indeed, it is not unusual for older men or women to refer to their spouse in daily conversation long after death has occurred. The memories of a long life together are powerful and sustaining. For some individuals they seem to provide the emotional foundation on which to build a new life in the future. However, not all memories are happy ones. Human relationships are very complicated, and over a long lifetime many events occur. Therefore, for some persons death is a release, and the grieving is abbreviated.

## Possible Warning Signs for Abnormal Grief Reactions

There is no right way to grieve. The way we grieve is as personal as the way we show our love, anger, or friendship. After the patient has died, many different factors may complicate the process of mourning. The way death occurs may have a major impact on the ability to grieve, especially if there is an accidental death or apparent suicide. Personality traits of surviving family members which have nothing to do with the patient, such as a depressive personality, may place certain individuals at high risk of long-term complications. The nature of the relationship between the deceased and various family members also has a profound influence on how people deal with their grief. Finally, the inability to express feelings related to the loss is a powerful predictor of problems sometime in the future. Although the individual at highest risk is a surviving spouse, anyone who has been close to the patient can be affected.

Knowing the complicating factors which prolong the grieving process may help family members be watchful for possible problems. "Pathological mourning" occurs when individuals do not deal with their initial reaction to death and do not resolve their feelings of loss. If several months after a death life still seems empty and devoid of meaning and if there is no enjoyment of any activity, professional attention should be sought.

Pathological mourning is not a disease, but it can lead to a serious depression. Families should not feel embarrassed to seek help if the grief persists over months. Caring for someone with dementia and dealing with the complex feelings it arouses before and after death is highly stressful. It is not a sign of personal weakness or a character flaw to need help. We are all vulnerable at different times in our lives.

A number of complicating factors which may prolong mourning are related to the psychological makeup of the survivors rather than to their relationship with the deceased patient. Individuals may be particularly susceptible to problems if they have had a lifelong tendency toward depression or difficulties in expressing anger or sadness. Aged widows or widowers may develop abnormal reactions if they are very old, frail, and chronically ill, have limited finances, or are socially isolated, since all of these factors serve to limit one's options in changing to a new lifestyle. Individuals who are extremely dependent on others to meet their emotional and social needs may also be at risk. The spouse who has tried to manage a husband's or wife's total care and who experiences excessive guilt about failure to do enough may need help if he or she cannot come to terms with such feelings.

Sometimes the family may create a situation in which a mother or father or child cannot grieve, by consciously or unconsciously blocking the process, by actively insisting that he or she "stop crying" or "carrying on." Abnormal reactions may result when people are not able to express feelings related to loss. There are many potential complications. Some individuals may simply not be able to tolerate the intense pain surrounding the death of a loved one, or, on the other hand, they may hide their feelings completely in an effort to protect others around them. It is not uncommon for family members and friends to act in ways that do not acknowledge a person's need to grieve. Families may do great harm if they insist that a spouse or other individual manage grief in very specific ways.

## Legal and Financial Steps after Death

Several legal and financial matters must be taken care of soon after death. These range from immediate problems to longer-range issues. The information in this section is intended to guide family members who have the responsibility to tend to the deceased's legal affairs:

- If the deceased is named in your will, contact your attorney and revise the will.
- Examine your insurance policies to check whether the deceased was designated as a beneficiary; if so, have the policies changed.
- Cancel all credit cards; when appropriate, arrange for them to be reissued in the spouse's name.
- Individuals often have several insurance policies. When bills arrive in the mail, check whether there is any life insurance coverage of the sort tied to major purchases or time payments. It is also a good idea to examine canceled checks for the past two or three years for evidence of payments on insurance premiums.
- It is important to ask a friend, clergyman, or attorney to help you make a checklist of other financial issues important for you to resolve.

Someone in the family should investigate what death benefits the survivors may be eligible to receive in addition to life insurance. The Social Security Administration and the Veterans Administration (VA) offer benefits, as do many business, church, and fraternal organizations. Survivors are often eligible for Social Security benefits if the deceased was employed. These benefits may be paid to the surviving spouse if they were living together at the time of death, or, if the spouse is not alive, the money may be given to the person responsible for the burial expenses. When there is no surviving spouse, survivors may request the Social Security Administration to send the payment, a maximum of $255, to the funeral director for burial costs.

The Veterans Administration provides a qualified veteran with $300 toward funeral expenses. Like the one with the Social Security Administration, the claim must be filed within two years. You must complete special VA forms, which are available from the VA or the mortuary you choose. In addition, VA benefits include a plot in the nearest VA cemetery or a sum of $150 toward burial in a private cemetery, a memorial marker for the grave, and an American flag for the casket. If the surviving spouse does not remarry, he or she may be buried in an adjoining plot in the VA cemetery.

Table 6 identifies what documents are needed when filing for Social Security, veterans', and other benefits.

## Preparing for the Funeral

Today, most funerals are handled by a licensed funeral service, which coordinates all the details. However, there is a range of alternatives, including cooperational groups to reduce the cost of burial, direct removal and burial without a formal ceremony, and cremation. Disposition of ashes is the decision of the family. They can be placed in a receptacle for the family to keep, or they may be buried or placed in a solumbarium. The family may also have the ashes scattered where doing so is not prohibited by law. Although cremation is usually handled by the funeral home, various groups will dispose of the body without any ceremonies if the family wishes.

The donation of the body is another alternative. Most medical-research institutions will allow time for the family to have a funeral service before the body is delivered to the hospital. Families may also request that the remains of the body be returned to them after they have been studied by the institution. The body, or the ashes of the body after cremation, may be returned.

A memorial service without the body is another alternative. Although the memorial service may meet the needs of the family, the decision should be made carefully. It should not be done because it is convenient or because the family is trying to avoid the reality of what has happened. Funeral practices may evoke strong emotions among family members. This is natural. It is important to have someone who has been with the family throughout the disease—friend, clergyman, or health professional—help plan the funeral.

Many families are prearranging and prefinancing funerals. This is another area in which professional advice is necessary. The payment of money in advance for services is controlled by law in most states. If there are no such laws in your state, the prepaid funeral agreement should provide for a trust fund, and the person making the payment should control the account. The fund should include all money paid in advance—for coffins, services, burial vaults. The prearranged agreement should allow the person controlling the trust to receive interest earned, which may be applied to the principal to offset inflation. Finally, the person should have the right to terminate the contract at any time and receive all funds, including interest earned.

Table 6. What You May Need When Filing for Death Benefits

| | Social Security Benefits | Veterans' Benefits | Life Insurance | Credit Life Insurance | Casualty Insurance | Railroad Benefits | Teachers' Benefits | Civil Service Benefits | Other Benefits |
|---|---|---|---|---|---|---|---|---|---|
| 1. Death certificate or equivalent | x | x | x | x | x | x | x | x | x |
| 2. Birth certificate or proof of age of | | | | | | | | | |
| a. deceased | x | x | | | | x | | x | |
| b. survivor | x | x | | | | x | | | |
| c. children | x | x | | | | x | | x | |
| 3. Social Security number of | | | | | | | | | |
| a. deceased | x | x | | | | x | | x | |
| b. survivor | x | x | | | | x | x | | |
| c. children | x | | | | | | | | |
| d. dependent parents | x | | | | | | | | |

| | | | | | |
|---|---|---|---|---|---|
| 4. W2 forms and income tax returns for past three years | x | x | | | x |
| 5. Marriage license | x | x | | x | x |
| 6. Divorce documents | x | x | | x | x |
| 7. Military records (ID number, hon. discharge, etc.) | x | x | | x | x |
| 8. Adoption documents | x | x | | x | |
| 9. Evidence of unborn child | x | x | x | x | x |
| 10. Receipted, itemized funeral bill | x | | | x | x |

Note: This information was generously provided by Riverside Memorial Chapels, Bronx, New York.

## The Postmortem Examination

The decision to have an autopsy performed can be a difficult and emotional issue. Mrs. Jarvis describes how she changed her mind about a postmortem examination:

As you know, Jim died this afternoon at two-ten. Shortly after his death the nurses let me sit alone with him to say good-bye. He was so peaceful. He even seemed to smile.

So many memories are with me tonight. We were married fifty-two years this January. Two weeks ago, when I started to leave him at the nursing home, he asked, "Are we married?" When I said yes, he asked, "Why are you leaving me here?" The look in his eyes broke my heart. I told him, "You are very sick and you must be here. I cannot take care of you by myself." He told me, "I am not sick. But go home now. You look very tired." I left and had a good cry. I will never forget that day as long as I live. Jim was a good husband and a good father. He worked hard all his life. Why should he end up like this? What caused his brain to change?

The doctors wanted to do an autopsy. I was against it for a long time. Jim had lost his ability to do everything for himself. His mind was gone, but his body was pure. And he had suffered too much. I didn't want anybody to touch him.

When I saw Jim dead, I suddenly changed my mind. I thought back to our last sailing trip before Jim became sick. We had decided to take the boat out together. The last night out we lay in the cabin listening to the sounds of the sea. I remember we made love or at least tried. He held me tightly and cried. "I hate this growing old. Something is very wrong, but I don't know what it is. I wish I knew. Whatever happens I want to give you and the kids everything you deserve. You are what I live and die for. As long as I can move or breathe, I will care for you." After Jim spoke those words, he looked at me in the strangest way for several minutes. He smiled the same smile when we said good-bye for the last time.

I signed the papers for the doctors to study his brain. Jim cared so much for everybody that I know he would want to help others with this awful disease. Jim's self is not lost. He has left a part of himself in all of us.

Donating the brain after death for scientific study is a gift to humanity. Unless they have brain tissue from victims of dementia, scientists will be unable to carry out investigations to study the causes of Alzheimer's disease and related disorders. Without this research there can be little hope of curing the disease.

Autopsy studies have already helped us learn a great deal about the brain. Some scientists have described the brain changes in Alzheimer's disease as "generalized cerebral atrophy" because with time most of the brain atrophies or deteriorates. But the process is not uniform in all parts of the brain. Just as memory is lost in bits and pieces, so are the brain cells lost. This cell loss is the ultimate basis of the dementia. However, the very fact that the changes are so slow may also carry with it a slight ray of hope. If we can discover what is causing brain cells to degenerate and die, we may be able to develop chemical agents to halt or reverse the process. And if we can detect the disease early enough, we may be able to prevent further destruction. Early detection, intervention, and prevention are the goals for which we strive. Until we reach these goals, brain autopsies are essential for research.

## Autopsy Planning

Your doctor may ask you to sign papers for an autopsy, or, if you are a member of a family-support group, you may be approached by a campaign to enroll patients for autopsies. Scientists may visit your family group to describe the research that can be done when brain tissue is available. Publications from the National Alzheimer's Association as well as newsletters from the local chapters may contain information about the dementia brain banks which have been established in several medical centers throughout the country. The Alzheimer's Disease and Related Disorders Association (ADRDA) has helped support the establishment of brain banks on the East Coast, on the West Coast, and in the Midwest to ensure the availability and careful storage of tissue. At the moment, brain banks exist in New York at the Montefiore Medical Center and at the Albert Einstein College of Medicine, in Boston at the McLean Hospital, in California at the University of California at San Diego, and in Ohio at Ohio State University. Specific information about how to donate brains to these banks can be obtained from the national office of ADRDA or one of its local chapters (Appendix 1).

When and how do you involve patients themselves in a discussion about their willingness to consent to an autopsy? There is no right way or right time. Since family members usually know the patient far better than the doctors do, a family meeting is often a useful means of airing the thoughts and feelings of everyone involved. Discussions about autopsies are not a kiss of death. They are a healthy way to think about and plan for the future, however distant that future. Writing a will, buying life insurance, selecting a burial plot, and several other legal and financial decisions require meetings and decisions to anticipate personal and family needs.

Many patients will sign the autopsy consent form as easily as they sign the organ donation statement on the back of a driver's license. Some may refuse to discuss the possibility, while others may have family members who will not allow them to talk about it. A significant number of patients ask many questions, and you may want to involve a doctor, clergyman, or close friend. Still others want to think carefully about the decision, and several meetings and phone conversations may be necessary before the patient consents. In certain situations religious law and convictions complicate or prohibit decisions about an autopsy.

If discussions and decisions do not occur early in the disease, at a time when the patient has the ability to participate in the decision making, family members will be in the position of signing consent forms in the late or terminal phases of the dementia. If this occurs, candid discussions with the doctors and a confidant are helpful. Sometimes it is best to have several family members participate in this process; at other times it is appropriate for one family member to assume leadership.

Regardless of the situation, the following points of information will help you know what is involved in autopsy planning as well as what to do at the time of death.

### THE COST-ABSORBED AUTOPSY

When you meet with the doctor to sign the consent form, ask him or her to tell you where the autopsy will be performed. Find out whether that hospital or research center will absorb all the costs of the autopsy. Autopsies are expensive, and you should not have to pay for them. Several steps need to be taken ahead of time, so that the necessary information can be given to doctors and nurses in the hospital or nursing home. Patients are often eligible for a cost-absorbed autopsy at a hospital where they have been inpatients.

Most hospitals and medical centers specializing in Alzheimer's research have an arrangement whereby they absorb the total cost of the autopsy. If you live a great distance from an Alzheimer's research center, ask your doctor to help you both get a cost-absorbed autopsy and ensure that the brain is sent to the center you designate. A few suggestions may be useful:

- Tell your physician the names of the doctors conducting the research in Alzheimer's disease who have asked you and your relative to arrange for an autopsy.
- Ask the doctor to place an autopsy request in the patient's medical records which says that your relative has the doctor's consent for autopsy.
- Ask the doctor to write two specific items in the written request form: first, that the patient needs a neurological and diagnostic autopsy; second, that your relative has Alzheimer's disease or a related disorder and that you have made or would like to make arrangements with researchers in the field of dementia to have the brain used for special research.

If there are any questions about any of this in your or your doctor's mind, call the scientists at the center where your relative's brain will be studied and ask them to speak with your doctor and explain the situation.

Some hospitals have a rule which states that a person must die in the hospital in order to qualify for autopsy. This means that if your relative dies at home or in a nursing home, he or she will not be eligible for a cost-absorbed postmortem examination. If this is the case, consult your doctor or the national Alzheimer's Disease and Related Disorders Association (Appendix 1) to help you find centers which will cooperate with you.

MORTUARIES

Contrary to what some people fear, autopsies do not prohibit an open-casket funeral or any other type of funeral you may wish your relative to have. However, it is important to choose a mortuary which will take your plans into consideration ahead of time so that you will not have to deal with these decisions when death occurs. One of the services which some mortuaries can supply is the transportation of the deceased from the place of death to an area where the body can be kept cool until the hospital is ready to do the autopsy. When choosing mortuaries, ask whether they provide such services and inquire about the cost. If the cost is high or if they do not have the service, ask your doctor for advice. Many researchers also have grants and will pay the costs for you.

NURSING HOMES

If your relative is in a nursing home the medical, administrative, and nursing staffs will probably know what to do at the time of death to ensure that your plans are carried out, but they should know your wishes. The doctor must write a statement in the patient's nursing-home chart to state that an autopsy has been requested and agreed to. Ask your doctor to talk with the nurses so that they will know what to do when death occurs. You yourself may wish to speak with the head nurse as well. Indicate which mortuary is to provide transportation from the nursing home to the hospital or other facility until the autopsy can be performed. If this makes you uncomfortable, ask the doctor or administrator to help see to these arrangements.

## What to Do at the Time of Death

At the time of death several phone calls need to be made. Survivors will need to contact the minister, priest, or rabbi tending the patient, the doctor or site of the autopsy, and close relatives and friends. Keep a list of important phone numbers in an accessible place. Furthermore, your relative's doctor—that is, the attending physician who made the official medical request for the autopsy—must be called if he or she did not sign the death certificate. If that doctor is unavailable, there should be someone else at the hospital who covers for him or her. Tell whoever is on call that your relative has died and that you would like to initiate the autopsy arrangements. Finally, the mortuary needs to be called and asked to transport the deceased from the place of death to an appropriate holding area until the autopsying hospital is ready to admit.

Even when the patient has given prior permission, in many states an autopsy permit must be signed by the legal next of kin after the death of the patient. If necessary the hospital will arrange a call to you and allow you to grant permission over the phone. In such instances a second member of the hospital staff will also be on the line to witness your permission.

The hospital may need to complete certain arrangements before it can admit the patient's body for an autopsy. This is why it sometimes helps to arrange for a mortuary service that will hold the deceased until the hospital is ready to receive the body. In most situations the hospital will need to call you (you do not have to call them) about the permit. We suggest, however, that you call them anyway (or have someone else do so) to say that the deceased is in the mortuary waiting to be admitted for autopsy. Also inform them of your location and give them your phone number, so that they know where to reach you when they are ready to call about the permit. This helps to ensure that the body is handled as carefully and quickly as possible.

When you call or are called to sign the permit, indicate that there are two very important points that you wish to be made clear on the autopsy permit. First, this is a neurological and diagnostic autopsy, not a donation of the brain to general science. Second, the patient has Alzheimer's disease, and you wish the brain to be given or sent to scientists conducting research on Alzheimer's disease or dementia.

There are two circumstances in which the autopsy permit may be signed in advance of the patient's death and held until the time comes. If the next of kin has legal guardianship, he or she can sign the autopsy permit in advance of death. The usual legal order of next of kin is spouse, children, parents, siblings, legal guardians, and then closest next of kin. In some states the patient can also sign his or her own permit if legally competent.

## Preparing for the Future

Death is not a challenge unique to the patient with dementia and the family. However, brain diseases rob victims of their ability to think, act, and participate in the decisions which must be made. At the same time the family members must watch and struggle with their own anguish and relate to a loved one who has changed from a former self. Alzheimer's disease destroys the quality of life which gives meaning to the quality of death.

The key is to discover how to live life "one day at a time" with the patient and cope with changes. There are ways to maximize comfort throughout the illness. Much can be done even in the final stages when the patient is bedridden, semiconscious, and laboring to live. Karen Russell, aged seventy-eight, sat by her husband's bedside in a nursing home for fifteen weeks as he grew progressively weaker but his body refused to succumb to pneumonia. She watched and tended him from eleven in the morning until eight at night. This constant attendance was a natural and necessary activity for her, since both she and her husband had always spent most of their time together. When the staff sensed his final hours, he went on the critical list and she was allowed to keep her vigil at any time of the day or night. Mrs. Russell had the support of friends, doctors, staff, her children, and her grandchildren. She lived with him emotionally to the end. She visited the hospital several weeks after his death and shared an hour with us. She spoke softly, and seemed at peace with herself. "It is hard to put love away," she said. "We spent fifty-four years together. My son and I will not forget him. Jewish writings say that we shall continue to live as long as we are not forgotten and as long as we have loved and have been loved."

There are many ways families can work together to help patients develop a legacy, to maximize comfort and dignity, and to reconstruct family life for the future. Families continually show us the strength and power of their love. In *The Bridge of San Luis Rey*,

Thornton Wilder wrote these words of consolation, which ring close to the thoughts of Mrs. Russell: "There is a land of the living and a land of the dead and the bridge is love; the only survival, the only meaning."

# 12

# WHAT SCIENTISTS KNOW ABOUT THE CAUSES OF DEMENTIA

THIS chapter is written in response to the many questions asked by individuals who want specific details about the causes of Alzheimer's disease and multi-infarct dementias. It is more technical than other parts of this book; its aim is to provide useful information for those who wish to broaden their scientific knowledge. Research efforts have intensified, and, it is to be hoped, we will soon witness a biological and medical revolution. Someday we may learn what causes Alzheimer's disease and related disorders. New technological advances should improve methods for diagnosis, and perhaps we will in the near future find ways to treat the dementias of later life and arrest or even reverse the savage destruction of the self.

## Changes in the Alzheimer's Brain

The size and weight of the brain are significantly reduced in Alzheimer's disease as a result of the loss of brain cells. Although this loss occurs throughout the brain, certain areas may be more affected than others. Significant cell loss occurs throughout the outer mantle of the brain, known as the cerebral cortex. The normal brain has a rugged, almost mountain-like appearance. It is full of grooves known technically as fissures; the elevated parts between these fissures are called gyri. In Alzheimer's disease the mountains appear more rugged. The gyri are narrowed, and the fissures or grooves are widened as a result of cell loss.

These gross brain changes, which are obvious to the naked eye, in and of themselves do not prove that the deceased patient had Alzheimer's disease. The diagnosis actually rests on the results of the microscopic examination of brain tissue which has been chemically treated to stain a number of anatomical structures. The diagnosis is established when a large number of anatomical lesions known as tangles and plaques are found. These structural changes are also found to some degree in the brains of older persons without dementia, but they are far more numerous in Alzheimer's disease. The density of these tangles and plaques is used to arrive at a definitive diagnosis.

The tangles are technically called neurofibrillary tangles. They resemble hairlike hooks or teardrop-like structures when they are stained and photographed under a powerful microscope. If we observe these tangles using the very high magnification of the electron microscope, we can see that they are composed of many bundles of little hairlike structures called filaments. These filaments may occur alone or in pairs. When they are paired, they are wrapped around each other in a helix, and not surprisingly they are called "paired helical filaments of the Alzheimer type." They are structually different from any other filaments in normal brain cells.

The plaques called neuritic plaques or senile plaques are spherical structures composed of a protein called amyloid. They are most often seen in the cerebral cortex but also develop in other areas of the brain. A small number of neuritic plaques are seen in the brains of most older people. However, what distinguishes the Alzheimer's brain from others is the extraordinary number of plaques per volume of brain tissue examined. The presence of a few plaques in the brain is not unusual, but the presence of many is abnormal.

The cortex, the most highly evolved part of the brain, is responsible for what are called higher brain functions—thinking, judgment, reasoning, speech, and language. Different locations in the cortex also have specialized functions which affect such behaviors as mood and sexual expression as well as language and thinking. Therefore, as more and more of the brain cells are destroyed in Alzheimer's disease, all aspects of intellectual functioning become worse, and normal behavior disintegrates.

Underneath the many thick layers of the cerebral cortex is a part of the brain known as the limbic system, which contains many different structures. One of these structures is a small group of cells shaped somewhat like a sea horse. Hence the name hippocampus. Autopsy studies have shown that in Alzheimer's disease the plaques and tangles are very dense in the hippocampus, especially in the bottom half. This widespread destruction of hippocampal cells significantly disrupts attention and memory. Damage in the hippocampus and other parts of the limbic system also affects the way emotions are expressed. Ferocious rage, extraordinary irritability, or their opposite, apathy and docility, may occur. The loss of cells in the limbic system probably accounts for the changes in emotional control and personality which occur in Alzheimer's disease.

Certain cells in the hippocampus undergo another change characteristic of Alzheimer's disease. Using special dyes to stain the hippocampus cells, we can show what is called granulovacuolar degeneration. The cells of the hippocampus are pyramid shaped, and they contain small spherical vacuoles, or holes with a small granule in the center of the hole. Alzheimer's disease is distinguished by the high density of these vacuoles. This granulovacuolar degeneration is quite rare in persons under the age of sixty but is seen with increasing frequency in the aging brain after the age of sixty. By the age of eighty, more than three-quarters of all brains show some amount of granulovacuolar degeneration. A high density of such change is indicative of disease at any age.

Autopsy studies have shown degeneration in other parts of the brain. The spinal cord connects with the base of the brain and runs into the brain stem, which looks like a flattened part of the spinal cord. Many critical functions are regulated by groups of cells in the brain stem, including breathing and the beating of the heart. Thus, damage to the brain stem is usually quite dangerous.

The brain stem contains several structures, including a group of nerve cells which have been named the locus coeruleus. Many of these cells are destroyed in Alzheimer's disease. "Locus coeruleus" means "blue place," and if the brain is cut and the locus coeruleus examined, it actually appears to have a blue color. This region is the site of a large number of nerves, some of which reach up into the cerebral cortex and some of which run down into a place in the brain called the cerebellum. The cerebellum sits on the back of the brain like a small head of cauliflower. It is responsible for coordinating the many muscle movements which allow us to walk, bend, and move about in our world. The destruction of the locus coeruleus probably contributes to the changes in awareness, the emotional outbursts, and perhaps the motor coordination problems observed in Alzheimer's disease.

The brain stem ascends into the brain and joins the cortex in a structure called the hypothalamus, which is also affected in Alzheimer's disease. The hypothalamus controls the functions of many of the body's internal organs. It regulates the pituitary gland and can stimulate this "master gland" to release into the bloodstream many hormones essential for life and growth. These hormones in turn affect other glands, causing them to secrete other essential hormones. The hypothalamus also has special centers of activity like the hippocampus that seem to be involved in the ability to control emotions as well as in the experience of such emotions as pleasure, hunger, and satiety, the sensation of fullness one gets after enjoying a meal.

## Causes of Alzheimer's Disease

These structural changes in the brain do not cause Alzheimer's disease. They are the result of something else. The great challenge is to discover what causes the degeneration.

### NEUROTRANSMITTER CHANGES: THE CHOLINERGIC SYSTEM

The brain contains chemicals known as neurotransmitters, and one of these neurotransmitters is significantly altered in Alzheimer's disease. In order to understand what these changes mean, it is useful first to review how neurotransmitters play a role in the way the brain works. There are more than $10^{10}$ nerve cells, or neurons, in the brain —that means 10,000,000,000 cells. These nerve cells form many interconnections allowing them to communicate with each other through a combination of electrical and chemical events. Nerve cells generate electrical impulses which travel along the length of the nerve, much the way an electrical current is carried by a wire. When the nerve impulse has reached the end of the nerve, it triggers the release of chemical substances known as neurotransmitters.

Neurotransmitters are discharged from the nerve endings into an area between the nerves which is called the synaptic cleft. When these chemical substances reach the nerve on the other side of the synaptic cleft, they cause the next cell(s) in the sequence to become excited and carry on the impulse. Since many neurons are clustered at each synaptic cleft, entire groups of nerve cells may become excited. Different groups of nerves become activated when we smell the aroma of a freshly baked pizza, hear the sounds of a jazz band, watch a ball game, read a novel, write a letter, or try to solve a problem. Entirely different parts of the brain are active when we sleep and when we are awake. Thus, the neurotransmitters of the brain are essential for learning, memory, and all those behaviors and actions that make us human.

Most individual nerve cells use or respond to only one type of neurotransmitter. However, there are many different neurotransmitters in the brain. Today we recognize hundreds of substances which may act as neurotransmitters. This area of science, known as neurochemistry, is growing rapidly and giving us profound insights into the way the brain works.

Acetylcholine is the neurotransmitter which appears to be most altered in Alzheimer's disease. Neurons that contain acetylcholine are known as cholinergic neurons, and many of these neurons are bunched together into clearly defined groups called brain tracts. The cholinergic tracts radiate throughout the entire brain. A large group of cholinergic nerves come together deep in the brain in a region called the nucleus basalis of Meynert, which may be one of the first parts of the brain affected in Alzheimer's disease. Autopsy examinations show that not all, but a significant number, of the nerve cells are destroyed in this nucleus and that there is an associated loss of large numbers of cells in cholinergic tracts throughout the entire brain.

From autopsy and laboratory studies we know that chemical changes occur in the cholinergic nerves sometime before they die. It is clear that the ability of these affected cells to produce acetylcholine is altered in several ways. Two substances, choline and acetyl CoA, are joined together by an enzyme to form acetylcholine. This enzyme, like other enzymes, is a special type of protein. It is called choline acetyltransferase and is often abbreviated as CAT.

One of the important recent research findings is that in the brains of Alzheimer's patients there is a dramatic reduction in the amount of choline acetyltransferase (CAT). Furthermore, this reduction is greatest in those areas of the brain where the well-recognized plaques and neurofibrillary tangles occur in the greatest numbers.

A decrease in CAT activity is not the only change observed in the cholinergic system of Alzheimer's brains. The synthesis or formation of acetylcholine has also been measured directly in brain material taken from Alzheimer's patients by means of a brain biopsy procedure. Brain samples containing plaques and tangles show more than a 50 percent reduction in the production of acetylcholine. However, brain samples without plaques and tangles retain their ability to synthesize acetylcholine.

These findings are exciting and important. They suggest that not all cholinergic nerve cells lose their ability to produce acetylcholine in Alzheimer's disease. The existence of healthy tissue provides a basis for hope. Research is urgently needed to understand how to chemically stabilize or improve cholinergic functioning in the brain.

Once the production of acetylcholine within many of the cholinergic nerves has fallen off greatly, much less is available to be discharged into the synaptic cleft. However, if ways can be found to increase the amount of acetylcholine secreted into the synapse, a nerve impulse should be generated. This is theoretically possible because the receiving apparatus of the cholinergic neurons and their capacity to fire a nerve impulse are not affected, at least not in the early stages of Alzheimer's disease.

This finding has been the basis for attempts to find drugs to increase the amount of choline in the synaptic cleft. Unfortunately, the use of drugs and compounds which contain acetylcholine, such as lecithin, has not been successful—for reasons we do not yet understand. Too much acetylcholine may have been lost for it simply to be replaced. Or it is possible that the compounds and drugs under investigation today may not be getting into the right areas of the brain. Other neurotransmitters may also be altered in Alzheimer's disease, and we have yet to discover how they exert their control on the cholinergic system. Many structural changes could also be occurring in the nerve, and they might affect its ability to use acetylcholine even if the chemical is available. Finally, intellectual functioning is a complex phenomenon and therefore a complex target for simple drug treatment.

One additional change in the cholinergic system merits discussion. Acetylcholinesterase is another important enzyme whose activity is diminished in Alzheimer's disease, but the reduction is not as severe as that observed for the CAT enzyme. The function of acetylcholinesterase is to break down the acetylcholine after it has been secreted into the synaptic cleft. The altering of a neurotransmitter after it has done its job is essential. Our bodies have a mechanism to remove or chemically change neurotransmitters in the synapse so that we end the stimulation of the nerve to prepare for the next transmission.

Drugs which prevent the deactivation of acetylcholine are also being studied for their potential value in Alzheimer's disease. Physostigmine, one of these drugs, has received substantial publicity. The assumption here is that it is possible to prolong the activity of whatever limited supply of acetylcholine is available. Some results have shown a limited, short-term value to this approach.

Although specific changes in certain cholinergic neurons are well established, it is not possible to say at this time that cholinergic changes *cause* Alzheimer's disease. It seems more likely that these cells are a target for something. We still need to find the bullet. Many important questions remain to be answered. We know many pieces of the puzzle, but we have to conduct more research to assemble the pieces and see the full picture.

CHANGES IN PROTEIN SYNTHESIS

Other chemical processes are necessary for the healthy functioning of nerve cells besides neurotransmitter synthesis and inactivation. One of the most important of these is protein synthesis, which

is significantly disrupted in the Alzheimer's brain. The brain manu-
factures many proteins, and they are used to build internal structures
within the nerve cell. These proteins form a skeleton-like framework
of multiple filaments, and they appear as a group of pipelines within
the cell. These filaments not only provide a skeleton for the cell but
also serve as conduits that transport nutrients and other chemicals
throughout the entire nerve.

The discovery of unusual twisted filaments in the neurofibrillary
tangles of Alzheimer's brain prompted research to determine how
protein metabolism is disrupted. Nerve cells containing these
strangely twisted filaments as well as neurons not containing them
have been studied carefully. The protein-synthesizing capacity of
cells from Alzheimer's brains is greatly reduced regardless of whether
or not the cells contain twisted filaments. Exactly how these abnormal filaments are formed is still a mystery. Some evidence suggests
that an anomalous protein may be produced in the brain of the
Alzheimer's patient and that the presence of this atypical protein
leads to the formation of abnormal filaments.

ACCUMULATION OF ALUMINUM

Does the accumulation of excess aluminum in the brain play a role
in Alzheimer's disease? A careful examination of research results
from many laboratories does not provide a clear answer. Several
investigators have reported that higher concentrations of aluminum
are present in the brains of patients with Alzheimer's disease than
in those of healthy older persons without dementia. The highest
concentration of aluminum was initially reported to be in those areas
of the brain with the highest density of neurofibrillary tangles. Many
investigators have reported elevated concentrations in the brains
both of healthy older persons and of Alzheimer's patients. They have
also found that the amount of aluminum in the brain varies with
geography. In some parts of the country, where the soil contains
more aluminum, everyone has higher aluminum levels, but there is
no evidence of a greater prevalence of Alzheimer's disease.

Using special techniques, scientists have been able to actually
measure the concentration of aluminum in different parts of the
nerve cell. Nerves containing a high density of tangles appear to be
richer in aluminum compared with cells without tangles. High con-

centrations of aluminum have also been reported in the brains of patients with other types of dementias. Therefore, the uptake of aluminum is probably not specific to Alzheimer's disease. It may be that aluminum and other chemicals surrounding the neurons may be taken into damaged or partially impaired cells.

The role of aluminum in Alzheimer's disease is puzzling. Aluminum may be associated with other forms of dementia. Patients with kidney disease who must use dialysis for many years have been known to develop a condition called dialysis dementia. They show intellectual deterioration, muscle tremors, and seizures. Autopsy studies have demonstrated a heavy accumulation of aluminum in the cortex of their brains, which probably comes from solutions used in the dialysis treatments. What is significant is that the brains of these dialysis patients do not show the rich concentration of plaques and tangles seen in Alzheimer's disease. Furthermore, the aluminum does not seem to accumulate inside the nucleus of the nerve cells of dialysis patients, as it does in those of Alzheimer's victims.

In sum, it appears unlikely that aluminum accumulation by itself causes Alzheimer's disease. On the other hand, if the patient has Alzheimer's disease, aluminum is probably taken into the already defective neurons and may cause further damage to the cell. Aluminum may also form a chemical bond with the protein filaments manufactured by the brain. This complex of aluminum-protein material could then interfere with the normal assembly of microfilaments in the brain. The result might then be the obstruction of the normal functions of the nerve cell involved.

Since aluminum is the most abundant metal in our environment, composing 8 percent of the earth's crust, its presence in the brain is not surprising. The selective deposit of aluminum inside nerve cells with tangles that has been observed in different forms of dementia is a mystery which remains to be solved.

POLYPEPTIDE CHANGES IN THE HYPOTHALAMUS

In Alzheimer's disease specific chemical changes may occur in the cells of the hypothalamus, a structure in the brain which controls the functions of many of the body's internal organs. The hypothalamus contains special clusters of nerve cells involved in the control of emotions, such as our experiences of joy, sexual pleasure, and hunger.

Certain cells in the hypothalamus are capable of manufacturing and secreting chemicals called neuropeptides. These neuropeptides are known to affect a wide range of behavior, including sex drive and sexual activity, mood changes, sensitivity to pain, and intellectual functioning. Scientists believe that neuropeptides affect behavior by the way they control or modulate the action of other neurotransmitters in the synapse. The discovery of these peptides is relatively recent, and the list has lengthened from a handful to well over a hundred within the past few years. Research on the role of neuropeptides in Alzheimer's disease is in its infancy. Many investigators have already shown that several neuropeptides may be deficient in Alzheimer's disease. Although the precise meaning of these changes remains to be discovered, further research on neuropeptides may explain why the simple replacement of acetylcholine is not an effective treatment.

ALTERATIONS IN THE IMMUNE SYSTEM

The body's immune system is crucial for good health because is has many mechanisms for fighting germs, bacteria, viruses, and other foreign invaders which may injure the body and cause disease. Although a great deal is known about how the immune system functions in most of the body, its activity in the brain is not well understood. In several diseases, such as multiple sclerosis, schizophrenia, and Huntington's chorea, scientists have reported the presence of a chemical substance called an "antibody" to nerve tissue. Antibodies are produced by white blood cells known as lymphocytes, and the production of large quantities of these antibodies is one of the major defense mechanisms of the immune system. The body is capable of manufacturing special antibodies to fight specific diseases. The value of these specific antibodies is that they make it possible to vaccinate people against many infectious viral diseases. Vaccination with a modified form of a particular virus leads to the production of special antibodies. Therefore, if and when individuals are exposed to the real thing, in most cases they will be able to resist the illness.

Occasionally, the production of antibodies can actually be stimulated to react against the body's very own cells. Antibodies produced to fight certain germs may also react to parts of the body. Because of similarities between the invaders and body tissue, the antibodies do not recognize that the cells of the body belong to the body. They react to them as if they were invaders. This is called an autoantibody reaction—a reaction against one's self. Furthermore, autoantibodies may cause serious diseases. One of the dangers of a "strep throat" in childhood is the creation of an antibody to a specific type of streptococcus germ which may in some people then affect the heart or other organs. Rheumatic heart disease is a consequence of this reaction in the heart.

Autoantibodies may also be produced as a result of another mechanism. Since many of the cells of the body die and are replaced, certain types of antibodies serve to destroy and remove the altered material now seen as debris by the body. In rare instances this process may stimulate autoantibody production when for some reason the cells being lost are not recognizable for what they are but instead are seen as new invaders. Since the specific antibody being produced is designed to destroy material which is so close in structure to normal tissue, the autoantibody effect is likely to occur.

Autoantibody reactions occur in the Alzheimer's brain, but little is known about them. The antibodies may be generated in response to neurofibrillary tangles or other structural changes in the dying neurons. One of the many questions to be answered is whether specific antibodies are produced in Alzheimer's disease which attack and destroy the brain tissue. These antibodies could also be manufactured to fight a virus or a virus-like particle which may be the cause of Alzheimer's disease.

THE VIRAL HYPOTHESIS

There has been a great deal of speculation about the possible role of a virus or a virus-like particle as the cause of Alzheimer's. Although there is no direct proof that a virus or virus-like particle causes Alzheimer's disease, similar diseases causing dementia in humans have been discovered to be the result of transmissible virus-like agents. Two of these diseases are kuru and Creutzfeldt-Jakob's disease.

Kuru is the name of a brain disease which has been observed in a group of people living in Papua New Guinea. Although individuals may carry the "kuru agent" for a long period without symptoms, once the disease appears, it progresses fairly rapidly and causes death in six to twenty-four months. As the illness worsens, individuals have severe dementia and a number of other neuromuscular signs, such as uncontrolled muscle twitches, tremors, and problems in walking. Dr. D. Carleton Gajdusek received a Nobel Prize for discovering that kuru was caused by a virus-like particle that was transmitted, probably through food and primarily to women and children who participated in cannibalistic rituals. Men have also been known to get kuru, but they were usually excluded from consuming the infected brains of the deceased in funeral rites. Women and children were entitled to the brains as reward for preparing the bodies.

Creutzfeldt-Jakob's disease is named after the two people who described the neuropathological changes in the brains of patients with this dementia. Unlike kuru, it occurs throughout the world, but it is relatively rare, compared with Alzheimer's disease. The chemical structures of the kuru and Creutzfeldt-Jakob's viruses are being identified, but the evidence for a viral etiology is clearly based on transmissibility tests in the laboratory. Brain samples from deceased patients are injected into animals who are watched for the neurological symptoms of the disease and later examined for brain changes at autopsy.

To date there is no evidence that Alzheimer's disease can be transmitted directly from human to human or from human to animal. However, there are clinical similarities between Alzheimer's disease and Creutzfeldt-Jakob's disease, and some scientists have used these similarities as a rationale for looking for a possible viral etiology or cause for Alzheimer's disease. Both disorders have similar ages of onset. The duration of illness is usually longer for Alzheimer's disease, but there is an overlap in the time from onset to death for the two disorders (1 to 120 months for Creutzfeldt-Jakob's disease and 10 to 300 months for Alzheimer's disease). Sometimes the clinical symptoms throughout the course of illness are so similar that the autopsy is the only way to make the definitive diagnosis. Myoclonus, which is muscle-jerking and twitching of the body as well as the arms and legs, was once thought to distinguish Creutzfeldt-Jakob's from Alzheimer's disease. However, myoclonus has been observed in a number of Alzheimer's patients.

There have also been a few reports of Creutzfeldt-Jakob's and Alzheimer's diseases occurring together in the same individual. Furthermore, Creutzfeldt-Jakob's and Alzheimer's diseases have been observed to occur in the same family. Both of these observations have been used as evidence for the view that these two brain disorders may be related.

Scrapie, a disease in sheep transmitted by a virus-like particle, has been known to cause degeneration of the sheep's central nervous system. The brains of sheep who die from scrapie show many of the changes observed in Creutzfeldt-Jakob's disease. Some scientists think that there are similarities between the agents which cause scrapie and Creutzfeldt-Jakob's disease and that there may be a modified scrapie-like agent which causes Alzheimer's disease.

In a number of experiments goats and other animals have been inoculated with scrapie or preparations from the brains of people who died with Creutzfeldt-Jakob's disease. Within three to four years the goats developed severe neurological symptoms and died, regardless of whether they received scrapie or the brain preparation. The symptoms—muscle tremors and twitching—as well as the lesions in the brains at autopsy were identical. Monkeys will react to both scrapie and the brains of Creutzfeldt-Jakob's patients. Curiously, chimpanzees are susceptible only to experimental Creutzfeldt-Jakob's disease, not to scrapie. At the moment, there is no evidence that the scrapie agent can infect human beings.

The scrapie agent acts differently from viruses and viroid-like particles. Because of its unusual properties it is known as a prion, a small *pro*tein *in*fectious particle. Using very specialized techniques, scientists have tried to purify brain samples of prions from patients with Creutzfeldt-Jakob's disease and from animals inoculated with scrapie or Creutzfeldt-Jakob's brains. When these purified samples are stained with a special colored dye, they resemble the amyloid found in the plaques of the Alzheimer's brain. Currently, some scientists think that the amyloid plaques in Alzheimer's disease may be composed of prions. Clearly, this is an exciting and complex area of investigation.

GENETIC FACTORS

Is Alzheimer's disease hereditary? For most persons the answer is probably no. Others may be at a higher risk than the average individual. In a relatively few instances there is a strong family history of the disease. However, family history does not necessarily mean that a disease will be transmitted to all members of that family.

Some family trees show a large number of persons with dementia. These families provide us an important opportunity to study the genetics of the disease. They allow us to look for a pattern in the way the disease is transmitted. Who gets the disease and in what generation of descendants? In a few cases, high-risk individuals can be identified. If there is a strong family history of Alzheimer's—if the disease frequently occurs before the age of sixty and if both a parent and a sibling (brother or sister) have the disease—the risk is high. In these situations it is possible that 50 percent of the family members in a single generation will develop Alzheimer's disease.

Some scientists have estimated that 12 percent of the total population carries the "Alzheimer's gene." Unfortunately, we do not yet have a way to identify the gene. We have not even confirmed that it exists, let alone identified the people who may carry it, so that any such notion is speculation at best. However, an important point should be considered. The presence of a gene for a disease does not always mean that the gene will express itself and that the disease will develop. It is conceivable that many individuals possess the "Alzheimer's gene," if it exists, yet that they will never develop dementia, because they are not exposed to the set of conditions which will trigger the disorder.

ONE CAUSE OR MANY CAUSES? ONE DISEASE OR MANY?

This is an age-old debate regarding many major diseases like cancer, heart disease, and schizophrenia and many other afflictions which have plagued humanity. It is entirely conceivable that there are many causes of Alzheimer's disease. Indeed, there may be multiple forms of Alzheimer's disease. Several experiments have shown biochemical and structural differences in the brains of patients who developed Alzheimer's early in life and of those who developed it after the age of sixty. This is important and provocative research.

## Related Disorders

Although Alzheimer's disease is the dominant theme of this book, it is not the only major form of dementia. The former belief that all late-life dementias were caused by circulation problems in the brain was wrong. It is accurate to state, however, that about 15 to 25 percent of the irreversible dementias are caused primarily by problems of circulation to the brain and that an additional small group of patients have a mixed dementia, that is, a combination of an Alzheimer's type of dementia and a vascular dementia. This section focuses on the diseases of the blood vessels in the brain which can lead to dementing illness.

The principal disorder of brain circulation appears to be strokes. Strokes are the second major cause of death in the United States and a leading cause of death throughout the world. Strokes do not always kill. They often cripple individuals and affect their ability to walk, talk, and carry out many activities of daily life. They may also cause dementia. At one time doctors thought that when people showed significant intellectual deterioration in later life, it was the result of disease in the arteries of the many blood vessels in the brain. Only a decade or so ago Alzheimer's disease was believed to be a rare disorder which affected only people in their middle years. For that reason it was classified as a presenile dementia.

In the late 1960s and early 1970s, it became evident that arteriosclerosis was not the major cause of dementia in the aged. Hundreds of brains were examined in autopsy studies at several medical centers, and the results were clear. More than half of the brains examined showed the concentration of plaques and tangles characteristic of Alzheimer's disease. However, approximately 25 percent showed clear evidence that the brain's blood vessels were damaged. Some had changes consistent with both Alzheimer's disease and cerebrovascular disease.

"Multi-infarct dementia" is the general term now used to refer to the group of diseases in which the blood vessels of the brain are affected and progressive intellectual deterioration occurs. Patients with multi-infarct dementia appear to suffer the equivalent of small strokes which destroy many areas of the brain. When the brains are examined during autopsy, small holes can be seen in the brain where the tissue has been destroyed. Hence the name "multi-infarct," or "many holes." Studies at many hospitals have confirmed that multi-infarct dementia may be responsible for 15 to 25 percent of the nonreversible dementias.

Many books have been written by people who have had strokes; many others describe what happens in strokes or cerebral hemorrhages. These are listed in the reference list in the back of the book. Some of the best include *A Stroke in the Family,* by Valarie Eaton Griffith, and *Stroke: A Doctor's Personal Story of His Recovery,* by Dr. Charles C. Dahlberg and Joseph Jaffe.

INFARCTIONS

Infarcts appear to be caused by a series of ministrokes in the brain. But what causes these strokes? We do not know. It may be helpful for our discussion to divide them into three clinical groups. Those in the first group are due to one or more strokes caused by the blockage of large or medium-sized blood vessels in the brain. The second clinical group comprises those in which the small arteries are affected, resulting in lacunar strokes. "Lacunae" is the Latin word for "holes." Lacunae are very small areas of tissue loss in the brain. In patients with multi-infarct dementia these lacunae or infarcts are shown at autopsy. What causes them? Perhaps the same factors that cause major strokes. Something clogs or blocks a small artery in the brain, causing a loss of circulation beyond the blocked area. When the blood supply is cut off for a long enough time, the cells die, leaving a hole. Individuals with a history of arrhythmias, irregular heart rhythms, may be particularly vulnerable to this type of problem.

There is a third form of multi-infarct disease. In this case the disorder affects the smallest blood vessels in the brain, and it is sometimes called micro-infarct dementia. It is difficult to distinguish this disease from Alzheimer's disease. Patients are not necessarily hypertensive, they may not have heart disease or irregular heart rhythms, and their blood vessels do not show clear evidence of arteriosclerosis.

Although the exact cause for cerebrovascular disease is not apparent, we do know a great deal about risk factors. A famous study in Framingham, Massachusetts, has helped us understand risk factors for stroke—high blood pressure, impaired cardiac functioning, diabetes, high levels of cholesterol in the blood, and cigarette smoking. High blood pressure is a major culprit, occurring in about half of all individuals who suffer a stroke. The risk for stroke also increases if several cardiovascular abnormalities are present in the same individual.

Well-identified large blood vessels and many small tributaries circulate the blood throughout the brain. The pattern of these arteries and the territory of the brain which each supplies are fairly similar, though not identical, in all people. If the blood flow is interrupted in a specific artery, it will usually cause similar deficits in most individuals. Therefore, the symptoms a patient displays can tell us what part of the brain has been affected by the blockage of a particular vessel. For example, problems in speech or the use of the right hand or leg will help us localize the stroke on the left and identify the areas of the brain involved, and the arteries which feed blood to those areas are implicated.

The major blood vessels which connect the heart to the brain are the vertebral and the carotid arteries. They emanate from the major arteries leaving the heart and travel into the neck, where they feed into the base of the brain. Many different arteries branch out from these major vessels to ensure that the blood circulates to all parts of the brain. Some arteries branch deep into the interior of the brain as well as to the outside of the brain.

Arteriosclerosis, or the narrowing of the arteries, is one of the most conspicuous changes in the blood vessels of the brain. The vessels may be blocked because of the buildup of foreign material or fat droplets. If the arteriosclerosis is severe, the artery will even have a yellow color.

"Aneurysms" are another indication of cerebrovascular disease. Aneurysms appear as small balloons or blisters in the blood vessels where the vascular wall has become thinned. If they break, blood flows into the brain, damaging brain tissue and sometimes even causing death. Such a bursting also interrupts the flow beyond the rupture and leads to starvation of the affected brain tissue.

The blood supply can be interrupted permanently when a stroke occurs. When the artery is blocked, the area of the brain that the artery usually supplies becomes impaired and surrounding areas also become swollen. In most cases people with strokes recover some lost functioning. This is because with time the swelling subsides and circulation from other vessels may supply some of the areas affected. However, the areas of dead tissue remain as scars, and their functions are lost.

Strokes usually occur rapidly and are generally painless. Many happen during sleep. Some occur over several days and may be accompanied by a headache. If the individual survives, the worst deficits occur between the third and tenth days after a stroke because the brain swelling is worst at this time. As the swelling subsides, some recovery of abilities takes place.

## Transient Ischemic Attacks

There are several other forms of cerebrovascular disease which may be early warning signs of an impending stroke.

The word "ischemia" means "without blood," and transient ischemic attacks, sometimes called TIAs by physicians, are conditions in which the blood supply in the brain is interrupted briefly and persons lose their ability to function temporarily. They may even lose consciousness and often do not remember what happened. After several minutes they can usually function again, but they may not feel quite like themselves for another day. Over time these attacks may become more frequent. Without treatment about 25 percent of all people with transient ischemic attacks will develop a serious stroke within a year.

What causes TIAs? They are a sign that there may be arteriosclerosis in the brain's blood vessels. Sometimes these attacks can be caused by a change in the heart rhythm or by a brief drop in blood pressure.

### DIAGNOSIS OF TIAS

Transient ischemic attacks can usually be diagnosed after a thorough neurological examination and a careful history. Since TIAs are thought to be warning signs of a stroke, further studies are normally recommended. The routine examination usually includes a special electrocardiogram. The heart rate is monitored for twenty-four hours in an attempt to identify an arrhythmia which might be causing the symptoms. An electroencephalogram, a record of the electrical activity of the brain, is also done in order to locate any abnormal activity in the brain itself.

Several specialized techniques may also be used to identify exactly where arteries are clogged. Some of these tests do carry a slight risk and should be done in patients only after a careful evaluation. In some types of arterial disease, surgery may be possible.

After a clinical diagnosis is made, therapy may be recommended to decrease the risk of future strokes. Although TIAs occur for short periods of time, people may fall, strike their head, or even fracture a hip during an attack. When surgery is not appropriate or desirable, medications may help. When supervised by a physician, the use of aspirin appears to be an effective therapy. Newer medications such as Anturane or Persantine may be used by people who cannot tolerate aspirin, although careful medical management is needed. It is important to emphasize that aspirin may have serious side effects when not properly prescribed and monitored.

Surgery may be possible. The surgeon may perform what is called a carotid endarterectomy. In this operation the carotid artery in the neck is opened briefly to remove the arteriosclerotic plaques. Even when done by the most skilled doctor, this procedure carries a risk. It can be of great benefit, however, if there is blockage in the artery.

Another surgical technique is promising for individuals with lesions inside the arteries which lie deep in the brain. Using a special microscope, the surgeon operates to do a bypass procedure. When a lesion is inoperable, the surgeon may be able to connect an artery outside the brain with another brain artery. Blood then flows into the brain from an outside vessel, bypassing the blocked area which cannot be operated on.

PREVENTION

Although we are just beginning to learn about the risk factors for stroke with dementia, there is one significant vascular disease in which recognition and treatment may significantly reduce the potential for multi-infarct dementia—high blood pressure. Each year high blood pressure is a factor in two-thirds of all first heart attacks and three-quarters of all first strokes. If the 23 million individuals in the United States estimated to have high blood pressure could be screened to detect and treat it early, the overall death rate from strokes and heart attacks would decrease about 20 percent.

Available treatments for high blood pressure are effective. Unfortunately, only about 12.5 percent of all people with hypertension are receiving adequate treatment. What about the others? Another 12.5

percent know they have high blood pressure but are not receiving adequate therapy. Some 25 percent know they have hypertension but are not being treated at all. The remaining 50 percent of the 23 million people who have high blood pressure are unaware of it.

These facts are frightening! Having a doctor check your blood pressure is a painless procedure. It seems such a small price to pay when discovery and proper treatment may save your life and protect your future.

## Course of Vascular Dementia

The diagnosis of multi-infarct dementia carries with it certain important considerations. Patients with vascular dementias appear to have a more variable course to their illness than do victims of Alzheimer's disease. At times the dementia seems to clear up, or, at least, there are fairly lucid periods. Memory seems better for a while, and everyone gets optimistic and thinks that the disease is cured. Occasionally, this natural event, in the course of the illness, happens right after some new treatment or new doctor is brought into the case. Then comes the next series of microstrokes and a loss of function. This up-down, up-down course with a general progressive downhill trend can be very upsetting. Indeed some clinicians feel that increased anxiety is a hallmark of the disorder and that it stems from the more variable course.

Clearly, a careful differential diagnosis and qualified clinical management are crucial for multi-infarct patients and their families. Much of the discussion in this book is as relevant to these related dementias as to Alzheimer's disease. But special attention to the vascular system is, of course, a special issue for these patients and families.

# 13

# THE
# COST
# OF
# CARING

---

CARING is expensive not only emotionally but also financially. The costs of hospitalization, intensive care, major surgery, and life-support systems may run into the thousands of dollars for a single day of care. Indeed, the total amount spent on health care in this country is now more than 10 percent of the gross national product, and the costs are rising at the phenomenal rate of more than 9 percent per year. Thus, the nation is fast approaching a time of crisis in the affordability of medical care. Medicare and Medicaid costs have become serious problems affecting both state and federal budgets, and despite government efforts to limit cost escalations, Medicare and Medicaid expenditures have been doubling every four years. However, there are still segments of the population, such as patients with dementia, who do not have access to the health care they need.

In this era of escalating health costs and economic crisis, the responsibility for patients with dementia places a special financial burden on the family. Government programs and private insurance together do not cover the types of care these patients need. Therefore, as new approaches to health care financing and delivery are proposed, families of dementia patients need to become educated advocates for policy changes which will meet their health needs. The focus of health policy debates in the 1980s is clearly on changing the delivery and financing of medical care in order to lower costs. National pressure for limits on health expenditures and government cutbacks in health care may further jeopardize the already restricted availability of health care for dementia victims.

## The Economics of Health Care

A brief overview of relevant health financing issues and the history of health insurance may help explain why dementia patients have been excluded. For every complicated problem, H. L. Mencken once remarked, there is a simple solution, and that solution is invariably wrong. The financing of health care is inherently complicated. However, at the risk of oversimplification, we will try to explain it as clearly as possible.

Payment systems for health care in the United States can be divided into three categories: (1) care of the aged, (2) care of the poor, and (3) care of everyone else. This simply means that the financing of health care services for the aged and the poor is different from that for the rest of the population. In 1965 Medicare was established to pay for medical care services for persons sixty-five years and older, and Medicaid was also introduced to pay for the needs of the poor and disabled. Both the aged and the poor had been excluded from the private health insurance plans available to the rest of the population through their jobs.

Although the concept of public health insurance was first introduced in Germany in 1883 to meet the needs of a population whose major problems arose from childbirth complications, accidents, trauma, tuberculosis, and other infectious diseases, public pressure for health insurance coverage did not build in the United States until the early 1900s. While there were repeated efforts in Congress to introduce some form of national health insurance, they faced strong opposition from the American Medical Association.

Nevertheless, private health insurance became very popular. The introduction of Blue Cross in 1929 to cover hospital bills, and later of Blue Shield to pay physician fees, made health insurance available to younger people through their jobs. Work-related group plans became widespread largely as a result of the demands of labor unions for more and better benefits. In 1945 some 25 percent of the U.S. population was covered, and after World World II private insurance companies aggressively followed Blue Cross's lead to market primarily union or employer-sponsored plans as well as coverage for those wealthy enough to buy individual insurance. It was clear that private health insurance was available to the middle and upper working classes and not to those who were poor, unable to work, and aged.

A wide variety of work-related health care plans currently exist. The employer usually pays a major part of the health policy premium and receives substantial tax benefits for doing so. In most instances employees have options about the kind of plan they may purchase. Benefits and costs vary in different policies. In addition to Blue Cross and Blue Shield, the choice of plans usually includes participation in health maintenance organizations (HMOs). These are group plans in which premiums are prepaid on a regular basis and care is provided by an organized group of doctors and hospitals. Except in rare circumstances, there are no additional bills beyond the premium for individual visits or hospitalization in the HMO.

Health insurance plans provide different levels of financial coverage for outpatient visits to a doctor's office or clinic as well as for inpatient or in-hospital care. With few exceptions, insurance plans cover the major portion of the cost of acute care. Acute care is an important concept, referring to medical services for sudden and relatively short-term illnesses or operations. Insurance plans make a clear distinction between acute-care conditions and long-term-care or chronic conditions.

The benefit schedule in some plans may exclude conditions and diseases which existed before the policy was purchased, whereas in others a higher premium is imposed. Many plans accept all new employees and their dependents as part of the group coverage. Regardless of the medical plan, the insurance pays the doctor, the hospital, or the patient for acute illnesses of relatively brief durations.

Some policies offer what is known as a catastrophic-illness supplement for a small surcharge, or individuals may purchase a separate catastrophe insurance policy and add it to their regular medical coverage. Catastrophe insurance pays for specific conditions like cancer or stroke which may require long periods of care with special nursing and rehabilitation programs. Unfortunately, most of these programs do not provide the type of care needed by patients with dementia, and none that we know of assist the family in its day-by-day problems of managing the patient.

## Medicaid

Medicaid is a public assistance program in which the federal government contributes dollars to match state funds for programs of medical assistance to individuals otherwise unable to afford such care. Although the size of the Medicaid program is awesome, limitations on eligibility have kept many poor people from receiving Medicaid benefits. Estimates are that perhaps up to two-third of the nation's poor are ineligible because of the way state requirements are worded. The federal government established only basic guidelines for the implementation of the program by defining who was "categorically needy." The original intent was to make it possible for even the poorest states to offer medical assistance through the matching program.

Medicaid policies vary from state to state, as do eligibility and benefits. Eligibility for Medicaid is determined by a means test, in which a ceiling is placed on the maximum earnings and other assets that individuals and their dependents may have in order to qualify for assistance. Eligibility levels vary according to the size of family, the number of dependents in the household, benefits available from other sources (such as the Veterans Administration, union or pension funds, unemployment insurance), and the income of one's spouse or, in some states, the income of children.

"Benefits" refer to the type of help and services available under a health insurance plan. A key feature of Medicaid, important for the Alzheimer's family, is the nursing-home benefit—Medicaid pays for long-term skilled nursing care. In some states Medicaid even pays for home-based services for patients who are medically certified for home care, since they would otherwise be in a hospital or skilled nursing home.

Medicaid was intended to allow the poor and the poor aged to receive health care from the same medical care system as did the population with higher incomes. However, many physicians discriminate against Medicaid patients. Twenty percent of all doctors see no Medicaid patients, and 6 percent of all doctors see one-third of all the Medicaid patients. Benefits are paid directly to hospitals and doctors, but the payments are less than the usual private rates for the same services. These payment rates are determined by the states in accordance with local and regional economics. The current trend in most states is to tighten up eligibility and reduce the scope of benefits whenever possible.

Medicaid was also intended primarily to carry the burden of paying for the acute medical care of the poor younger patient. However, because of the way Medicare was structured, to meet only the acute-care needs of the aged, and because of the virtual absence of private insurance for long-term care in the United States, Medicaid has become the principal payer for long-term institutional care in the United States. Approximately 55 percent of the cost of nursing-home care is paid by Medicaid. Only 2 percent is paid by Medicare and about 1 percent by private insurance. It is important to emphasize that about 42 percent of long-term-care costs are still being paid by families.

Since an individual's assets include savings, insurance benefits, and home and property equity, many families with small or modest incomes may find that they simply are not eligible for Medicaid benefits. It is usual for individuals entering long-term-care institutions to pay private rates until they have "spent down" to a level of indigency which makes them eligible for Medicaid support. The average cost of nursing-home care is between $2,000 and $3,000 per month or more. When personal funds run out, the patient (and spouse) may apply to the state welfare department to receive Medicaid. However, since this is a complicated procedure and since a substantial number of patients need Medicaid, it often takes a long time to process the application.

A recent congressional survey reported that patients without financial means have a difficult time getting admitted into nursing homes. It is not surprising, though distressing, to learn this sad bit of medical economics. In many states nursing-home beds are not readily available, and overall, Medicaid pays less than the private rate for care. Individuals responsible for running nursing homes argue in their defense that since Medicaid rates are lower than the actual cost of care provided in the facility, they can provide quality care only by "averaging out" the income of private and Medicaid patients.

There is another unfortunate piece of medical economics. Patients with Alzheimer's disease and other related dementias will be able to get only those medical benefits for which they are eligible by virtue of an existing private insurance plan or by proving that they are too poor to pay for care. Virtually no private plan has any provision either for long-term home-based care or for extended nursing-home care.

## Medicare

Congress enacted the Medicare legislation in 1965 to make older Americans eligible for health care benefits. Medicare was designed to reduce the financial burden of older persons and their families by paying the cost of needed acute and expensive medical or hospital care, including surgery. Congress clearly intended to avoid dealing with the financial burden of long-term care, which was not a high priority in 1965. Medicare was never designed to cover long-term care, and it therefore provides only very limited nursing-home benefits. There was concern about the open-ended nature of long-term care and about a precise definition of what custodial or medical benefits would be expected. As a result, benefits for two types of illnesses associated with chronic care, tuberculosis and mental illness, were severely limited. Benefits were also defined in such a way as to apply only to episodes or "bouts" of acute illness, so that chronic disease or long-term institutional care would not be covered.

In Medicare, as in most private insurance coverage, certain costs have to be paid by the patient or family. These out-of-pocket costs are called deductibles. Initially, the first $40 per year of hospital costs were covered by the individual. By 1979 the patient was responsible for the first $160 of the hospital bill. By 1984 that amount had increased to $356 for each hospital stay and applied to a period of 60 days after discharge. Thus, if the patient was readmitted to a hospital 61 days after leaving, another deductible charge was levied.

Medicare pays for in-hospital care of up to 60 days in a semiprivate room. After 60 days, however, another deductible payment is charged to the patient. This year it is $89 a day for the 61st to 90th day. There is a provision that after 90 days one may draw against a lifetime allotment of 60 days. During this period a larger deductible is levied (at this time it is $178 per day). Although such a long hospital stay may be rare, it can happen. Finally, after 150 days Medicare pays nothing. And if a person must go into a long-term-care facility, Medicare will pay only for certain types of skilled nursing care, not for management or custodial care. Therefore, it predictably pays only 2 percent of the long-term-care bills in the United States per year.

Part A of Medicare pays for hospital benefits; physician's services are covered by a separate Medicare provision—Part B. However, Part B requires the payment of a small monthly premium, now $14.60 a month. The initial deductible is $75 per year, after which Medicare pays 80 percent of the amount determined to be reasonable by Medicare authorities. If the doctor accepts this assignment, the patient may still need to pay 20 percent of the bill. However, some doctors do not accept assignment and insist on a fee higher than that approved by the local authorities who handle Medicare payments. In this instance, the patient may bill Medicare for the Part B payment on the basis of proof of payment (or billing) to the doctor but has to cover out-of-pocket the difference between the physician's actual fee and that deemed reasonable by Medicare. Although there is increasing governmental pressure on physicians and hospitals to control rates and generate universal agreement to accept assignment, at the moment it is important to find out early whether your physician does or does not accept assignment. Many physicians feel that the rate set by Medicare is not at all reasonable.

The complex pattern of Medicare deductibles and Part A/Part B costs has given rise to new private insurance policies, coinsurance, to pay for the deductible portions of Part A and/or Part B. These policies have also come to be known as Medigap insurance because they can play a valuable role in filling "gaps" in the insurance coverage for the aged. There are, unfortunately, some individuals and companies who promote Medigap insurance which is worthless because the language disguises the fact that the coverage it offers duplicates that of Medicare. These policies are often sold by a high-pressure salesperson who frightens older persons or their families into believing that multiple insurance policies are needed. Medigap fraud has been estimated to deprive the elderly of billions of dollars per year in premiums for worthless policies.

In sum, although acute episodes of illness of the older patient with dementia are often covered, long-term care, chronic care, and family services are simply not reimbursed under Medicare. Furthermore, Medicare does not pay for special diets, eyeglasses, dentures, hearing aids, or medications. To inquire about Medicare benefits and to apply, call or write the local Social Security office. Each region has a private contractor like Blue Cross or another insurance company which acts as the local intermediary for the federal government in handling claims. If you are homebound, you may complete the application over the telephone or send a representative to the office. Once you have qualified for Medicare and you visit the doctor, it is important that you and the doctor fill out the Medicare forms correctly. Before you receive a treatment from your doctor, ask what she or he charges. Since Medicare pays only a certain amount of the charges, individuals are responsible for the additional costs.

Several Medicare terms are important to understand. A *beneficiary* is a person who receives Medicare. The *deductible* is the money you must pay before you can be covered by Medicare. *Premiums* are monthly payments which you must make in order to receive Medicare if you do not qualify for Social Security. *Copayment* is the monthly payment necessary to receive Medicare Part B. *Carriers* are organizations that process the claims for physician's fees and services under Part B. Finally, the *Medicare-approved* amounts are those charges determined by the Medicare carrier in each local area. Each July 1 new approved-fee levels are established. The maximum amount Medicare will pay is 80 percent of the approved fee.

## Medicare Supplemental Policies

If you can afford to, you should supplement your Medicare because it pays less than half of the average bill. There are several places you can contact for information on Medicare supplemental insurance. Two federal publications are updated every year. *Your Medicare Handbook* is put out by the Health Care Financing Administration (HCFA) and the Social Security Administration (SSA). The second, entitled *Guide to Health Insurance for People with Medicare,* is published by the HCFA and the National Association of Insurance Commissioners (NAIC). You can obtain both of these from your local Social Security office or from your state insurance department. The guidebook *How to Use Private Health Insurance with Medicare* is available from the Health Insurance Association of America (1850

K Street, NW, Washington, DC 20006). Finally, many state insurance departments have their own guidebook. Write to them. The address should be under state listings in the phone book. Not only will they probably have the most up-to-date information, but some state insurance departments will tell you which companies have had complaints filed against them.

There are a series of specific questions you can ask as you compare supplemental policies. In addition to going through the checklist below, you should consult *Best's Insurance Reports,* a highly regarded reference work available in most libraries, which rates the financial solvency of most insurance companies from A+ to C. You should consider only companies with an A or A+ rating. Blue Cross and Blue Shield plans are not rated but would qualify for an A rating.

- What is the annual premium you must pay? You must be the judge of the quality of the policies and decide what you can afford.
- Does the premium increase as you get older? Some policies have a single premium regardless of age, whereas others automatically charge more as you get older.
- Does the policy repay the initial deductible of Part A?
- Does it repay Part A copayments for days 61 to 90 and reserve days?
- Are there Part A benefits beyond 150 days?
- Does it repay Part A copayments for nursing-care days 21 to 100?
- Does it repay Part A copayments for nursing-care days 101 to 365?
- Does the policy repay the Part B deductible?
- What percentage of the provider's charge is paid?
- Does the policy provide benefits which cover the actual cost or only the Medicare approved charge?
- What is the maximum benefit from Part B charges?
- What is the policy's deductible?
- Does the policy cover expenses for pre-existing medical conditions? The maximum period a company can make you wait for coverage to begin is six months, but many policies have shorter waiting periods.
- What are the conditions for renewal of the policy? The best designation is "guaranteed renewable," which means that the company cannot cancel your policy if you pay your premiums. Although this is not an option with most Blue Cross and Blue

Shield plans, officials of Blue Cross and Blue Shield have said they would never cancel Medicare supplemental policies.
- What are the items covered by the policy which are *not covered* by Medicare?
- Can you get a rider for optional coverage?

If you do not have Medicare supplemental insurance, you should purchase a policy, *but only one*. More than one is likely to be a waste of money, so examine the policies carefully, using our checklist of questions, and weigh your options carefully. Even when you have only small medical expenses, the difference between policies in payments for benefits may be hundreds of dollars. When you have large medical bills, the difference in payments may be substantial—in the thousands of dollars.

Many of the best plans have been issued by Blue Cross and Blue Shield organizations. It is useful to use at least the Blue Cross plan in your region as a standard by which to judge other policies. However, do not assume immediately that the Blue Cross plan is always the best.

What are the alternatives to a Medicare supplemental policy? They include Medicaid, continuation of your work group coverage to an individual policy, major medical insurance, and health maintenance organizations (HMOs). If you qualify for Medicaid, do not waste money on Medicare supplemental policies. Long before your retirement you should investigate whether your work group insurance plan continues benefits after the age of sixty-five and whether the premium changes. Check with your benefits department. If your group policy can be converted to an individual one, compare it with the supplemental policies, using the checklist.

Major-medical insurance is intended to cover large medical bills. In many parts of the United States it is almost impossible for individuals sixty-five and older to acquire major-medical insurance; if it is available, the premium may be very high. It also may not cover the Medicare deductibles and copayments; if it does, the premium may be even higher. If major medical is indeed available, examine the costs and benefits very carefully. You may wish to purchase only catastrophe coverage for major bills, an option which may keep the premium low.

Health maintenance organizations may be an effective way to

meet medical care needs, but they are not inexpensive for older individuals, and some HMOs do not enroll people over sixty-five. These plans deserve thorough research if there is one close enough to you and if it is affordable.

## Personal Issues Confronting the Family

There are many arguments about what or who is responsible for the increased cost of medical care, which is growing faster than inflation and already represents a significant percentage of the U.S. gross national product. Whether the argument focuses on hospital inefficiencies, doctor's bills, the high cost of new technology, the expenses of intensive efforts to extend life in its final days (25 to 30 percent of all Medicare funds go to persons who will die within twelve months), the growth of an aged population more in need of medical care, or other issues, one thing is certain. State and federal governments will continue to make vigorous efforts to control the cost of health care—both acute care and long-term care. The burden will be borne not only by those providing care but by those needing care and by their families.

A letter to a cousin from the wife of an Alzheimer's patient contains the following passage: "I am a little worried about the future. The nursing home is expensive, and Seth's graduate education is still ahead of him. I want my husband to have the best care possible, but I am not sure how long I can afford it. What price is love?"

In most places little relief is in sight for the Alzheimer's family. A careful examination of the personal financial issues in caring is thus an essential part of living with the patient at home or in an institution. Legal and financial assistance may be helpful. It is tragic to think of couples who consider divorce in order to sever assets and allow one partner to go into long-term care without pauperizing the healthier spouse. Forcing children to move out of states where they are legally responsible for their parents represents another equally undesirable approach. Are there other ways of dealing with the problem? Perhaps.

State laws vary, since community-property legislation in some states leads to fiscal constraints different from those in others. It may be possible to set aside assets in a trust to deal with the long-term needs of spouse or younger children. Consult a lawyer or legal services (see Appendix 4).

Spending down before becoming eligible for Medicaid, in order to establish eligibility for benefits, is illegal unless the assets are spent months or even years before the Medicaid assistance is required, though the legality varies from state to state. Remember, however, that the patient with dementia is in the position of spending years at home, unemployed and of questionable (legal) competence. This period of time may enable the family, in concert with the patient and financial advisers, to plan intelligently for the future. Clearly, long-term planning is absolutely necessary for exploring various options and for examining what, if any, legal arrangements could and should be undertaken.

For these reasons we urge that, as soon as possible after the diagnosis is confirmed, and during the same time the family is working out its plan for medical and social care, the family also obtain the advice of a good lawyer or accountant. This is an instance where planning not only is helpful but may be essential if certain goals are to be realized.

## Health Policy Issues Confronting the Family

As we have already stated, caring for someone with dementia can be expensive. As the disease progresses, the cost of medical care, home health attendants, and other supportive services can become prohibitive. If and when institutionalization occurs, the costs may reach well over $30,000 a year. Until such a time when long-term-care health insurance is widely available at affordable premiums, the health care costs for patients with dementia will continue to threaten all but the wealthiest of families. One of the greatest challenges now facing us is to find ways to provide and pay for the long-term health care needs of the impaired aged.

Patients with dementia rely much more on their families than on formal medical services. Indeed, families carry this enormous burden with little help from anyone. At the moment, many areas of the country do not have the community or hospital-based services that families need to help them care for the patient at home (see Chapter 7). And where these programs are available, families normally must pay out-of-pocket since Medicare does not reimburse for them.

Families usually care for their relatives at home until their emotional and financial resources are exhausted. Although relatives will swear they will never surrender a loved one to an institution, sickness, desperation, and exhaustion often force the decision. Many, unfortunately, regard institutionalization as a defeat rather than as an appropriate decision to provide the best care for the patient as the patient's health and custodial needs increase. Thus, when family members place a relative in a nursing home, they become involuntary members of a large group of Americans. In 1984 there were over 1.3 million nursing-home beds in the United States, and that number will continue to grow every year. Of the 1.3 million it is estimated that at least 600,000 patients have Alzheimer's disease. Perhaps another 300,000 have dementia caused by strokes or other brain disorders.

Nursing homes are costly, and they are not necessarily the best way to care for Alzheimer's patients. However, for the moment they have become the only available option for many families. In 1979, nursing-home expenditures amounted to $17.9 billion, and the cost of such care is projected to be over $75 billion in 1990 (in 1980 dollars).

Why has Medicare failed to provide for older persons who need long-term care? The answer is simple. Our health care system developed primarily to meet the needs of our young and middle-aged population with acute illnesses and disorders which could be diagnosed, treated, and cured in a short period of time. However, recent changes in the age structure of our population have led to the emergence of a different disease pattern in our society. The aged are now the fastest-growing segment of the population, and chronic illnesses are much more common among the older old.

Chronic diseases like Alzheimer's are by definition not curable, although they are treatable and manageable. Medicare does not pay for most of the services involved in treating chronic illness. For patients with Alzheimer's disease, much of the care needed is not primarily biological. Usually, a combination of physical and social assistance, emotional support, cognitive-rehabilitation efforts, family support, and occasional medical intervention are helpful; except for the last, such services are disallowed by Medicare.

Until recently, policymakers have not invested in studies of the benefits of such alternatives to nursing homes as home care, day-care, respite care, and other programs. The increasing numbers of older persons in nursing homes, many of whom have dementia, and the economic problems we face in the high cost of health care are finally forcing government officials and health care professionals alike to examine the need for reform in long-term care.

In looking at this problem, we should remember two things. First, cost aside, Medicare (and Medicaid) have enjoyed great success. If anything, the problem is that we are suffering from the fulfillment of the promise to make health care available to everyone in this country without regard to age or ability to pay. Statistics all confirm the achievement; the problem is that after twenty years we are now looking at the cost of that commitment and recognizing that we cannot do business in the same old way.

The second point is that not all old persons are sick. The aged are not a homogeneous group of sick old people who are draining society's resources. Forty-two percent of the Medicare-enrolled population received *no* reimbursements for care in 1979, and 36 percent received none in 1982. Only 4.5 percent of the aged are in long-term care, and most are able to manage well at home with no assistance.

Although most Americans would agree that older persons should get the care they need, the changing age structure of the population, the significant health needs of the aged, and the economics of providing health services all tend to increase the need for services and associated costs. Can we afford to care for the aged? The answer is yes, but we must find a better way than the one we have at the moment.

## The Challenge to the Family

Families of patients with Alzheimer's disease have a special responsibility to understand proposals for health policy changes, so that they can become advocates for policies that help provide appropriate care. It has become apparent that Medicare as it now exists, however costly, is not adequate to meet the needs of our aged population and their families.

Initiatives are needed to examine the possible role of catastrophe insurance for Alzheimer's disease. Alternative forms of group coverage may also be possible. Special legislation should be tried to support families, through tax relief, who care for demented patients at home as an alternative to institutionalization. Since family care is far and away the most cost-effective way of helping patients, it should be supported and encouraged. Today, families receive virtually no help in their difficult task.

Social and community services as a component of a health insurance program—or prepaid group plans—should be developed as another approach to helping maintain the Alzheimer's patient at home. Since such services can also be preventive in nature and help keep patients out of costly institutions, this is an investment which could lead to important savings as well as an improved quality of life for the family. The role of respite care, in which families caring for patients can have relief for one or two weeks with needed vacations, hospice care as an alternative to dying in isolated, high-technology hospital settings, trained geriatric social workers working as a team with doctors and nurses to help provide care at home, day-care centers, sheltered housing, and similar social and environmental supports have all been successful in keeping patients out of nursing homes. Eventually, a plan to organize such community and medical services will have to be undertaken. This linking of social services and preventive care will do much to alleviate the burdens of cost and of caring. It demands only that we take on these initiatives.

There is a new role for advocacy by families and groups, who need to make their feelings known and to indicate where legislative and government investment is needed. The value of financial aid and of support services to the family, at home, as means of preventing the illness of the care giver should also be appreciated. There is good evidence (described elsewhere in this book) which clearly shows the stressful burden of caring as well as the potential pathological consequences to care givers and eventually to the patient. Remember, when the family collapses, so does the patient!

In sum, we need to recognize that a new and special effort is required if more and more Americans are not to be pauperized or made ill while trying to care for their loved ones. Sadly, though not surprisingly, it is the families themselves who need to place these issues before the decision makers.

# AFTERWORD

# THE
# GIFT
# OF
# LOVE

FAMILIES and patients live in a delicate balance, watching and reacting to the changes in one another. The challenge is to have a realistic understanding not only of the patient's needs and changing capacities but also of the needs, desires, and preferences of the family. There are no golden rules when you are caring for someone you love who has Alzheimer's disease.

In the opening chapter of this book we quoted a haunting passage by James Thomas. The lives of Mr. Thomas, his family, and millions throughout the world are symbols of hope. Although it defies scientific measurement, love seems to be the liberating force in families. Trust, patience, honesty, respect, and love create an environment in which the patient and family enjoy feelings of mastery, a sense of belonging, and a sense of self.

In one of the last pages of his diary, James Thomas, with the help of his wife, made the following entry:

Dear Self,
    These may be my last written words. It is becoming very difficult to think

and write. Although the last years have been spent in sorrow, and you have wasted away, so be it. There was nothing we could do about it. But we sure raised hell together before this brain problem started.

I have been very lucky. My wife has been my rock. I wouldn't have made it without her. Losing you has been tough, but I hope I don't lose her before this is over.

I am tired and must stop now. Before I end, and I am afraid I may not be able to say this again, I want to thank you for being there and say good-bye.

Your best friend

J.T.

# EPILOGUE

This book was started several years ago after the successful publication of a pamphlet entitled "A Family Handbook on Alzheimer's Disease." We wanted *The Loss of Self* to be a comprehensive, factual and personal resource for families. The experiences and feelings of our patients and families were described in the hope that others could learn that there are many ways to cope with these brain disorders. For us, a powerful message emerged from working with families. By dealing with their hurt, many family members and patients achieved a special maturity—a maturity that came from living each day with dignity, and doing their best in face of overwhelming emotional and financial pressures.

During the period in which *The Loss of Self* was written, we witnessed three major changes relevant to the book: an increased popular recognition of the importance of dementia as a serious public health problem, a significant increase in research support, and a change in the financing of hospital-based health care in this country. These changes have both eased and increased the family's burden of caring. Heightened public awareness and political concern have resulted in more research, including the development of centers for the study of Alzheimer's disease in a number of universities, as well as more news coverage, with reports of imminent scientific breakthroughs and cures. Although progress is being made, the emotional see-saw of the family afflicted with the disease is a sad price to pay for journalistic or scientific overstatement. While we are learning much more about Alzheimer's disease, there is still no immediate prospect of uncovering cause(s), cure(s), or prevention.

Financing is still a major problem affecting care. With increased technological advances in medicine, we are prolonging life and exacerbating still further the personal and economic issues discussed in this book. They remain more relevant today than ever and, for many, the pressures are even more intense. Yet, as more families deal with the disease openly, as there is a sharing of experience, and as more knowledge and professional help become available, there are avenues of relief.

Any book reporting on scientific or medical research will suffer from not having the latest work on the day it is printed. We believe that *The Loss of Self* is as current as our last-minute alterations allow, and we thank our editor and publisher for helping. Our editor was a treasured guide over the period in which we wrote this book. Many others—friends, colleagues, staff, and families—throughout the country helped by educating us about the disease, by reading parts of the book and criticizing them, andy by working with us on the manuscript. Those who have contributed to this effort over the years are legion. Our feelings about confidentiality, in some instances, and our concern that we omit any one of you have led us to the difficult decision that recognition of all of you as a group is the most fitting. Our deeply felt thanks for your help.

As we conclude *The Loss of Self*, we hope we have been able to do more than write a technical resource. The stories of our patients and families describe human beings who have refused to be dehumanized by the devastation of disease. We hope that their pain and their triumphs will inspire all of us to have the courage to meet the challenge of caring for ourselves and one another.

# SELECTED
# READINGS
# AND
# REFERENCES

These references and materials have been chosen for their usefulness to family members and care givers.

*General References*

Cohen, D., and C. Eisdorfer. *Family Handbook on Alzheimer's Disease.* New York: Health Advancement Services, 1982. (1700 Peoples Bank Building, 1500 Fifth Avenue, Seattle, WA 98101)

Harnett, E. R., ed. "Alzheimer's disease." *Pride Institute Journal of Long Term Home Health Care* 3 (Fall 1984). (*Pride Institute Journal,* 153 West 11th Street, New York, NY 10011)

Heston, L., and J. White. *Dementia: A Practical Guide to Alzheimer's Disease and Related Illness.* (ADRDA, 360 N. Michigan Avenue, Chicago, IL 60601)

Mace, N. L., and P. V. Rabins. *The 36-Hour Day: A Family Guide for Persons with Alzheimer's Disease, Related Dementing Illnesses, and Memory Loss in Later Life.* Baltimore: Johns Hopkins University Press, 1981.

Powell, L. S., and K. Courtice. *Alzheimer's Disease: A Guide for Families.* Reading, Mass.: Addison-Wesley, 1983.

Roach, M. *Another Name for Madness.* Boston: Houghton Mifflin, 1985.
Seymour, C. *Precipice: Learning to Live with Alzheimer's Disease.* New York: Vantage Press, 1984.

*Bibliotherapy: Manuals*

Brown, E. F. *Bibliotherapy and Its Widening Applications.* Metuchen, N.J.: Scarecrow Press, 1975.
Rubin, R. J., ed. *Using Bibliotherapy: A Guide to Theory and Practice.* Phoenix, Ariz.: Oryx Press, 1978.

*Bibliotherapy: Book Suggestions*

Bateson, M. C. *With a Daughter's Eye: A Memoir of Margaret Mead and Gregory Bateson.* New York: William Morrow, 1984.
Bellow, S. *Mr. Sammler's Planet.* Greenwich, Conn.: Fawcett, 1971.
Cooper, W. *Scenes from Married Life and Scenes from Later Life.* New York: E. P. Dutton, 1984.
Crawford, O. *The Execution.* New York: Popular Library, 1978.
Farnan, D. *Auden in Love.* New York: Simon and Schuster, 1984.
Plain, B. *Evergreen.* New York: Dell, 1979.
Updike, J. *Poorhouse Fair.* Greenwich, Conn.: Fawcett, 1964.
Welty, E. "A Worn Path." In J. R. McCuen and A. C. Winkler, eds., *Readings for Writers.* New York: Harcourt Brace Jovanovich, 1980.
———. *One Writer's Beginnings.* Cambridge: Harvard University Press, 1983.

*Care givers*

Calder, A., and J. Watt. *I Love You But You Drive Me Crazy: A Guide for Caring Relatives.* Vancouver, Canada: Fforbez, 1981. (Fforbez Publications, 2133 Quebec Street, Vancouver, Canada V57)
Edwards, H. *What Happened to My Mother?* New York: Harper and Row, 1981.
Eyde, D. R., and J. A. Rich. *Psychological Distress in Aging: A Family Management Model.* Rockville, Md.: Aspen, 1983.
Fall Creek, S., and M. Mettler, eds. *A Healthy Old Age: A Sourcebook for Health Promotion with Older Adults.* New York: Haworth Press, 1984.
Silverstone, B., and A. Burack-Weiss. *Social Work Practice with the Frail Elderly and Their Families.* Springfield, Ill.: C. C. Thomas, 1983.
Sloan, B. *The Best Friend You'll Ever Have.* New York: Crown, 1980.

*Cerebrovascular Disorders*

Toole, J. F. *Cerebrovascular Disorders.* New York: Raven Press, 1984.

*Cognitive Training*

Wilson, B. A., and N. Moffat, eds. *Clinical Management of Memory Problems.* Rockville, Md.: Aspen, 1984.

*Death*

Barton, D. *Dying and Death: A Clinical Guide for Caregivers.* Baltimore: Williams and Wilkins, 1977.
Feifel, H. *New Meanings of Death.* New York: McGraw-Hill, 1977.
Garfield, C. A. *Psychological Care of the Dying Patient.* New York: McGraw-Hill, 1978.
Kübler-Ross, E. *On Death and Dying.* New York: Macmillan, 1969.
Shneidman, E. S. *Deaths of Man.* New York: Quadrangle, 1973.

*Drugs*

Graedon, J. *The People's Pharmacy: Two.* New York: Avon, 1980.
*Physicians' Desk Reference.* Oradell, N.J.: Litton Industries (published yearly).
*The Physicians' Desk Reference for Nonprescription Drugs.* New York: Van Nostrand Reinhold, 1981.
*The Pill Book.* New York: Bantam Books, 1982.
Simonson, W. *Medications and the Elderly: A Guide for Promoting Proper Use.* Rockville, Md.: Aspen, 1983.

*Ethical Issues*

Jonsen, A. R., M. Siegler, and W. J. Winslade. *Clinical Ethics.* New York: Macmillan, 1982.

*Family-Support Groups*

Adelstein, H. *Educating Medical Professionals: A Manual for Lay Persons Planning and Implementing Training Programs on Alzheimer's Disease and Related Disorders.* (Harriet S. Adelstein, 2758 Prairie, Evanston, IL 60201)
Aronson, M., ed. *Help Line Resource Manual.* (ADRDA, 360 N. Michigan Avenue, Chicago, IL 60601)
Gwyther, L., and B. Brooks. *Mobilizing Networks of Mutual Support: How*

to Develop Alzheimer Caregivers' Support Groups. (Lisa Gwyther, ADRDA, Duke Family Support Network Chapter, Room 153, Civitan Building, Duke University Medical Center, Durham, NC 27710)

Lieberman, M. A., L. D. Borman, and Associates. Self-Help Groups for Coping with Crisis. San Francisco: Jossey-Bass, 1979.

Roback, H. B., ed. Helping Patients and Their Families Cope with Medical Problems. San Francisco: Jossey-Bass, 1984.

Family Support Groups: Training Materials

Buckley, K. D., J. S. Kleinbaum, and R. Johnson. Peer Counselor Workbook. University of Minnesota, 1980. (Older Adult Program, Continuing Education and Extension, University of Minnesota, Minneapolis, MN 55455)

Herr, J. J., and J. H. Weakland. Counseling Elders and Their Families. New York: Springer, 1980.

Olson, D. H., H. I. McCubbin, and Associates. Families: What Makes Them Work. Beverly Hills, Calif.: Sage, 1985.

Puryear, D. A. Helping People in Crisis. San Francisco: Jossey-Bass, 1979.

Sargent, S. S., ed. Nontraditional Therapy and Counseling with the Aging. New York: Springer, 1980.

Financial Costs

Brody, S. J., and N. A. Persily. Hospitals and the Aged: The New Old Market. Rockville, Md.: Aspen, 1984.

Callahan, J. J., and S. S. Wallack. Reforming the Long-Term-Care System. New York: Lexington Books, 1981.

Department of Health and Human Services (Write to Department of Health and Human Services, Health Care Financing Administration, Baltimore, MD 21207):

Guide to Health Insurance for People with Medicare. Pub. No. HCFA-02110.

Hospice Benefits under Medicare. Pub. No. HCFA-02154.

Medicaid/Medicare: Which Is Which? Pub. No. HCFA-02129.

Your Medicare Handbook. Pub. No. HCFA-10050.

Estes, C. L., et al. Political Economy, Health, and Aging. Boston: Little, Brown, 1984.

"Medicare-supplement Insurance." Consumer Reports, June 1984, pp. 347–55.

Sidel, V. W., and R. Sidel, eds. Reforming Medicine. New York: Pantheon Books, 1984.

*Home Care*

Murphy, L. B. *The Home Hospital.* New York: Basic Books, 1982.
Perlman, R., ed. *Family Home Care.* New York: Haworth Press, 1983.
Trocchio, J. *Home Care of the Elderly.* Boston: CBI, 1981.

*Housing Environments*

Koncelik, J. A. *Aging and the Product Environment.* New York: Van Nostrand Reinhold, 1984.
Raschko, B. B. *Housing Interiors for the Disabled and Elderly.* New York: Van Nostrand Reinhold, 1984.

*Legal Issues*

"Law and Aging." *Generations* 8 (Spring 1984).
Ziegenfuss, J. T. *Patients' Rights and Professional Practice.* New York: Van Nostrand Reinhold, 1984.

*Long-Term-Care Programs and Services*

Blues, A., and J. V. Zerwekh. *Hospice and Palliative Nursing Care.* Orlando, Fla.: Grune and Stratton, 1983.
Cleland, M. *Senior Respite Care Program.* (Senior Respite Care Program, Good Samaritan Hospital and Medical Center, 1015 NW 22d, Portland, OR 97210)
Dush, D. M., ed. *The Hospice Journal.* New York: Haworth Press, 1985.
Gelfand, D. E., and J. K. Olsen. *The Aging Network: Programs and Services.* New York: Springer, 1980.
Hall, B. A., ed. *Mental Health and the Elderly.* Orlando, Fla.: Grune and Stratton, 1984.
The Hospital Research and Educational Trust. *Health Promotion and Wellness Programs for Older Adults.* Chicago: Hospital Research and Educational Trust, 1984.
National Institute of Mental Health. *A Resource Guide for Mental Health and Support Services for the Elderly.* Pub. No. DHHS 81-985. Washington, D.C.: U.S. Government Printing Office, 1981.
Norback, J., ed. *Sourcebook of Aid for the Mentally and Physically Handicapped.* New York: Van Nostrand Reinhold, 1984.
Sayer, A. *Planning Home Care with the Elderly.* Cambridge, Mass.: Ballinger, 1983.
Zawadski, R. T., ed. *Community-Based Systems of Long Term Care.* New York: Haworth Press, 1984.

*Medical Handbooks*

Abreu, B. *Physical Disabilities Manual.* New York: Raven Press, 1981.

Berkow, R., ed. *Merck Manual of Diagnosis and Therapy.* Rahway, N.J.: Merck. (For most recent edition write to Merck & Company, P.O. Box 2000, Rahway, NJ 07065.)

Villaverde, M. M., and C. W. MacMillan. *Ailments of Aging: From Symptom to Treatment.* New York: Van Nostrand Reinhold, 1984.

*Medical Dictionaries*

*Blackiston's Gould Medical Dictionary.* New York: McGraw-Hill, 1979.

*Blackiston's Pocket Medical Dictionary.* New York: McGraw-Hill, 1979.

Brace, E. R. *A Popular Guide to Medical Language.* New York: Van Nostrand Reinhold, 1984.

*Dorland's Illustrated Medical Dictionary.* Philadelphia: W. B. Saunders, 1974.

*Dorland's Pocket Medical Dictionary.* Philadelphia: W. B. Saunders, 1977.

*Pocket Medical Encyclopedia and First Aid Guide.* New York: Simon and Schuster, 1979.

*Nursing—Basic Manuals*

Brunner, L., et al. *Lippincott Manual of Nursing Practice.* New York: Lippincott, 1978.

Burnside, I. M. *Nursing and the Aged.* New York: McGraw-Hill, 1981.

Campbell, C. *Nursing Diagnosis and Intervention in Nursing Practice.* New York: John Wiley, 1978.

Flaherty, M. O. *The Care of the Elderly Person: A Guide for the Licensed Practical Nurse.* St. Louis: C. V. Mosley, 1980.

O'Hara-Devereaux, M., L. H. Andrus, and M. I. Gary, eds. *Eldercare.* Orlando, Fla.: Grune and Stratton, 1981.

*Nurse's Aides and Home Aides*

Brooks, L. *The Nurse Assistant.* New York: Van Nostrand Reinhold, 1978.

Isler, C. *The Nurses' Aide.* New York: Springer, 1973.

Stolen, J. H. *The Health Aide.* Boston: Little, Brown, 1972.

*Nursing at Home*

American National Red Cross. *American Red Cross Home Nursing Textbook.* New York: Doubleday, 1979.

American National Red Cross. *Family Health and Home Nursing.* New York: Doubleday, 1979.

*Home Nursing Handbook.* New York Metropolitan Life Insurance Company, 1976. (Health and Welfare Division, Metropolitan Life Insurance Company, One Madison Avenue, New York, NY 10010)

## Nursing Homes

Bowker, L. H. *Humanizing Institutions for the Aged.* Lexington, Mass.: Lexington Books, 1982.

Brody, E. *Long-Term Care of Older People.* New York: Human Sciences Press, 1980.

Moss, F. E., and V. J. Halamandaris. *Too Old, Too Sick, Too Bad.* Rockville, Md.: Aspen, 1977.

Rausch, E., and M. M. Perper. *Resident Care Management Systems.* New York: Van Nostrand Reinhold, 1984.

Tobin, S. S., and M. A. Lieberman. *Last Home for the Aged.* San Francisco: Jossey-Bass, 1978.

West, K. L. *What Do I Do?* 1981. (Amata Graphic, P.O. Box 12313, Portland, Or 97212)

## Nutrition

Burgess, A. *Nurse's Guide to Fluid and Electrolyte Balance.* New York: McGraw-Hill, 1979.

Community Nutrition Institute Training Center. *Nutrition Service Provider's Guide.* Washington, D.C.: U.S. Department of Health and Human Services, Administration on Aging, 1981.

Natow, A. B., and J. Heslin. *Geriatric Nutrition.* New York: Van Nostrand Reinhold, 1984.

Natow, A. B., and J. Heslin, eds. *Journal of Nutrition for the Elderly.* New York: Haworth Press, 1984.

## Parkinson's Disease

Duvoisin, R. C. *Parkinson's Disease: A Guide for Patient and Family.* New York: Raven Press, 1984.

## Rehabilitation

Breuer, J. *A Handbook of Assistive Devices for the Handicapped Aged.* New York: Haworth Press, 1982.

"The Disabled Older Person." *Generations* 8 (Summer 1984).

Gallender, D. *Eating Handicaps: Illustrated Techniques for Feeding Disorders.* Springfield, Ill.: C. C. Thomas, 1979.

Hopf, P. S., and J. A. Raeber. *Access for the Handicapped.* New York: Van Nostrand Reinhold, 1984.

Sacks, O. "The Lost Mariner." *The Man Who Mistook His Wife For a Hat and Other Clinical Tales.* New York: Summit Books, 1985 (pp.22–41).

Wilder, C. N., and B. E. Weinstein, eds. *Aging and Communication: Problems in Management.* New York: Haworth Press, 1984.

Williams, T. F., ed. *Rehabilitation in the Aging.* New York: Raven Press, 1984.

Taira, Ed. D., ed. *Physical and Occupational Therapy in Geriatrics.* New York: Haworth Press, 1984.

## Stroke Guides and Personal Experiences

Dahlberg, C. C., and J. Jaffe. *Stroke: A Doctor's Personal Story of His Recovery.* New York: W. W. Norton, 1977.

DeMille, A. *Reprieve: A Memoir.* New York: Doubleday, 1981.

Downey, J. A. *Stroke: A Guide for Patient and Family.* New York: Raven Press, 1981.

Freese, A. S. *Stroke: The New Help and the New Life.* New York: Random House, 1980.

Griffith, Valerie A. *A Stroke in the Family: A Manual of Home Therapy.* New York: Delacorte, 1970.

Hess, L., and R. Bahr. *What Every Family Should Know about Strokes.* New York: Appleton, 1981.

## Therapeutic Strategies

Chermak, J. *Activities for Patients with Alzheimer's Disease and Related Disorders.* (The Hillhaven Corporation, Regional Office, 1835 Union Avenue, Suite 100, Memphis, TN 38104-3994)

Epstein, C. *Learning to Care for the Aged.* Reston, Va.: Reston, 1977.

Karr, K. L., and J. D. Karr. *What Do I Do: How to Care For, Comfort, and Commune with Your Nursing Home Elder.* New York: Haworth Press, 1985.

Killeffer, E. H. P., R. G. Bennett, and G. Gruen, eds. *Handbook of Innovative Programs for the Impaired Elderly.* New York: Haworth Press, 1984.

Weiss, J. C. *Expressive Therapy with Elders and the Disabled.* New York: Haworth Press, 1984.

# APPENDIX 1

# ALZHEIMER'S DISEASE SELF-HELP GROUPS

National Office—Alzheimer's Disease and Related Disorders Association, 70 East Lake Street, Suite 600, Chicago, IL 60601, 312–853–3060

*Colorado*

ADRDA-Denver, Rose Medical Center, 4567 East 9th Avenue, Denver, CO 80220, Janice DeTemple, 303–393–7675

*District of Columbia*

ADRDA–Metro Washington, 819 Aster Boulevard, Rockville, MD 20850, Helen Chambers, 301–424–9420

*Florida*

ADRDA–Greater Daytona Beach, 1282 Mayflower Drive, Daytona Beach, FL 32019, Mrs. Thomas K. Warke, 904–767–3757

ADRDA–Fort Myers (Lee County), Lee Mental Health Center, Inc., 2789 Ortiz Avenue, SE, P.O. Box 06137, Ft. Myers, FL 33906, Susan Workman or Suzanne Christ, 813–334–3537

ADRDA–Greater Jacksonville, 848 Glynlea Road, Jacksonville, FL 32216, Catherine Lester, 904–724–1447

ADRDA–Broward County (Florida), 9301 Sunrise Lake Boulevard, #109, Sunrise Lake, FL 33322, Esther Rothchild, 305–741–3984

ADRDA–Manatee-Sarasota Counties, 6303 Sun Eagle Lane, Bradenton, FL 33507, Eva Davis, 813–755–4331; 585 Yawl Lane, Longboat Key, FL 33507, Bernice Braznell, 813–383–7870

*Georgia*

ADRDA-Atlanta, Wesley Woods Campus, 1817 Clifton Road, NE, Atlanta, GA 30029, Carolyn French, 404–633–8759; 4764 La Vista Road, Tucker, GA 30084, Martha Sanders, 404–491–8969

*Hawaii*

ADRDA-Honolulu Chapter, Inc., Ward Warehouse, Building D, Upper Level, 1050 Ala Moana Boulevard, Honolulu, HI 96816, Helen Mac-Bride, 808–521–3771

*Illinois*

ADRDA-Chicago, Eths, Room S-217, 1600 Dodge Street, Evanston, IL 60204, Carol Kallish, 312–864–0045

*Indiana*

ADRDA–St. Joseph County (South Bend, Indiana), 2113 Beverly Place, South Bend, IN 46616, Sadie Mager, 219–233–4444

*Iowa*

ADRDA–Des Moines, Iowa Methodist Medical Center, 1200 Pleasant Street, Des Moines, IA 50308, Linda Simonton, M.S.W., 515–283–6431

*Kansas*

ADRDA–Greater Kansas City Area, 10108 West 96 Street, #B, Overland Park, KS 66212, Evelyn Sidner, 913–492–5228

*Kentucky*

ADRDA-Louisville, 6607 Watch Hill Road, Louisville, KY 40228, Ed Schmidt, 502–239–9329

*Maryland*

ADRDA-Baltimore, P.O. Box 9751, Baltimore, MD 21204, Glenn Kirkland, 301–792–7800, ext. 7224

*Massachusetts*

ADRDA-Massachusetts, Boston University School of Medicine, 80 East Concord Street, Boston, MA 02118, F. Marott Sinex, Ph.D., 617–247–5941

*Michigan*

ADRDA–Greater Ann Arbor, 1225 Astor Drive, #222, Ann Arbor, MI 48104, Alma L. Ford, 313–662–6638

ADRDA-Detroit, 725 S. Adams, Suite L-6, Birmingham, MI 48011, Nancy Lombardo or Sarah Glover, 313–540–2373 or 313–332–4110

ADRDA–Flint & Genessee County, 514 East Main Street, Flushing, MI 48433, John Tomaszweksi, 313–659–4435

ADRDA–Grand Rapids Area (Serving West Michigan), P.O. Box 1646, Grand Rapids, MI 49505, General Information 616–245–5735; Elly Lenihan, 616–456–5664; Michael L. Hale, 616–243–0231

ADRDA–Mid-Michigan, 9470 Rosebush Road, Mt. Pleasant, MI 48858, Mary Spierling, 517–465–6602

*Minnesota*

ADRDA-Association for Alzheimer's and Related Diseases, 2501 West 84 Street, Bloomington, MN 55431, Audrey Lindahl, 612–888–7653

*Missouri*

ADRDA–St. Louis, Washington University, School of Medicine, P.O. Box 8111, 660 S. Euclid Avenue, St. Louis, MO 63310, Warren Danziger, Ph.D., 314–454–2384

*Nebraska*

ADRDA-Lincoln, 4600 Valley Road, Lincoln, NE 68510, Marilyn Baalhorn, 402–489–6513

ADRDA-Omaha, P.O. Box 14933, Omaha, NE 68124, Cheryl McKay, 402–334–0506; Ralph Peppard, 402–399–9069

*Nevada*

ADRDA–Las Vegas, Charleston Convalescent Center, 2035 Charleston Boulevard, Las Vegas, NV 89102, Janna Benkelman, 702–386–7980

*New Mexico*

ADRDA-Albuquerque, 1027 Pampas Drive, SE, Albuquerque, NM 87108, Nance Dancy, 505–299–8223; Marian Knapp, 505–266–6621

*New York*

ADRDA–Capital District (Albany), 87 Brookline Avenue, Albany, NY 12203, Barbara Vickers, 518–438–4929

ADRDA–Alzheimer's Disease Society, 32 West Broadway, New York, NY 10004, Lonnie E. Wollin, Esq., Mailing Address: 1435 Tenth Street, Ft. Lee, NJ 07024, 212–736–3670 or 201–224–0388

ADRDA-Manhattan, 125 West 76th Street, New York, NY 10023

ADRDA–Nassau and Suffolk Counties, 579 Monroe Street, Cedarhurst, NY 11516, Ellen Tolle, 516–569–2310

ADRDA-Rochester, 24 Harvard Street, Rochester, NY 14607, Jim Reveley, 716–473–1634(H) or 716–442–3820

ADRDA-Westchester, 785 Mamaroneck, White Plains, NY 10605, Renee Pollack or Marilyn Herman, 914–428–1919

ADRDA–Western New York (located in the Buffalo area), Dent Neurological Institute, Millard Fillmore Hospital, 3 Gate Circle, Buffalo, NY 14209, Barbara Galus, 716–873–2988

*North Carolina*

ADRDA–Duke Family Support Network, Room 153, Civitan Building, Duke University Medical Center, Durham, NC 27710, Lisa Gwyther, 919–684–2328

*Ohio*

ADRDA-Athens, 37 Pleasant View Drive, Athens, OH 45701, Dr. Anne Samaan, 614–592–2013(H) or 614–592–1913(W)

ADRDA-Canton, 1509 Howenstine Drive, SE, East Sparta, OH 44626, Lynn Wasnak, 216–484–5878

ADRDA-Cincinnati, 8995 Tripoli Drive, Cincinnati, OH 45239, Elizabeth Bolles, 513–729–3271

ADRDA-Cleveland, 1801 Chestnut Hills Drive, Cleveland, OH 44106, Carolyn Lookabill, 216–721–8457

ADRDA–Alzheimer's Disease Association, Martin Janis Senior Center, 600 East 11 Avenue, Columbus, OH 43211, Dr. Gerland Robinson, 614–299–2327

ADRDA–Dayton Area, 157 Shenandoah Trail, West Carrollton, OH 45449, Doris Palm, 513–435–0151

ADRDA-Youngstown, 344 S. Broad Street, Canfield, OH 44406, Diana Williams, 216–533–7234

*Oklahoma*

ADRDA–Oklahoma City Area Chapter, 1613 Andover Ct., Oklahoma City, OK 73120, Jerry Robinson, 405–843–4680

*Oregon*

ADRDA–Columbia-Williamette (located in the Portland area), Neurological Sciences Center, Good Samaritan Hospital, 1015 NW 22 Avenue, Portland, OR 97210, Sharon Moody, 503–232–0306

*Pennsylvania*

ADRDA–Cobs, 1201 Arrott Building, 401 Wood Street, Pittsburgh, PA 15222, Martha Fenchak Bell, 412–355–5248 or 412–469–1567

ADRDA–Greater Philadelphia, 821 Clifford Avenue, Ardmore, PA 19003, Peggy Morscheck, 215–649–3198; George Bates, 215–485–4528, or 2424 Easton, #D3, Willow Grove, PA Pennsylvania 19090; Ed Mello, 215–441–4614

*Rhode Island*

ADRDA-Providence, Gerontology Center, Rhode Island College, 600 Mt. Pleasant Avenue, Providence, RI 02908, Sylvia Zaki, 401–456–8276

*Tennessee*

ADRDA-Memphis, 4060 Southlawn Avenue, Memphis, TN 38111, Dot King, 901–744–1165

*Texas*

ADRDA-Amarillo, Route 6, Box 760, Amarillo, TX 79106, Becky McGee, 806–381–1010

ADRDA-Dallas, 11216 Dumbarton, Dallas, TX 75228, Jo Ann Ray, 214–270–9604(H) or 214–948–7973(W)

ADRDA–El Paso, 6545 Fiesta Drive, El Paso, TX 79912, Grace Braly, 915–581–4926

ADRDA-Tarrant County (Fort Worth), 2925 Conejos Drive, Fort Worth, TX 76116, Bill Walters, 817–244–1085

ADRDA-Houston, 8101 Amelia, #304C, Houston, TX 77055, Lois Mullen, 713–465–9505(H) or 713–869–5546(W)

*Utah*

ADRDA–Greater Ogden, 232 Polk Avenue, Ogden, UT 84404, Pat Sackett, 801–392–5588

*Virginia*

ADRDA–Hampton Roads, Comprehensive Mental Health Service, Pembroke Three, Suite 109, Virginia Beach, VA 23462, Terry Jenkins, 804–490–0583

ADRDA–Northern Virginia, P.O. Box 2715, Springfield, VA 22152, John Dingle, 703–273–5453

ADRDA-Richmond, Counseling & Psychological Services, P.O. Box 3185, Richmond, VA 23235, Nan Wentzel, 804–794–9723, or 1163 Southam Drive, Richmond, VA 23235, Paul Gerhardt, 804–320–3365

ADRDA–Roanoke/Salem, VA Medical Center, Salem, VA 24153, Jean Taylor, 703–982–2463, ext. 2477

*Wisconsin*

ADRDA–Greater Milwaukee, Wisconsin Regional Geriatric Center, Family Hospital, 2711 West Wells Street, Milwaukee, WI 53208, Barbara Keyes, 414–933–6769; Dorothy Heydinger, 414–547–6406

# APPENDIX 2

# NATIONAL ORGANIZATIONS ON AGING

THIS is a listing of organizations and people you can write to in Washington, D.C. Let them know what you think should be done to improve community resources to help you provide better care for your relatives.

1. U.S. Department of Health and Human Services
   Office of Human Development
   Administration on Aging
   HEW N. Building
   330 Independence Avenue, SW
   Washington, DC 20201
   202–245–0724
   Associate Commissioner of Program Development: Dr. Joyce Berry
2. U.S. House of Representatives
   Select Committee on Aging
   Room 712 House Annex #1
   Washington, DC 20515
   202–226–3375
   Staff Director: Jorge J. Lambrinos

Chairperson: Edward R. Roybal
Ranking Minority: Matthew J. Rinaldo R–N.J.)
3. U.S. Senate
Special Committee on Aging
SD-G 33
Washington, DC 20510
202–224–5364
Deputy Chief Council: Steve McConnell
Chairperson: Senator John Heinz (R–Penn.)
4. National Centers for Long-Term Care
2131 "O" Street, NW
Washington, DC 20037
202–785–2576
President: Clay P. Herron
5. Veterans' Administration (VA)
810 Vermont Avenue., NW
Washington, DC 20420
General Information Office on VA Programs: 202–389–3781
Geriatrics and
Long-Term Care: Dr. John Mather

The following is an extensive list of national organizations on aging. Write to these groups. Find out whether they have a staff member or committee knowledgeable about Alzheimer's disease and disorders. If they do not, educate them about the importance of the problem and the implications of more research, training, and improved health care.

A number of these organizations will have offices in your part of the country. Most have a publication or magazine that may be useful to you. Care givers play important roles in advocacy and education.

1. Administration on Aging
330 Independence Avenue
Washington, DC 20201
General Information: 202–472–7257
PURPOSE: Serves as the principal agency for implementing programs of the Older Americans Act. Developed information package on Alzheimer's disease for distribution through all local area Agencies on Aging.
2. Alzheimer's Disease and Related Disorders Association, Inc.
70 East Lake Street, Suite 600

Chicago, IL 60601
Executive Director: Thomas M. Ennis
3. American Academy of Family Physicians
1740 West 92nd Street
Kansas City, MO 64114
Committee on Aging: Charlotte Krebs
4. American Association of Homes for the Aging
1050 17th Street, N.W., Suite 770
Washington, DC 20036
202–296–5960
President: William R. Thayer
   PURPOSE: Organization of 2,200 nonprofit long-term-care institutions that provide housing, skilled nursing, and related services.
5. American Association of Retired Persons
1909 K Street, N.W.
Washington, DC 20049
202–872–4700
President: Cyril Bickfield
   PURPOSE: To provide services, including group discount and insurance plans and educational and informational programs, to persons 55 and older.
6. American College of Health Care Administration
4650 East West Highway
P.O. Box 5890
Bethesda, MD 20814
301–652–8384
President: Mardell Brandt, CFACHCA
   PURPOSE: Serves as a professional society for individuals who administer long-term-care facilities.
7. American Council of the Blind
1211 Connecticut Avenue, N.W.
Washington, DC 20036
202–833–1251
National Representative: Oral Miller
8. American Dental Association
211 East Chicago Avenue
Chicago, IL 60611
312–440–2500
Executive Director: Dr. M. John Coady
9. American Federation for Aging Research (AFAR)
335 Madison Avenue
New York, NY 10017

212–503–7600
President: Dr. Irving S. Wright
10. American Geriatrics Society, Inc.
10 Columbus Circle
New York, NY 10019
212–582–1333
President: Dr. Knight Steel
11. American Health Care Association
1200 15th Street, N.W.
Washington, DC 20005
202–833–2050
President: Harold J. Moffie
PURPOSE: Serves as a nonprofit federation of 48 state associations serving more than 8,500 nursing homes and related facilities.
12. American Medical Directors Association
1200 15th Street, N.W.
Washington, DC 20005
202–833–2050
President: Dr. G. William Nice
PURPOSE: Serves as a nonprofit organization of 1,500 physicians long-term-care facilities.
13. American Nurses' Association, Inc.
2420 Pershing Road
Kansas City, MO 64108
Executive Director: Dr. Judith Ryan
14. American Occupational Therapy Association
1383 Piccard Drive, Suite 300
Rockville, MD 20850
Executive Director: James J. Garibaldi
15. American Osteopathic Association
212 E. Ohio Street
Chicago, IL 60611
312–280–5800
Executive Director: John Perrin
16. American Psychiatric Association
1400 K Street, N.W.
Washington, DC 20005
Medical Director: Dr. Melvin Shabshin
17. American Society on Aging
833 Market Street, Suite 516
San Francisco, CA 94103
415–543–2617

Executive Director: Gloria Cavanaugh

PURPOSE: To bring researchers, practitioners, older persons, and business leaders into a supportive network working toward the preservation and enhancement of independence and dignity through education, training, applied research, and participation in decision making.

18. American Society for Geriatric Dentistry
271-11 76th Avenue
New Hyde Park, NY 11040
212–343–2100, ext. 260
Dr. Saul Kamen

19. American Society of Consultant Pharmacists
2300 9th Street South
Arlington, VA 22204
703–920–8492
Executive Director: Tim Webster
PURPOSE: Serves as a national professional society of pharmacists in nursing homes, home health care, and other institutions.

20. American Speech–Language–Hearing Association
10801 Rockville Pike
Rockville, MD 20852
301–897–5700
Executive Director: Dr. Frederick T. Spahr
PURPOSE: Serves as a professional organization for speech–language pathologists and audiologists.

21. Asociacion Nacional pro Personas Mayores
(National Association for Hispanic Elderly)
1730 W. Olympic Boulevard
Los Angeles, CA 90015
213–487–1922
Executive Director: Carmela G. Lacayo
PURPOSE: To present the needs of the Hispanic elderly and to encourage their participation in social service programs. Conducts research and disseminates information to interested persons and organizations.

22. Association for Gerontology in Higher Education
600 Maryland Avenue, SW
West Wing 204
Washington, DC 20024
202–484–7505
Executive Secretary: Elizabeth B. Douglass
PURPOSE: To promote research, education, and training for careers in gerontology. Focal point for information and referral services and

for cooperation among public agencies, organizations, and other professionals interested in aging and education.
23. Consultant Dietitians in Health Care Facilities
2041 West Wesley Road
Atlanta, GA 30327
404–352–1943
Chairman: Judy Ford Stokes, R. D.
PURPOSE: Serves as a practice group for dietitians working in nursing homes and other long-term-care facilities.
24. Dietary Managers Association
4410 W. Roosevelt Road
Hillside, IL 60612
312–449–2770
Executive Director: Jean Denwood
PURPOSE: Serves as an organization for dietary managers who work in the food service departments in long-term-care facilities.
25. The Gerontological Society of America
1411 K Street, NW, Suite 300
Washington, DC 20005
202–393–1411
Executive Director: John M. Cornman
PURPOSE: To promote education and scientific study of aging for professionals and other interested groups.
26. Gray Panthers
2480 16th Street, NW, Suite 903
Washington, DC 20009
202–332–6117
Executive Director: Thelma V. Rutherford
PURPOSE: To promote group consciousness-raising and activism among the aging and young people to combat age discrimination.
27. Health Care Financing Administration
200 Independence Avenue, S.W.
Washington, DC 20201
202–245–6726
28. Hillharen Foundation
1835 Union Avenue, Suite 100
Memphis, TN 38104-3994
901–274–8428
President: Dorothy Brodnax
29. Home Health Services and Staffing Association
815 Connecticut Avenue, N.W., Suite 206

Washington, DC 20006
202–331–4437
Director of Government Affairs: Susan Pettey
30. Legal Research and Services for the Elderly
925 15th Street, N.W.
Washington, DC 20005
202–347–8800
Executive Director: David Marlin
31. National Association for Home Care
519 C Street
Stanton Park
Washington, DC 20002
202–547–7424
President: Val J. Halamandaris
32. National Association for Human Development
1620 Eye St., NW, Suite 517
Washington, DC 20006
202–331–1737
President: Jules Even Baker
PURPOSE: To promote physical and mental health among persons aged 60 and over through demonstration projects, education, training programs, and research. Monitors and comments on legislation affecting the health and well-being of older adults.
33. National Association of Area Agencies on Aging (N4A)
600 Maryland Avenue, SW
West Wing Suite 208
Washington, DC 20024
202–484–7520
Executive Director: Raymond C. Mastalish
PURPOSE: To promote cooperation and communication within the national aging network, federal government, and other interested persons and organizations; to provide technical and administrative assistance to Area Agencies on Aging in response to federal legislation and regulations.
34. National Association of County Aging Programs (NACAP) An affiliate of the National Association of Counties (NACo)
440 1st Street, NW, 8th Floor
Washington, DC 20001
202–393–6226
Executive Director: Matthew B. Coffey
PURPOSE: To provide technical assistance to county officials interested in establishing or improving services to the elderly.

35. National Association of Jewish Homes for the Aged
    2525 Centerville Road
    Dallas, TX 75228
    214-327-4503
    Executive Vice-President: Dr. Herbert Shore
    PURPOSE: To serve nonprofit, charitable homes, medical and long-term-care facilities, and other special facilities for the Jewish elderly and chronically ill.
36. National Association of Nutrition and Aging Services Programs
    c/o Aging Projects, Inc.
    Reno County Courthouse
    Hutchinson, KS 67501
    316-669-8201
    President: Kathryn Helsel
    PURPOSE: To promote professional growth and standards, effective communication, and the development of resources for aging service programs.
37. National Association of State Units on Aging
    600 Maryland Avenue, SW
    West Wing, Suite 208
    Washington, DC 20024
    202-484-7182
    Executive Director: Daniel Quirk
    PURPOSE: To serve as coordinating body for State Units on Aging to collect, analyze, and disseminate information among the different state units, federal agencies, and national organizations; to develop training and program models.
38. National Caucus and Center on Black Aged
    1424 K Street, N.W., Suite 500
    Washington, DC 20005
    202-637-8400
    President: Dr. Dolores A. Davis-Wong
39. National Citizens' Coalition for Nursing Home Reform
    1825 Connecticut Avenue, N.W., Suite 417B
    Washington, DC 20009
    202-797-0657
    Executive Director: Elma L. Griesel
40. National Council of Senior Citizens
    925 15 St., NW, 1st Floor
    Washington, DC 20005
    202-347-8800

Executive Director: William Hutton

PURPOSE: To foster health, education, service programs, social/ political action, and legislation on behalf of the elderly for members of senior associations, clubs, and other groups.

41. National Council on Black Aging
Box 8813
Durham, NC 27707
919–489–2563
Director: Jacquelyne J. Jackson
PURPOSE: To inform interested persons of research conducted on and public policies affecting black and other minority aged.

42. National Council on the Aging
600 Maryland Avenue, SW
West Wing 100
Washington, DC 20024
202–479–1200
Executive Director: Jack Ossofsky
PURPOSE: To conduct research and develop programs for the aging; to serve as an information, training, and consultation center for all professionals and organizations concerned with aging and services to the elderly.

43. National Homecaring Council (NAC)
235 Park Avenue South, 11th Floor
New York, NY 10003
212–674–4890

44. National Hospice Organization
1901 N. Fort Myer Drive, Suite 402
Arlington, VA 22209
703–243–5900
Executive Director: Jay Mahoney
PURPOSE: To promote the concept and program of hospice care; to ensure quality care through development of standards, programs, and national policies in the care and treatment of the terminally ill and their families.

45. National Indian Council on Aging, Inc.
P.O. Box 2088
Albuquerque, NM 87103
505–766–2276
Executive Director: Alfred G. Elgin
PURPOSE: To advocate improved comprehensive services and other concerns of the Indian and Alaskan native elderly with the public and

federal agencies, through information, training, and consultation services.

46. National Institute of Handicapped Research
200 Maryland Avenue, S.W.
Washington, DC 20202

47. National Institute on Aging
National Institute of Health
9000 Rockville Pike
Bethesda, MD 20014
301–486–9265
Director: Dr. T. Franklin Williams

48. National Institute of Senior Centers
National Council on the Aging, Inc.
600 Maryland Ave.,
West Wing 100
Washington, DC 20024
202–479–1200 ext. 252
Coodinators: Robert Cosby, Betty Ranson
PURPOSE: To create program materials giving training and assistance to a nationwide network of senior centers, clubs, and groups; to provide counsel in the planning, design, and operations of senior centers; to assist center personnel through research, conferences, and seminars.

49. National Pacific/Asian Resource Center on Aging
811 First Avenue
Colman Building, Suite 212
Seattle, WA 98112
206–622–5124
Executive Director: Louise Kamikawa
PURPOSE: To facilitate and improve the delivery of health and social services to the Pacific/Asian elderly community by providing advocacy, training, program consultation, and technical assistance, and by developing policy recommendations. A national project funded by the Administration on Aging (DHHS).

50. National Senior Citizens Law Center
1302 18th St., NW, Suite 701
Washington, DC 20036
202–887–5280
Executive Director: Burt Fretz
PURPOSE: To provide technical, consultative, and other assistance to lawyers serving the poor elderly and to state and area agencies on aging to improve and expand legal-service delivery.

51. Southern Gerontological Society
    Box 3003
    Duke Medical Center
    Durham, NC 27710
    919–684–3058
    President: Dr. Erdman Palmore
    PURPOSE: To encourage education, research, communication, and service development and delivery throughout the southern region of the United States as well as nationally; to assist in research, training, model, and demonstration projects on behalf of the elderly and service providers.

52. United States Conference of Mayors Aging Program
    1620 Eye Street, NW
    Washington, DC 20006
    202–293–7330
    Director: Larry McNickle
    PURPOSE: To assist mayors and local officials in identifying effective administrative approaches to planning, developing, and coordinating efficient programs to meet the needs of their older constituents. Conducts training sessions, develops and distributes resource tools, and provides technical assistance to mayors and their staffs regarding administrative and programmatic issues concerning the elderly.

# APPENDIX 3

# SOURCES OF HELP

*State Agencies on Aging*

Many state agencies on aging provide free information about state, county, and city services for older people. They also often have information about private agencies. The addresses and phone numbers for each state agency on the aging is listed below. In this country there are currently 662 area agencies on aging, which were established under the Older Americans Act. The Select Committee on Aging of the House of Representatives has put together a directory of all these agencies. It can be purchased from the U.S. Government Printing Office, Washington, DC 20402 (Stock No. 052-070-05816-1), for $6.50.

*Alabama*
  Commission on Aging, 2853 Fairlane Drive, Building G, Suite 63, Montgomery, AL 36130; 205–832–6640
*Alaska*
  Older Alaskan Commission, Department of Administration, Pouch C-MS-0209, Juneau, AK 99811; 907–465–3250
*Arizona*
  Office on Aging and Adult Administration, P.O. Box 6123, 1400 West Washington Street, Phoenix, AZ 85007; 602–255–4446

*Arkansas*

Office of Aging and Adult Services, 1428 Donaghey Building, Suite 1428, 7th and Main Street, Little Rock, AR 72201; 501–371–2441

*California*

Department on Aging, Health and Welfare Agency, 1020 19th Street, Sacramento, CA 95814; 916–322–5290

*Colorado*

Department of Aging and Adult Services, 1575 Sherman Street, Denver, CO 80203; 303–866–2586

*Connecticut*

Department on Aging, Room 312, 80 Washington Street, Hartford, CT 06115; 203–566–3238

*Delaware*

Department of Health and Social Services, Division of Aging, 1902 North Dupont Highway, New Castle, DE 19720; 302–421–6791

*District of Columbia*

Suite 1106, Office of Aging, 1012 14th Street, NW, Washington, DC 20005; 202–724–5622

*Florida*

Aging and Adult Services, Department of Health and Rehabilitative Services, 1323 Winewood Boulevard, Tallahassee, FL 32301; 904–488–8922

*Georgia*

Office of Aging, Department of Human Resources, 618 Ponce de Leon Avenue, NE, Atlanta, GA 30308; 404–894–5333

*Hawaii*

Executive Office on Aging, Office of the Governor, State of Hawaii, Room 307, 1149 Bethel Street, Honolulu, HI 96813, 808–548–2593

*Idaho*

Idaho Office on Aging, Statehouse Room 114, Boise, ID 83720; 208–334–3833

*Illinois*

Illinois Department on Aging, 421 East Capitol Avenue, Springfield, IL 62706; 217–785–3356

*Indiana*

Indiana Department on Aging and Community Services Suite 1350, 115 North Penn Street, Indianapolis, IN 46204; 317–232–7006

*Iowa*

Iowa Commission on Aging, 415 West 10th Street, Jewett Building, Des Moines, IA 50319; 515–281–5187

*Kansas*
Kansas Department of Aging, 610 West 10th Street, Topeka, KS 66612; 913–296–4986

*Kentucky*
Kentucky Division for Aging Services, Bureau of Social Services, 275 East Main Street, Frankfort, KY 40601; 502–564–6930

*Louisiana*
Louisiana Office of Elderly Affairs, P.O. Box 80374, Capital Station, Baton Rouge, LA 70898; 504–925–1700

*Maine*
Bureau of Maine's Elderly, Department of Human Services, State House Station 11, Augusta, ME 04333, 207–289–2561

*Maryland*
Maryland Office on Aging, State Office Building, 301 West Preston Street, Baltimore, MD 21201; 301–383–5064

*Massachusetts*
Massachusetts Department of Elder Affairs, 38 Chauncey Street, Boston, MA 02111; 617–727–7751

*Michigan*
Michigan Office of Services to the Aging, 300 East Michigan, P.O. Box 30026, Lansing, MI 48909; 517–373–8230

*Minnesota*
Minnesota Board on Aging, 204 Metro Square Building, Seventh and Robert Street, St. Paul, MN 55101; 612–296–2544

*Mississippi*
Mississippi Council on Aging, 201 Executive Building, 802 North State Street, Jackson, MS 39201; 601–354–6590

*Missouri*
Missouri Office of Aging, Department of Social Services, Broadway State Office Building, P.O. Box 570, Jefferson City, MO 65101; 314–751–3082

*Montana*
Community Services Division, Department of Social and Rehabilitation Services, P.O. Box 4210, Helene, MT 59601; 406–449–3865

*Nebraska*
Nebraska Department on Aging, P.O. Box 95044, 301 Centennial Mall South, Lincoln, NE 68509; 402–471–2306

*Nevada*
Division of Aging Services, Department of Human Resources, 505 East King Street, Room 600, Kinkead Building, Carson City, NV 89710; 702–885–4210

*New Hampshire*
New Hampshire Council on the Aging, 14 Depot Street, Concord, NH 03301; 603-271-2751
*New Jersey*
Department of Community Affairs, P.O. Box 2768, 363 West State Street, Trenton, NJ 08625; 609-292-4833
*New Mexico*
New Mexico State Agency on Aging, La Villa Rivera Building, 224 East Palace Avenue, Santa Fe, NM 87501; 505-827-7640
*New York*
Office for the Aging, Agency Building 2, Empire State Plaza, Albany, NY 12223; 518-474-5731
*North Carolina*
Division on Aging, Department of Human Resources, Raleigh, NC 27603; 919-733-3983
*Ohio*
Ohio Commission on Aging, Ninth Floor, 50 West Broad Street, Columbus, OH 43215; 614-466-5500
*Oklahoma*
Special Unit on Aging, Department of Human Services, P.O. Box 26352, Oklahoma City, OK 73125; 405-521-2281
*Oregon*
Senior Services Division, Human Resources Department, Room 313, Public Services Building, Salem, OR 97301; 503-378-4728
*Pennsylvania*
Pennsylvania Department of Aging, Room 404, Finance Building, Harrisburg, PA 17101; 717-783-1550
*Rhode Island*
Department of Elderly Affairs, 79 Washington Street, Providence, RI 02903; 401-277-2858
*South Carolina*
South Carolina Commission of Aging, 915 Main Street, Columbia, SC 29201; 803-758-2576
*South Dakota*
Office of Adult Services and Aging, Division of Human Development, Department of Social Services, Richard F. Kneip Building, Illinois Street, Pierre, SD 57501; 605-773-3656
*Tennessee*
Tennessee Commission on Aging, 703 Tennessee Building, 535 Church Street, Nashville, TN 37219; 615-741-2056

*Texas*
  Texas Department of Aging, P.O. Box 12786, Capital Station, Austin,
  TX 78704; 512–475–2717
*Utah*
  Division of Aging Services, Room 326, 150 West North Temple, Salt
  Lake City, UT 84103; 801–533–6422
*Vermont*
  Vermont Office on the Aging, 103 South Main Street, Waterbury, VT
  05676; 803–241–2400
*Virginia*
  Virginia Office on Aging, Suite 950, 830 East Main Street, Richmond,
  VA 23219, 804–786–7894
*Washington*
  Bureau of Aging and Adult Services, Department of Social and Health
  Services, Olympia, WA 98504; 206–753–2502
*West Virginia*
  Commission on Aging, State Capitol, Charleston, WV 25303; 304–
  348–3317
*Wisconsin*
  Department of Health and Social Services, Room 686, 1 West Wilson
  Street, Madison, WI 53703; 608–266–2536
*Wyoming*
  Commission on Aging, Room 139, Hathaway Building, Cheyenne, WY
  82002; 307–777–7986

# APPENDIX 4

# MONEY MATTERS: LEGAL AND FINANCIAL ISSUES

COMPLEX legal and financial problems face patients and their families. A great deal can be done to help individuals make wise decisions about their personal well-being, property, and other assets, but it is important to begin explaining these issues as soon as possible after the diagnosis of Alzheimer's disease. In addition to giving the families adequate time for deliberate discussions, beginning early enough will help ensure that the individuals suffering from dementia will not be deprived of the right to determine what will happen to them or their assets.

The information presented here is intended to help you understand the various options available, but it is not a substitute for sound legal advice. Laws vary from state to state, and only lawyers knowledgeable about protective services are aware of the legal alternatives in your area. Furthermore, legal arrangements need to be tailored to the individual's circumstances. However, regardless of the legal mechanisms used as the dementia progresses, some amount of control over the patient's assets should be given to someone who is trusted—a family member, a friend, or an institution.

In this appendix five general alternatives are discussed: (1) assistance with no legal responsibility, (2) power of attorney, (3) durable power of attorney, (4) living trust, and (5) conservatorship. Assistance without legal responsibility is the least restrictive, and a conservatorship is the most restrictive.

*Financial and Personal Assistance without Legal Responsibility*

In the beginning, family members may help patients manage money and assets without assuming legal power. This usually works well while the individual is minimally impaired. At least once a month sit down with your relative to go over bills, pay them, and balance the checkbook. It may be necessary to meet on other occasions to review more-complicated issues, such as Internal Revenue Service (IRS) forms, financial portfolios, and investments.

Monthly sessions provide the mechanism for discussing longer-term solutions. This initial assistance acknowledges your respect for the patient and your desire to involve him or her in preparations for the future. The transition to other legal solutions may be managed more easily if the patient is involved. However, this may not always be possible if the family waits too long and the individual develops significant cognitive deficits.

*Power of Attorney*

Power of attorney is the next recourse of relatives when patients are becoming too impaired to handle many of their financial tasks. It allows individuals to delegate certain powers to someone else, called the attorney-in-fact. In this situation the individual patient, called the principal, is stating in essence that although he/she could handle his/her own financial affairs, it is more convenient to let someone else handle them. The document must specify exactly what legal and/or financial responsibilities are being transferred. In reality, the attorney-in-fact may have very limited or very broad control over the patient's assets.

Power of attorney may be a valuable mechanism for assuming more control as needed over the patient's assets. It is a way for individuals to gradually relinquish control over an area they have managed successfully for many years. It leaves them the dignity of deciding what control they wish to delegate to others. There are two important restrictions when power of attorney is given to another party: first, it is valid only as long as the patient has mental capacity; second, it can be revoked by the patient at any time.

*Durable Power of Attorney*

In some states patients may sign a document for "durable power of attorney." A "durable power of attorney" is a little more restrictive than a "power of attorney" document. In order for a durable power of attorney to be legal the patient must sign the document while he/she still has substantial mental capacity and must also designate who is the "holder" of the durable power of attorney. The patient may give the power to two or more people and require that they act together as coholders. The holder or coholders control the patient's resources, but the papers can be written so that the holders must follow specific guidelines set forth by the patient. The papers can designate that the holder(s) get(s) the power of durable attorney immediately or only when two or more people, such as family members, clergy, or physician, say in writing that the individual has lost mental capacity.

The legal holder can make decisions about the patient's financial assets and living arrangements, including the right to sign checks or legal documents. If the holder does not handle the individual's assets properly, a court may revoke the power should a trusted party object.

There are several types of durable powers of attorney—a "durable power of attorney for persons" and a "durable power of attorney for property management." Durable power of attorney for property does not give the holder legal rights over persons. Therefore, if a patient refuses to go to a nursing home and is not manageable at home, the holder cannot place him/her in an institution against his/her will. This requires what is technically called a "durable power of attorney for health care," which allows the holder to make many health care decisions for the patient. This document can be written so that the holder can consent to diagnostic and treatment services, make decisions to halt the use of life-support machines when necessary, and decide whether to donate the patient's brain or other organs to research.

The holder of durable power of attorney for health care has the legal obligation to follow whatever wishes or preferences the patient made known before he/she lost mental capacity. Thus, the patient's preferences for medical treatment and placement can be written into the durable power of attorney document.

The same individual may be the holder of durable power of attorney for person, property management, and health care. It is important for the patient also to identify who should become the holder if the original designee dies or cannot function in that capacity.

### Living Trust

The area of trusts is extremely complicated. In certain situations, living trusts are set up to handle assets in an acceptable way that avoids estate taxes after an individual dies. A living trust is similar in some ways to a durable power of attorney. The patient signs a document known as a "trust instrument" or "trust agreement," prepared by an attorney to specify the patient's wishes about how his/her property is to be used during the patient's life as well as after his/her death. The patient usually chooses a family member, a trusted friend, or an institution such as a bank to be the "trustee." The patient should also designate a backup, in the event the first trustee cannot continue.

In creating a living trust, the patient signs a paper which gives the trustee title to the patient's assets. This means that the trustee is the "technical" owner of the assets, while the patient remains the "real" owner of the assets and their benefits. The document reflects exactly how the patient's assets are to be used. Trustees risk a lawsuit and penalties if they do not respect the patient's wishes.

A trust can be written in such a way that the patient may revoke it at any time, or it may be written so that it is revocable only until the patient loses mental capacity. The trustee does not have any control over the patient's "person." Therefore, the trustee will not be able to institutionalize the patient unless he/she agrees to go into a nursing home. This is true even if the patient has lost the capacity to know what he/she is doing.

*Conservatorship*

A conservatorship is a serious step for families to take. Although state regulations differ, it always involves a legal procedure. Medical testing must be presented in court, and on the basis of the evidence, the court will decide whether a conservator will be appointed. A family member or close friend must file a petition with the court requesting a hearing for conservatorship. The judge reads and hears evidence to determine whether a conservatorship is necessary. Close family members are notified about the hearing, and they may support or object to the petition.

Generally, a conservatorship of estate is designed to control and manage all of a patient's finances. However, under new laws the patient may retain control over certain financial matters, such as an allowance or the right to make a will deemed valid by the court. The conservator controls the patient's assets and must use them for the patient's benefit. A conservator of the state is appointed if the patient is shown to be unable to manage his/her finances or if the patient requests one and demonstrates a good cause, such as Alzheimer's disease. More than one person or an agency can be appointed to serve as "coconservators" of the patient.

The conservator usually must file an account of all financial transactions with the court at the end of the first year of the conservatorship and every two years thereafter. The report must show the patient's assets and document all transactions made by the conservator on behalf of the patient. The conservator is expected to protect the patient's assets.

A conservator of the patient's person could be appointed if the patient becomes unmanageable and abusive at home and must be placed in a nursing home. Even if the patient wants to be released, the nursing home can legally keep him/her if the patient's conservator placed him/her in the home. However, the patient retains the right to maintain state residence, to marry, and to give medical consent in non-life-threatening emergencies unless the court decides otherwise. The courts usually appoint the same individual as conservator of the estate and person. A conservator of person is appointed only when the individual is unable to provide for his/her personal needs.

### Get Legal Help

Remember, laws governing these various protective services differ among the states. Legal advice is necessary. When you do not have an attorney, contact your local area agency or commission on aging. Most have a legal office.

# INDEX

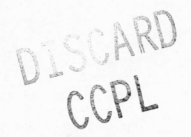